Ophthalmology in Small Animal Care

Editor

BRUCE GRAHN

VETERINARY CLINICS OF NORTH AMERICA: SMALL ANIMAL PRACTICE

www.vetsmall.theclinics.com

March 2023 • Volume 53 • Number 2

ELSEVIER

1600 John F. Kennedy Boulevard • Suite 1800 • Philadelphia, Pennsylvania, 19103-2899
http://www.vetsmall.theclinics.com

**VETERINARY CLINICS OF NORTH AMERICA: SMALL ANIMAL PRACTICE Volume 53, Number 2
March 2023 ISSN 0195-5616, ISBN-13: 978-0-323-93955-3**

Editor: Stacy Eastman
Developmental Editor: Axell Ivan Jade Purificacion

Veterinary Clinics of North America: Small Animal Practice (ISSN 0195-5616) is published bimonthly by Elsevier Inc., 360 Park Avenue South, New York, NY 10010-1710. Months of issue are January, March, May, July, September, and November. Business and Editorial Offices: 1600 John F. Kennedy Blvd., Ste. 1800, Philadelphia, PA 19103-2899. Customer Service Office: 3251 Riverport Lane, Maryland Heights, MO 63043. Periodicals postage paid at New York, NY and additional mailing offices. Subscription prices are $387.00 per year (domestic individuals), $844.00 per year (domestic institutions), $100.00 per year (domestic students/residents), $488.00 per year (Canadian individuals), $1049.00 per year (Canadian institutions), $528.00 per year (international individuals), $1049.00 per year (international institutions), $100.00 per year (Canadian students/residents), and $220.00 per year (international students/residents). To receive student/resident rate, orders must be accompanied by name of affiliated institution, date of term, and the *signature* of program/residency coordinator on institution letterhead. Orders will be billed at individual rate until proof of status is received. Foreign air speed delivery is included in all *Clinics* subscription prices. All prices are subject to change without notice. **POSTMASTER:** Send address changes to *Veterinary Clinics of North America: Small Animal Practice*, Elsevier Health Sciences Division, Subscription Customer Service, 3251 Riverport Lane, Maryland Heights, MO 63043. Customer Service (orders, claims, online, change of address): Elsevier Periodicals Customer Service, Elsevier Health Sciences Division Subscription **Customer Service 3251 Riverport Lane Maryland Heights, MO 63043. Tel: 1-800-654-2452 (U.S. and Canada); 314-447-8871 (outside U.S. and Canada). Fax: 314-447-8029. E-mail: journalscustomerservice-usa@elsevier.com (for print support); journalsonlinesupport-usa@elsevier.com (for online support).**

Reprints. For copies of 100 or more of articles in this publication, please contact the Commercial Reprints Department, Elsevier Inc., 360 Park Avenue South, New York, NY 10010-1710. Tel.: 212-633-3874; Fax: 212-633-3820; E-mail: reprints@elsevier.com.

Veterinary Clinics of North America: Small Animal Practice is also published in Japanese by Inter Zoo Publishing Co., Ltd., Aoyama Crystal-Bldg 5F, 3-5-12 Kitaaoyama, Minato-ku, Tokyo 107-0061, Japan.

Veterinary Clinics of North America: Small Animal Practice is covered in *Current Contents/Agriculture, Biology and Environmental Sciences, Science Citation Index, ASCA, MEDLINE/PubMed (Index Medicus), Excerpta Medica,* and *BIOSIS.*

Contributors

EDITOR

BRUCE GRAHN, DVM
Diplomate, American College of Veterinary Ophthalmologists; Diplomate, American Board of Veterinary Practitioners; Professor Emeritus, Prairie Ocular Pathology Service, Prairie Diagnostic Laboratory, Department of Small Animal Clinical Sciences, Western College of Veterinary Medicine, University of Saskatchewan, Saskatoon, Saskatchewan, Canada

AUTHORS

MARIE-ODILE BENOIT-BIANCAMANO, DMV, PhD, FIATP
Diplomate, American College of Veterinary Pathologists; Diplomate, European College of Veterinary Pathologists; Professor, Department of Pathology and Microbiology, Groupe de recherche sur les Maladies Infectieuses en Production Animale (GREMIP), Faculté de Médecine Vétérinaire, Université de Montréal, Quebec, Canada

BRUCE GRAHN, DVM
Diplomate, American College of Veterinary Ophthalmologists; Diplomate, American Board of Veterinary Practitioners; Professor Emeritus, Prairie Ocular Pathology Service, Prairie Diagnostic Laboratory, Department of Small Animal Clinical Sciences, Western College of Veterinary Medicine, University of Saskatchewan, Saskatoon, Saskatchewan, Canada

ELIZABETH M. JAMES-JENKS, BVSc (Hons)
Department of Clinical Studies, University of Guelph, Ontario Veterinary College, Guelph, Ontario, Canada

AMBER LABELLE, DVM, MS
Diplomate, American College of Veterinary Ophthalmologists; Practice Owner, Bright Light Veterinary Eye Care, Ottawa, Ontario, Canada

PHILIPPE LABELLE, DVM
Diplomate, American College of Veterinary Pathologists; Anatomic Pathologist, Antech Diagnostics, Mississauga, Ontario, Canada

MARINA L. LEIS, BSc, DVM, MVSc
Diplomate, American College of Veterinary Ophthalmologists; Associate Professor, Western College of Veterinary Medicine, Saskatoon, Saskatchewan, Canada

CHANTALE L. PINARD, DVM, MSc
Diplomate, American College of Veterinary Ophthalmologists; Associate Professor, Department of Clinical Studies, Ontario Veterinary College, University of Guelph, Ontario, Canada

LYNNE SANDMEYER, DVM, DVSc
Diplomate, American College of Veterinary Ophthalmologists; Professor, Veterinary Ophthalmology, Department of Small Animal Clinical Sciences, Western College of Veterinary Medicine, University of Saskatchewan, Saskatoon, Saskatchewan, Canada

MARIA VANORE, DMV, MSc
Diplomate, European College of Veterinary Ophthalmologists; Assistant Professor, Ophthalmology Service, Veterinary Teaching Hospital, Université de Montréal, Quebec, Canada

Contents

tear film deficiency, adnexal disease, corneal ulceration, and breed-related corneal pigmentation syndromes. Accurate etiologic diagnosis is critical to determining effective treatment.

Eosinophilic keratitis is a disease of the feline ocular surface. It is charac-terized by conjunctivitis, white to pink raised plaques on the corneal and conjunctival surfaces, corneal vascularization, and variable ocular pain. Cytology is the diagnostic test of choice. Identification of eosinophils in a corneal cytology sample usually confirms the diagnosis, although lym-phocytes, mast cells, and neutrophils are often present concurrently. Im-munosuppressives are the mainstay of therapy, topically or systemically. The role of feline herpesvirus-1 in the pathogenesis of eosinophilic kerato-conjunctivitis (EK) remains unclear. Eosinophilic conjunctivitis is a less common manifestation of EK and presents as severe conjunctivitis without corneal involvement.

Feline glaucoma is best categorized as either secondary, congenital and anterior segment dysgenesis associated, or primary. More than 90% of all feline glaucoma develops secondary to uveitis or intraocular neoplasia. The uveitis is usually idiopathic and assumed to be immune-mediated, whereas lymphosarcoma and diffuse iridal melanoma account for many of the intraocular neoplastic-induced glaucoma in cats. Several topical and systemic therapies are useful in the control of the inflammation and elevated intraocular pressures associated with feline glaucoma. Enucle-ation remains the recommended therapy for blind glaucomatous feline eyes. Enucleated globes from cats with chronic glaucoma should be sub-mitted to an appropriate laboratory for histologic confirmation of the type of glaucoma.

This article provides a simplified approach to diagnosis and clinical deci-sion making in cases of canine glaucoma for the general practitioner. An overview of the anatomy, physiology, and pathophysiology related to canine glaucoma is provided as a foundation. Classifications of glaucoma based on cause are described as congenital, primary, and secondary, and a discussion of key clinical examination findings is provided to guide appropriate therapy and prognostication. Finally, a discussion of emer-gency and maintenance therapy is provided.

Reports of glaucoma associated with anterior segment dysgenesis in dogs and cats are rare. Anterior segment dysgenesis is a sporadic, congenital syndrome with a range of anterior segment anomalies that may or may not result in congenital or developmental glaucoma within the first years of life. Specifically, the anterior segment anomalies that put the neonatal or juvenile dog or cat at high risk for the development of glaucoma are filtration angle and anterior uveal hypoplasia, elongated ciliary processes, and microphakia.

Episcleritis is synonymous with episclerokeratitis although the latter is most appropriate as the cornea is often affected as well as the episclera. Episcleritis is a superficial ocular disease characterized by inflammation of the episclera and conjunctiva. It responds most commonly to topical antinflammatory medications. In contrast scleritis is a granulomatous fulminant panophthalmitis that will progress rapidly and induce significant intraocular disease including glaucoma and exudative retinal detachments without systemic immune suppressive therapy.

Canine eyelid masses (tumors) should include the differential clinical diagnoses of neoplasia and blepharitis. They have many common clinical signs including tumor, alopecia, and hyperemia. Biopsy and histologic examination remains the most effective diagnostic test to establish a confirmed diagnosis and appropriate treatment. Neoplasms are typically benign (tarsal gland adenomas, melanocytomas, and so forth) with the exception of lymphosarcoma. Blepharitis is noted in 2 age groups including dogs aged less than 1.5 years and middle aged to older dogs. Most blepharitis cases will respond to specific therapy once an accurate diagnosis is established.

This article reviews the administration of common topical ophthalmic medications, in relation to factors influencing absorption including composition of topical ophthalmic preparations, and potential systemic effects. Commonly prescribed, commercially available topical ophthalmic medications are discussed with respect to pharmacology, their indications for use, and adverse effects. Knowledge of topical ocular pharmacokinetics is essential for the management of veterinary ophthalmic disease.

VETERINARY CLINICS OF NORTH AMERICA: SMALL ANIMAL PRACTICE

Preface

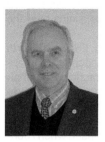

Bruce Grahn, DVM
Editor

It is an honor to edit an issue of *Veterinary Clinics of North America: Small Animal Practice* in Ophthalmology. I am humbled when I consider following the many distinguished guest editors in varied specialties of Veterinary medicine who have edited previous issues over the last five decades. *Veterinary Clinics of North America: Small Animal Practice* was first published in 1971, the year that I began my preveterinary program. At that time, specialties within veterinary medicine were in their infancy, and the creation of small review books that came in several issues dedicated to varied disciplines each year was far ahead of its time. However, it quickly gained favor with veterinary clinicians. In 1979, the success of *Veterinary Clinics of North America: Small Animal Practice* was obvious, and this publication split into a small animal practice issue and a large animal practice issue. In 1985, it further split along species lines, into equine, food animal, and exotic animal issues. For five decades now, many issues have lined the shelves of libraries within academia and veterinary hospitals across the world, and they continue to provide updates on the latest advancements and reviews of timely topics in the clinical diagnosis and treatment of animal diseases.

I first became acquainted with the *Veterinary Clinics of North America: Small Animal Practice* when I was in veterinary college. However, I only seriously started to read these publications when I entered clinical practice in 1977. I enjoyed each issue, as they were always an excellent resource for clinical, diagnostic, and treatment information in a variety of disciplines in varied species of animals. Later in that decade as I prepared for the American Practitioner Board examinations in small animal practice, I reread and studied 10 years of these issues and was surprised at how much I had forgotten since graduation. This was a significant factor for me in the passing of those specialty examinations and recognizing the importance of continuing education. As I entered the specialty of ophthalmology in the following decade, I agreed to author selected articles in small animal ophthalmology in *Veterinary Clinics of North America*. It was then that I began to appreciate the time, and effort, it takes to author and edit these publications so that they provide cohesive, current, and timely publications. In 2021, after retiring from academia, I received a small e-mail request from *Veterinary Clinics of North America: Small Animal Practice* asking me to consider guest

Vet Clin Small Anim 53 (2023) ix–xi
https://doi.org/10.1016/j.cvsm.2022.12.001
0195-5616/23/© 2022 Published by Elsevier Inc.

editing an issue on small animal ophthalmology. After a few months of ignoring their polite but persistent queries, I finally agreed to guest edit this issue. I thank the *Veterinary Clinics of North America: Small Animal Practice* for this opportunity and ask that they consider this as a token repayment for the many things I have learned from the *Veterinary Clinics of North America: Small Animal Practice* issues over the last five decades.

What can you expect that is unique from this issue of *Veterinary Clinics of North America: Small Animal Practice* in 2022? First, the senior authors of each of the chapters are all board-certified ophthalmologists who are currently practicing ophthalmology north of the 49th parallel in Canada. Canadian veterinarians owe much to the American-based specialty colleges. All the ophthalmologists that authored this issue were trained in America or in Canada in residencies approved by the American College of Veterinary Ophthalmologists. I was actually surprised when I contacted each of them, by their eagerness to contribute and create this Canadian-based issue. Each author selected his or her own topics. These are timely for small animal veterinary clinicians and those interested in, or already in training programs for, veterinary ophthalmology.

Dr Marina Leis provides current insight into the ocular microbiome based on her award-winning research in this area. In her second article, she introduces the reader to the relatively scantly described small animal early-onset glaucoma. She is an expert in both these conditions, a gifted teacher and writer, and I am most thankful that she agreed to author and coauthor these articles. She is back at the University of Saskatchewan, her alma mater, and enjoying an academic career.

Drs Maria Vanore and Marie-Odile Benoit-Biancamano, of the Faculté de Médecine Vétérinaire, Université de Montréal are introducing the readership to optical coherence tomography in its application to veterinary ophthalmology. This technology has been available to veterinary ophthalmologist for approximately a decade, and the data arising from this technology are rewriting our current knowledge in ophthalmology. I was fortunate to use this technology and author one of the first clinical articles in dogs with multifocal retinopathy many years ago. Therefore, I was particularly pleased that Maria chose this timely introduction to this advanced laser imaging technology that is revolutionizing our understanding of retinal and corneal diseases.

Dr Chantel Pinard, an associate professor at the University of Guelph, provides an excellent review of ophthalmic examination diagnostics. This is particularly timely for all veterinary practitioners, including the novice to the experienced ophthalmologist. She is a thorough, excellent writer and teacher. She also coauthored with Dr Lizzie James Jenks a second valued article on therapeutics of ocular disease. I am indebted to both of them for providing such timely and practical examination and therapeutic advice to small animal clinicians.

Drs Amber and Philip Labelle contributed the article on pigmentary keratitis, one of the most common and challenging corneal disorders to manage in the Pug and many brachiocephalic dogs. They also contributed a review of a less-common but important and commonly misdiagnosed feline ocular disease, eosinophilic keratitis. Amber owns a private ophthalmology referral practice in Ottawa, while her husband Phillip, a board-certified pathologist, works for Idexx.

Dr Lynne Sandmeyer is a professor at the Western College of Veterinary Medicine at the University of Saskatchewan. She shares her experience and expertise on one of the most challenging and often blinding disorders we see in the dog, glaucoma. I had the privilege of working with her for over two decades. She is a gifted writer and teacher, and I am very proud of all her accomplishments and her article on canine glaucoma.

Finally, I authored the article on feline glaucoma, canine episcleritis, and scleritis and the review of canine eyelid tumors and inflammation. I chose these three based on my experience over three decades as a referring ophthalmologist and a mentor of many ophthalmology graduate students. The nomenclature surrounding these areas of ophthalmology is confusing; the disorders are challenging to treat, and most of them involve significant contributions from ocular pathology, my second passion. I encourage all practicing small animal veterinarians to read this and future *Veterinary Clinics of North America: Small Animal Practice* issues as part of their continuing education. I trust that this issue will meet the expectations of the *Veterinary Clinics of North America: Small Animal Practice* staff, small animal veterinarians, and ophthalmologists who read it.

Bruce Grahn, DVM
Emeritus Professor
Western College of Veterinary Medicine
Prairie Ocular Pathology Service
Prairie Diagnostic Laboratory
Department of Small Animal Clinical Sciences
University of Saskatchewan
52 Campus Drive
Saskatoon, Saskatchewan S7N 5B4, Canada

E-mail address:
bruce.grahn@usask.ca

Diagnostic Tests Used During the Ocular Examination

Chantale L. Pinard, DVM, MSc*

KEYWORDS

- Tear production • Schirmer tear test • Ophthalmic dyes • Fluorescein stain uptake
- Intraocular pressure • Tonometry

KEY POINTS

- Ocular tests will help confirm the diagnoses in dogs and cats with ocular disease.
- The use of medication can influence values of the Schirmer tear test and tonometry.
- To limit variation of values and for better trending, measurements of tear production and intraocular pressure are best done in the same day period, with consistent materials and instruments, and by the same examiner.

SEQUENCE OF EVENTS FOR OCULAR TESTING

With respect to the ocular examination and associated tests, a systematic approach will best serve the patient. This is especially true when contemplating ocular tests such as the measurement of tear production with the Schirmer tear test (STT); the use of dyes for the detection of corneal lesions, patency of the nasolacrimal system, tear quality and quantity; and measurement of intraocular pressure (IOP) via tonometry. It could be argued that the STT should be performed before the neuro-ophthalmic examination because shining bright lights to induce reflexes could falsely increase the tear production value. Conversely, performing the STT, application of ocular dyes and tonometry, without a cursory examination of the cornea, could lead to disastrous consequences with descemetoceles or previously ruptured corneas.

MEDICATION THAT FACILITATE RESTRAINT AND THEIR POTENTIAL EFFECTS ON OCULAR TESTS

Patients who present with painful eyes, extreme anxiety, dominance or fear aggression can be challenging to examine. Restraint with the use of muzzles for dogs (making

Disclosure statement: The author has nothing to disclose.
Department of Clinical Studies, University of Guelph, Ontario Veterinary College, 50 Stone Road East, Guelph, Ontario N1G 2W1, Canada
* Corresponding author.
E-mail address: cpinard@uoguelph.ca

sure that the muzzle does not ride up too close to the eye and inadvertently put pressure on eyelids) and towel wrapping of cats can be done to help the examiner. Sedatives and other classes of medications can also be helpful in safely performing an ocular examination; however, knowledge of these medications and their associated ocular effects is necessary when interpreting ocular findings. Sedatives such as acepromazine, dexmetodomidine, and trazodone, as well as medications used to reduce pain such as gabapentin, buprenorphine, and nonsteroidal anti-inflammatory drugs (NSAIDS), may influence values obtained during ocular testing. Commonly used sedatives and pain-modulating medications, and their potential effects on ocular parameters are presented in **Table 1**. It must be noted that not all medications have been tested on both dogs and cats and not all ocular parameters have been investigated for each medication.

BASIC OCULAR TESTS

Basic ocular tests give adjunctive information and help the veterinarian narrow down differentials or confirm a diagnosis. Proper techniques are required to ensure that these tests give just values.

Schirmer Tear Tests

The STT 1 is performed routinely during the ocular examination to determine tear production per minute. The strip is folded at the notch and is typically inserted in the central ventral conjunctival fornix for 60 seconds (**Fig. 1**); should the dorsal fornix be used, the values are statistically different.[22] Care must be taken not to touch the folded area because skin lipids or applied skin lotions will affect tear absorption. The STT 1 measures the basal and the reflex tear production as compared with the STT II, which only measures the basal tear production following the application of topical anesthesia. **Table 2** reveals tear production values using standard STT and meniscometry strips as well as conditions that could alter values. Ideally, tear production measurement should be done before the neuro-ophthalmic examination because touching of the eyelids and shining bright lights could falsely elevate tear production. It is also customary to perform the STT before fluorescein stain application. Yet, the application of 0.5 ll fluorescein 10 minutes prior did not change the STT I results in dogs.[23] Consistent brands of STT strips is important because using differing manufacturers can vary canine values from 17.5 ± 3.4 mm to 26.5 ± 3.7 mm due to differing surface areas.[24] Room humidity but not temperature can play a factor in STT I measurements but this factor is unlikely to cause clinically significant effects.[25] Chemical restraint can also alter the tear measurements (see **Table 1**). Low repeated values with corroborating clinical signs (mucoid to mucopurulent discharge, conjunctivitis, corneal vascularization with or without pigmentation), strongly suggests a diagnosis of keratoconjunctivitis sicca (KCS).

In dogs, neonatal canine STT I and II increase with age until 9 to 10 weeks of age (see **Table 2**).[26,27] Tear production increases in a linear fashion by approximately 3 mm/min every week until 10 weeks of age, where values mirror adult tear values.[26,27] Tear production in adult dogs does decrease with every year of age (0.4 mm/y increased).[28] Diurnal variations have been documented in dogs with the highest values in late afternoon and lowest at midday[29] but one rigorous study revealed the highest values in the evening (20:00 hours) and the lowest in the early morning (08:00 hours).[30] It should be noted that the differences measured were not clinically relevant (2.31 mm/min).[30] Another study also documented that time of day can statistically but not clinically affect measurements (difference of 0.7 mm/min).[28] Gender does not seem to

Table 1
Medication effect on Schirmer tear test and intraocular pressure in cats and dogs

Medication (Species)	Dose	Effects on STT and IOP	References
Sedatives:			
Acepromazine (cats)	0.2 mg/kg IM	Decreased STT	Ghaffari M et al,[1] 2010
Acepromazine (dogs)	0.1 mg/kg IM	Decreased STT	Santos P et al,[2] 2013
Acepromazine + tramadol (dogs)	0.1 mg/kg ace + 2 mg/kg tramadol IM	Decreased STT	Santos P et al,[2] 2013
Acepromazine + oxymorphone (dogs)	0.03 mg/kg ace + 0.1 mg/kg oxy IM	Decreased STT	Dodam J et al,[3] 1998
Chlorpromazine (dogs)	1 mg/kg IM	Decreased STT	Ghaffari M et al,[4] 2011
Dexmetodomidine (dogs)	4 µg/kg IM	Decreased STT for 8 h	Di Pietro S et al,[5] 2021
Diphenhydramine (dogs)	2.2 mg/kg, PO, BID for 21 d	No effect on STT and IOP but decreased corneal sensitivity and TBUT in dogs	Evans P et al,[6] 2021
Medetomidine (cats)	100 µg/kg	No effect on IOP	Malmasi A et al,[7] 2016
Medetomidine (dogs)	0.033 mg/kg IM	No effect on IOP	Wallin-Hakanson N et al,[8] 2021
Medetomidine (dogs)	80 µg/kg IM	No effect on IOP	Kanda T et al,[9] 2015
Medetomidine (dogs)	10–15 µg/kg IV	Decreased STT	Sanchez R et al,[10] 2006
Medetomidine-butorphanol (dogs)	Medetomidine 10–16 µg/kg + butorphanol 10–16 mg/kg IV	Decreased STT	Sanchez R et al,[10] 2006
Metedomidine-bupernorphine (dogs)	medetomidine 20 µg/kg + buprenorphine 10 µg/kg IV	Decreased STT	Soontornvipart K et al,[11] 2003
Trazodone (cats)	50 mg per os once	No effect on STT, IOP	Klein A et al,[12] 2019
Trazodone (dogs)	5 or 9 mg/kg per os once	No effect on STT, IOP	Pelych L et a,[13] 2018
Trazodone (dogs)	5 mg/kg per os once	No effect on STT, IOP	Simmerman K et al,[14] 2018
Pain modulating medications			
Butorphanol (dogs)	0.5 mg/kg IM	Decreased STT	Dodam J et al,[3] 2021
Butorphanol (dogs)	0.2 mg/kg IM	Decreased STT and IOP (?)	Douet J-Y et al,[15] 2018

(continued on next page)

Table 1
(continued)

Medication (Species)	Dose	Effects on STT and IOP	References
Carprofen (dogs)	202 mg/kg BID per os for 7 d	No effect on IOP	Meekins M et al,[16] 2018
Etodolac (dogs)	10–15 mg/kg SID per os	Induced KCS	Klauss G et al,[17] 2012
Fentanyl (dogs)	10 μg/kg IM	Decreased STT	Biricik H et al,[18] 2004
Gabapentin (dogs)	10 mg/kg TID per os 3 d	No effect on STT Decreased IOP (?)	Shukla A et al,[19] 2020
Gabapentin (dogs)	10 mg/kg TID for 3 doses	Decreased in IOP	Rajotte S et al,[20] 2019
Meloxicam (dogs)	0.2 mg/kg once then 0.1 mg/kg per os for 2 d	No effect on STT, IOP	Shukla A et al,[19] 2020
Tramadol (dogs)	3 mg/kg per os TID 3 d	No effect on STT Decreased IOP (?)	Shukla A et al,[19] 2020
Tramadol (dogs)	2 mg/kg IM	No effect on STT	Santos P et al,[20] 2013
Tramadol (dogs)	4–6 mg/kg IM	No effect on STT, IOP	Ruiz T et al,[21] 2015

(?) Values within normal range and not considered clinically relevant; KCS: keratoconjunctivitis sicca.

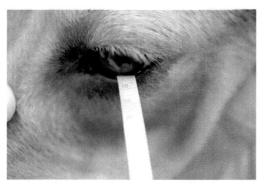

Fig. 1. The STT strip is inserted into the ventral conjunctival sac for 60 seconds before reading the millimeter recorded.

have an influence on STT[27,28,31] and neither does right eye compared with left.[31] Large breed dogs have a higher tear production,[32] with Labrador and golden retrievers having higher values than beagles and Shetland sheepdogs.[31] Skull conformation may influence tear production because one study revealed that brachycephalic dogs have lower tear production than non-brachycephalic dogs.[33] Diabetic cataractous dogs have lower STT I values compared with cataractous non-diabetic dogs.[34] In the same venue, low production was seen with dogs with endocrinopathy.[35] Lower tear values have also been document in canine patients in the intensive care unit,[36] whereas, as expected, dogs with corneal ulceration had higher STT values than controls.[37]

In cats, STT during 30 and 60 seconds showed good correlation between both time settings.[38] As seen with dogs, kittens have a lower STT than adults (STT under 6 months: 7.0 ± 2.6 mm/min; 7 months-2 years: 16.0 ± 3.3 mmin/min; 3-6 years 15.7 ± 4.2 mm/min).[39] In this same study, no gender difference was seen but intact status did statistically decrease STT values as compared with neutered cats. Interestingly, Persians had a higher STT values (16.5 ± 3.1 mm/min) than domestic shorthairs (14.6 ± 5.0 mm/min). This study also mentioned that several cats had STT less than 10 mm/min and were normal based on a complete ophthalmologic examination. This reinforces the notion that STT values alone may not be enough to diagnose KCS. The STT I should be performed on cats with ocular surface diseases and therapy with lacrimomimetics should be promptly initiated if STT I values were low.[40] Cats with feline herpesvirus infection have lower tear values than controls.[41]

A new version of the STT 1 with strips that only takes 5 seconds to record has been relatively recently introduced on the veterinary market. The strip meniscometry test (SMT) measures quantitative tear levels in the tear meniscus and does not measure reflex tearing. The meniscus strip's touch end contacts the tear film meniscus, and neither should it be placed under the eyelid, as in the case of an STT strip, nor should it touch the cornea or conjunctiva. In the veterinary literature, these strips have been studied in mice,[42] birds (amazon and macaw),[43] reptile (caiman),[43] and dogs.[44,45] Only one study has established reference values for cats.[46] Although a strong correlation between SMT and STT was shown in one canine study,[45] none was found in the feline study.[46] As seen with an STT greater than 15 mm/min, SMT greater than 5 mm/5 s was considered normal in dogs.[44] This same study reported that this test had a 98% sensitivity and 98% specificity in predictive value for clinical diagnosis of KCS, whereas the STT had a 96% sensitivity and 94% specificity. Interestingly, these strips did not show

Table 2
Schirmer tear test (1 and II) and strip meniscometry test values in dogs and cats

Species	STT 1 (mm/60 s)	STT II (mm/60 s)	SMT (mm/5 s)	References
Dogs				
Neonate (14–84 d old)	5.1 ± 2.4 at 14 d of age to 21.4 ± 2.8 at 84 d of age	2.3 ± 1.6 at 14 d of age to 15.8 ± 3.0 at 84 d of age		Verboven C et al,[27] 2014
Juvenile (21–139 d old)	~6 at 21 d of age to ~21 at 90 d of age	~3.5 at 21 d of age to ~11 at 76 d of age		Broadwater J et al,[26] 2010
Adult	20.25 ± 3.58 20.2 ± 0.1 18.89 ± 2.62–21.0 ± 4.2	NA NA 3.8 ± 2.7–11.6 ± 6.1	10.97 ± 2.93 11.2 ± 0.5	Miyasaka K et al,[45] 2019 Miller R et al,[44] 2017 Hamor R et al,[31] 2000, Gelatt KN et al,[47] 1995, Saito A et al,[48] 2001
	15.10 ± 3.06 18.89 ± 2.62 20.3 ± 3	9.52 ± 4.55 6.2 ± 3.1	9.66 ± 2.15	Rajaei A et al,[46] 2018 Saito A et al,[48] 2001 Hamor R et al,[31] 2000
Ventral vs dorsal conjunctival fornix placement	23.56 ± 3.98 (ventral) vs 20.44 ± 4.46 (dorsal)			Visser H et al,[22] 2017
Brachycephalic vs nonbrachycephalic	20.1 ± 3.4 vs 23.3 ± 5.7	13.0 ± 3.4 vs 16.9 ± 3.9	7.4 ± 2.0 vs 7.3 ± 2.4	Bolzanni H et al,[33] 2013
Diabetic cataractous	15.7 ± 6.5 OD; 15.5 ± 6.4 OS			Cullen C et al,[34] 2005
Diabetic	12.3 ± 5.3			Williams D et al,[35] 2007
Cushing	14.0 ± 4.0			Williams D et al,[35] 2007
Hypothyroid	12.3 ± 3.2			Williams D et al,[35] 2007
ICU patients	13.2			Chandler J et al,[36] 2013
Corneal ulcer vs control	20.2 ± 4.6 (ulcer) vs 16.7 ± 3.5 (control)			Williams D et al,[37] 2017
Cats				

			Reference
16.2 ± 3.8		13.2 ± 3.4	McLaughlin S et al,[49] 1988
13.7 ± 4.6; 13.7 ± 4.6 mm/30 s			Sebbag L et al,[38] 2020
11.00 ± 1.41	10.50 ± 0.7		Rajaei A et al,[46] 2018
14.9 ± 4.8			Rajaei S et al,[39] 2019
FHV	8 ± 4 (FHV) vs 14 ± 6 (control)		Lim C et al,[41] 2009

Abbreviation: FHV, feline herpes viral infection.

a difference between brachycephalic and nonbrachycephalic dogs as compared with the standard STT I, where a difference between skull conformity was detected.[33] The advantages of these strips are less time for each test, less "invasiveness" perceived by clients and more comfort in dogs with corneal ulceration. The use of these strips in dogs with poor eyelid conformation (ie, mastiffs) that do not allow for a good tear meniscus, or dogs with copious mucus may be problematic (Miller, personal communication). Additionally, uncooperative patients make this technique of tear measurement difficult to perform correctly.

Dyes: Fluorescein, Rose Bengal, and Lissamine Green Stains

Most practitioners will detect corneal ulceration with the aid of fluorescein stain uptake in both dogs and cats. Commercially available impregnated sterile paper strips of 1% fluorescein are commonly used in general practice as opposed to fluorescein solution. The moistened strips with saline are applied to the conjunctival surface; care must be take not to directly touch the cornea because this site could be interpreted as a false positive at the point of contact. Flushing of excessive stain minimizes false positives and only a thin rim of fluorescein stain should be seen adjacent to the lower eyelid. The subsequent use of a cobalt-blue filter in a darkened room will make the uptake of stain more visible. Fluorescein is lipophilic and hydrophilic, which entails that normal epithelial and conjunctival cells do not stain. Stain retention is only seen in exposed corneal stroma because Descemet membrane also repels this dye. That said, it can stain intercellular spaces and this can be seen as corneal erosions (stippling).[50] Although fluorescein has been shown to have antibacterial activity in an in vitro study,[51] an in vivo study demonstrated no significant decrease in the bacteria isolated in dogs following its application alongside topical propracaine and tropicamide.[52] The use of preservative-free fluorescein solution is not recommended because it can harbor bacteria if not properly handled.[51] The dilution of the commercially available strips into a 3 to 6 mL saline-filled syringe is also not recommended because the fluorescein may be too dilute to detect corneal defects.

Fluorescein can also be used to detect other ocular conditions. Its direct application to the cornea can detect aqueous leakage in cases of suspect corneal perforation (Seidel test). The instillation of undiluted fluorescein at the suspected site may reveal a green rivulet among an orange background, signifying a break in corneal integrity.

Patency of the nasolacrimal duct (Jones test) can also be achieved with this dye. The exit of fluorescein stain from the nasal puncta will confirm the patency of one of the lacrimal puncta, cannaliculi, and duct; flushing of both lacrimal puncta will be necessary to complete the full analysis of the nasolacrimal system in question. The interval of time for dye passage can range from several seconds to half an hour, pending nose conformation and amount of flush used. Brachycephalic dogs and cats usually have a negative Jones test due to anatomy. Because there are several explanations for a false-negative test, a negative test is only suggestive of a disease or congenital condition. To confirm lack of patency, a nasolacrimal flush and contrast-enhanced sectional imaging is often required.

This dye can also help assess tear film quality via the tear break up time (TBUT). By instilling concentrated fluorescein and letting it cover the corneal surface, seconds are counted until the fluorescein breaks up and a dark spot is noted. The patient is only allowed to blink once at the beginning to spread the fluorescein-stained tear film and the eyelids must be held open. The reference range for dogs is 19.7 ± 5 seconds to 21.53 ± 7.42 seconds[48] and 21 seconds $\pm$ 12 in cats.[53] The TBUT test is not generally performed in general practice.

Rose Bengal is also not commonly used in private practice. It is reserved for the evaluation of the tear film and presence of corneal epithelial defects, such as epithelial erosions.[50,54] This dye was originally used for staining devitalized cells in cases of KCS.[53] Care must be taken with the interpretation of this dye because healthy conjunctival and corneal epithelium will stain positive when a mucin cover is absent.[50] In other words, a negative stain uptake can signify that precorneal tear film components, such as mucin, are present.[50] Patients with a poor-quality tear film, such as a lack of mucin coming from conjunctival goblet cells, will likely stain positive.[50] Rose Bengal also has a slow diffusion into the corneal stroma as compared with fluorescein, and epithelium-denuded stroma may not retain this stain.[50] Its use has been discouraged because it is intrinsically toxic to cells.[54] Similar to fluorescein, this dye also has antibacterial activity and should not be applied before sampling the ocular surface for bacterial culture.[51,54]

Lissamine green is not commonly used in veterinary ophthalmology. It has similar corneal detection properties as Rose Bengal and similar antimicrobial properties.[51] Lissamine green has also been shown to have antiviral properties.[55] This dye can be used as an alternative to fluorescein when measuring TBUT in dogs.[56]

Tonometry

Tonometry determines the IOP of our companion animal patients. Veterinarians have access to several types of tonometers and each has its benefits and drawbacks. The 3 classes of tonometers commonly used in veterinary medicine are indentation, applanation, and rebound (**Fig. 2**). The indentation tonometer, Schiotz, is no longer widely used and has been largely replaced with applanation and rebound tonometers (**Table 3**).

The applanation tonometers have been available in veterinary medicine for some time and require topical anesthesia before their use. These tonometers can give a reading after 3 correct touches; acceptable readings are indicated by a clicking sound, and the final reading is signaled by a long beep. The footplate must contact the cornea without indenting it; however, the contact must flatten it. The Tono-Pen XL has been widely used in research and in private practice.

The rebound tonometers relatively recently entered the veterinary market. The probe deceleration after touching the cornea and rebounding is what calculates the IOP. Six measurements are performed before the mean average being displayed. Calibration for several species is found based on the manufacturer. The TonoVet is now widely used in veterinary practices for several reasons. Due to the small footplate and rapid influence (0.3 m/s), there is no need for topical anesthesia because the

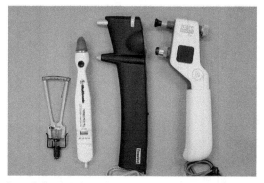

Fig. 2. Tonometers from left to right: Schiotz (indentation), TonoPen XL (applanation), TonoVet (rebound), and TonoVet Plus (rebound).

Table 3
Intraocular pressure measurements (mm Hg) with applanation (TonoPen) and rebound tonometers (TonoVet & TonoVet Plus) in dogs and cats

Species	TonoPen	TonoVet	TonoVet Plus	References
Dogs				
Neonate		5.6 ± 2.7 at 2 wk of age to 12.6 ± 1.8 at 12 wk of age		Verboven C et al,[27] 2014
Adult	19.2 ± 5.9	16.1 ± 2.9		Gelatt K et al,[69] 1998
	11.7 ± 2.5	14.2 ± 4.4 OD;		Tofflemire K, et al,[63] 2017
	13.7 ± 4.1 OD;	14.2 ± 4.5 OS		Nagata N et al,[61] 2011
	13.8 ± 4.8 OS	15.20 ± 6.47	19.01 ± 6.86	Shim J et al,[67] 2021
	12.8 ± 2.9 (AVIA)	15.0 ± 3.2	19.2 ± 3.1	Ben-Shlomo G et al,[66] 2021
	11.053 ± 3.451	9.158 ± 3.471		Leiva M et al,[75] 2006
Corneal ulceration vs control		11.9 ± 3.1 (ulcer) vs 16.7 ± 2.6 (control)		Williams D et al,[37] 2017
Cats				
Neonate		13.2 ± 2.4		Adelman S et al,[68] 2018
Adult	20 ± 6			Miller P et al,[76] 2018
	15.6 ± 4.1			Ghaffari M et al,[77] 2018
	19.86 ± 0.71 OD;	20.74 ± 0.49 OD;		Rusanen E et al,[78] 2010
	19.5 ± 0.75 OS	20.74 ± 0.47 OS		

corneal reflex is not engaged.[57] There is limited user error because the user presses a button and does not need to touch the cornea, as required with the applanation tonometers. False reading errors arise with the restraint of the patient, manual opening of the eyelids, and being too close or too far with the probe. Traction on feline eyelids has been shown to increase values and thus care must be taken not to inadvertently cause a dorsoventral or lateral eyelid extension when taking measurements.[58] In addition, careful manipulation of the instruments must take place because the probe must make perpendicular contact with the cornea at the right distance (4–8 mm) to limit the error message. Differences in values have been documented with varying distances.[59]

In cats, the TonoVet has been deemed more accurate than the Tono-Pen.[60] In dogs, a study between applanation and rebound tonometers revealed no significant differences in the normotensive eyes.[61] This same study reported the Tono-Pen measurements were lower than TonoVet in glaucomatous eyes, and the TonoVet was more accurate in hypertensive eyes but less than Tono-Pen in hypotensive eyes. In glaucomatous canine eyes, TonoVet gave higher values than Tono-Pen Vet with an average of 17.2 mm Hg difference.[62] A canine study comparing the TonoVet and TonoPen concluded that the TonoVet had higher readings but was more accurate when compared with manometric values.[63]

Recently, a new rebound tonometer appeared in the market, the TonoVet Plus. The advantage of this tonometer is that it has a green or red rim, which signals to the examinor if the tonometer is well placed in front of the cornea. The measurements can be done individually or in a sequence if the button is pressed continuously. The TonoVet Plus consistently and significantly had higher readings than the Tono-Pen AVIA and TonoVet but the readings were not deemed clinically relevant.[64] An ex vivo canine study found that the rebound tonometers (TonoVet and TonoVet Plus) were more accurate than applanation tonometers (Tono-Pen XL and Tono-Pen AVIA VET) but all tonometers were not significantly different in the physiologic IOP range.[65] Studies have shown that the TonoVet Plus had higher readings than the TonoVet.[66,67]

Several factors can influence tonometry readings (see **Tables 1** and **3**). Neonatal dogs will increase their IOP from 2 to 12 weeks of age,[27] similar to cats.[68] Age can influence readings over time because one study found a decrease of 2 to 4 mm Hg starting at 2 years of age.[69] A circadian rhythm is also noted with IOP, and this was seen with a diurnal acrophase.[29,70] To ensure consistency in measurements, body position should be recorded when measuring IOP because one study showed that the IOP decreased during a 5-minute interval in a sitting position but not in sternal recumbency.[71] This was also found in another study where repeated measurements of the designated eye did decrease on second measurement 15 minutes later.[72] This same study also noted that the IOP measured in the first eye has higher values than in the fellow eye. It must be noted that although both these studies had statistically significant differences, they were not clinically relevant. Care in restraint must also occur because an increase of 51.1% in values was seen with dogs having compression of their jugular veins by a collar; a return to baseline was recorded 1 minute after the force applied was released.[73] The angle and corneal location of the rebound probe must also be considered because values can be statistically different.[74] Surprisingly, corneal thickness did not show an impact on readings with 3 different types of tonometers.[64] Not surprisingly, corneal ulceration in dogs will decrease IOP measurements due to the presence of secondary uveitis.[37]

Gonioscopy

Gonioscopy is a tool used by veterinary ophthalmologists that may provide useful information regarding a diagnosis of glaucoma. Gonioscopy visualizes the canine pectinate ligament, the anterior part of the uveal trabeculae and opening of the ciliary cleft and can be performed on awake patients following the instillation of topical anesthetic drops.[79,80] Examination of the feline iridocorneal angle is possible with diffuse illumination and magnification and not require a goniolens.[81] For visualization of the canine iridocorneal angle, several types of direct and indirect goniolens exist. Direct lenses, such as the Koeppe, reveal a real and slightly magnified image from the opposite iridocorneal angle. Indirect lenses, such as the Karickhoff diagnostic lens, use prisms to form an image that the examiner sees from a frontal position. Gonioscopy is useful to confirm open/narrowed/closed iridocorneal angle, pectinate ligament dysplasia, and consolidation of pectinate ligaments into broad sheets with flow holes.[82–84] Gonioscopy's main aim is to help predict glaucoma because abnormal iridocorneal angles are at higher risk.[82,83,85–87] Gonioscopy may also reveal intraocular extension of limbal or uveal neoplasms.[88,89]

The main limitation of gonioscopy is that it is subjective and good levels of agreement can be challenging to obtain between examiners.[90] Furthermore, the restricted area seen on examination may not relate to function and may be soon replaced by ultrasound biomicroscopy.[91,92] Other limitations include the examination of eyes with ocular hypertension/glaucoma because the iridocorneal angle will narrow and the ciliary cleft will collapse with increasing pressure. Care must be taken during examination because pressure onto the goniolens could alter the appearance of the iridocorneal angle. Corneal edema, due to IOPs of 40 mm Hg or greater, may also prevent visualization of the angle. Although gonioscopy may not always predict postoperative hypertension following cataract surgery,[93,94] it should be considered in breeds with high prevalence of goniodysgenesis.[95–97]

Corneal Esthesiometry

The corneal reflex serves to protect the eye and is mediated by the ophthalmic branch of the trigeminal nerve, the abducens nerve, and facial nerve. Corneal esthesiometry is a quantitative estimation of corneal sensitivity and is measured by the corneal touch threshold (CTT).[98–100] To determine the CTT in veterinary medicine, the Cochet-Bonnet esthesiometer is the most commonly used instrument by veterinary ophthalmologists. This esthesiometer has a 0.12-mm nylon filament that ranges from 0.5 to 6 cm in length and values obtained are converted to grams per square millimeter via a manufacturer conversion table.[100] To record the CTT, the cornea is touched by the end of the fully extended filament until a minor bend in the filament is seen (**Fig. 3**). The filament

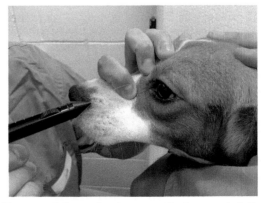

Fig. 3. The nylon filament of the Cochet-Bonnet esthesiometer is fully extended filament until a minor bend in the filament is seen.

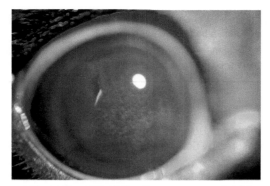

Fig. 4. A linear fluorescein stain uptake following measurement of the CTT.

is shortened by 0.5 cm each time until more than 50% of successive touches elicit a blink reflex. Once this is achieved, the filament's length is converted to the CTT.[100–103] In other words, a less-sensitive eye will have a shorter filament and lower CTT.[102] The central cornea has been determined to being the most sensitive and is the area of choice for this test.[103]

In dogs, normal CTT is reported to be 2.16 g/mm².[104] The CTT is decreased in brachycephalic breeds[105]; in patients with diabetes mellitus[100] and canine herpetic infection[106]; in patients with buphthalmos that underwent evisceration with intrascleral prosthesis[103]; and in patients under topical therapy with topical anesthetics[107] and systemically administered diphenhydramine.[6] Topical NSAIDS may not affect CTT[102] or have differing effects on CTT.[108] In the latter study, benzalkonium chloride was found to increase CTT in dogs.[108]

In cats, the CTT is reported to be 1.33 g/mm².[104] A decreased CTT was detected in patients with congenital glaucoma[109] and following administration of topical 0.5% proparacaine hydrochloride.[110] Interestingly, topical NSAIDs had no effect on feline CTT.[111] Limitations of this test include a spontaneous blink reflex that could be mistaken as a positive touch, inadvertent iatrogenic corneal trauma (**Fig. 4**),[19] the lack of calibration in veterinary patients,[102] and room humidity affecting the filament's rigidity.[102]

SUMMARY

Ocular tests can play a vital role in determining a diagnosis. Taken in conjunction with the ocular examination findings, ocular tests can confirm the path forward toward therapy for each canine and feline patient. Several factors such as medication, restraint, technique, and age can influence the values obtained.

CLINICS CARE POINTS

- Ocular tests must be accurately performed to optain optimum data for diagnosis of ocular diseases.[22,50,58]

- Sedatives and pain management medications can influence tear production and intraocular pressure measurements (**Table 1**).

- Fluorescein stain is used to detect ulcerative corneal disease, corneal perforation, nasolacrimal system patency and tear break up time.

- Age of patient must be factored when interpretating Schirmer tear tests and intraocular pressures.[27,26,31,39,46–48,61,63,66,67,68,69,75,76–78]

- Rose bengal and lissamine green dyes are not commonly used in private practice. Rose bengal dye has been shown be toxic to epithelial cells.[54]
- Tear break up time, gonioscopy and corneal estheiometry are usually performed by ophthalmic veterinary specialists due to instrumentation and expertise.

REFERENCES

1. Ghaffari M, Malmasi A, Bokaie S. Effect of acepromazine or xylazine on tear production as measured by Schirmer tear test in normal cats. Vet Ophthalmol 2010; 13(1):1–3.
2. Santos P, de Sousa K, Pinto R, et al. Comparison of pupil diameter and tear production in dogs treated with acepromazine, tramadol and their combination. Rev Ceres 2013;60(2):166–72.
3. Dodam J, Branson K, Martin D. Effects of intramuscular sedative and opioid combinations on tear production in dogs. Vet Ophthalmol 1998;1(1):57–9.
4. Ghaffari M, Madani S, Trbolova A, et al. Effects of intramuscular chlorpromazine alone and chlorpromazine–morphine combination on Schirmer tear test results in clinically normal dogs. Comp Clin Pathol 2011;20:413–5.
5. Di Pietro S, Giannetto C, Falcone A, et al. Dexmedetomidine and Tear Production: Evaluation in Dogs as Spontaneous Model for Ocular Surface Disorders. Vet Sci 2021;8(2):28–37.
6. Evans P, Lynch G, Labelle P. Effects of oral administration of diphenhydramine on pupil diameter, intraocular pressure, tear production, tear film quality, conjunctival goblet cell density, and corneal sensitivity of clinically normal adult dogs. Am J Vet Res 2012;73:1983–6.
7. Malmasi A, Ghaffari S. Lack of effects of intramuscular medetomidine on intraocular pressure in clinically normal cats. J Feline Med Surg 2016;18:315–7.
8. Wallin-Hakanson N, Wallin-Hakanson B. The effects of topical tropicamide and systemic medetomidine, followed by atipamezole reversal, on pupil size and intraocular pressure in normal dogs. Vet Ophthalmol 2001;4(1):3–6.
9. Kanda T, iguchi A, Yoshioka C, et al. Effects of medetomidine and xylazine on intraocular pressure and pupil size in healthy Beagle dogs. Vet Anaesth Analg 2015;42:623–8.
10. Sanchez R, Mellor D, Mould. Effects of medetomidine and medetomidine-butorphanol combination on Schirmer tear test 1 readings in dogs. Vet Ophthalmol 2006;9(1):33–7.
11. Soontornvipart K, Rau P, Kecova E, et al. Effect of Anaesthetic Premedication with Medetomidine-Buprenorphine on the Aqueous Tear Production in Dogs. Acta Vet Brno 2003;72:267–72.
12. Klein A, Salpeter E, Simons A, et al. Effects of Oral Trazodone on Ocular Parameters in Healthy Cats. Conference Proceedings 50th Annual Scientific Meeting of the American College of Veterinary Ophthalmologists. Maui (Hawaii). Nov 6-9, 2019.
13. Pelych L, MacLeese J, La Croix N. Effects of oral trazodone on canine tear production and intraocular pressure. Conference Proceedings 49th Annual Scientific Meeting of the American College of Veterinary Ophthalmologists. Minneapolis (Minnesota). Sept 26-29, 2018.
14. Simmerman K, Silva E, Murray J, et al. Effects of oral trazodone hydrochloride on tear production, intraocular pressure, pupil size, heart rate, and respiratory rate in healthy dogs. Conference Proceedings Annual Scientific Meeting of

the European College of Veterinary Ophthalmologists. Florence (Italy). May 10-13, 2018.

15. Douet J-Y, Regnier A, Dongay A, et al. Effect of sedation with butorphanol on variables pertaining to the ophthalmic examination in dogs. Vet Ophthalmol 2018;21(5):452–8.

16. Meekins M, Overton T, Rankin A, et al. Effect of oral administration of carprofen on intraocular pressure in normal dogs. J Vet Pharmacol Therap 2016;39:344–9.

17. Klauss G, Giuliano E, Morre C, et al. Keratoconjunctivitis sicca associated with administration of etodolac in dogs: 211 cases (1992–2002). J Am Vet Med Assoc 2007;230:541–7.

18. Biricik H, Ceylan C, Sakar M. Effects of pethidine and fentanyl on tearproduction in dogs. Vet Rec 2004;155:564–5.

19. Shukla A, Pinard C, Flynn B, et al. Effects of orally administered gabapentin, tramadol, and meloxicam on ocular variables in healthy dogs. Am J Vet Res 2020; 81:973–84.

20. Rajotte S, Salpeter, Martins B, et al. Effect of Gabapentin on Ocular Parameters Following Oral Administration in Healthy Dogs. Conference Proceedings 50th Annual Scientific Meeting of the American College of Veterinary Ophthalmologists. Maui (Hawaii). Nov 6-9, 2019.

21. Ruiz T, Peres T, da Silva Campos W, et al. Effects of tramadol on tear production, intraocular pressure, and pupil size in dogs: clinical study. Ciênc Rural 2015;45:724–9.

22. Visser H, Tofflemire K, Love-Myers K, et al. Schirmer tear test I in dogs: results comparing placement in the ventral vs. dorsal conjunctival fornix. Vet Ophthalmol 2017;20(6):522–5.

23. Iwashaita H, Wakaiki S, Kazama Y, et al. When should we measure the schirmer tear test? Conference Proceedgins 48th Annual Conference of the American College of Veterinary Ophthalmologists. Baltimore (Maryland). October 11-14, 2017.

24. Lewin A, Liu C, Yoon A, et al. Schirmer strip wetting length varies by commercial manufacturer. Vet Ophthalmol 2020;23:1031–5.

25. Yoon A, Liu C, Carter R, et al. Environmental relative humidity affects Schirmer tear test results in normal dogs. Vet Ophthalmol 2020;23:923–6.

26. Broadwater J, Colitz C, Carastro S, et al. Tear production in normal juvenile dogs. Vet Ophthalmol 2010;13(5):321–5.

27. Verboven C, Djajadiningrat-Laanen S, Teske E, et al. Development of tear production and intraocular pressure in healthy canine neonates. Vet Ophthalmol 2014;17(6):426–31.

28. Hartley C, Williams D, Adams V. Effect of age, gender, weight, and time of day on tear production in normal dogs. Vet Ophthalmol 2006;9(1):53–7.

29. Hakanason NW, Arnesson K. Temporal variation in tear production in normal beagles dogs as determined by Schirmer tear test. Vet Comp Ophthalmol 1997;7:196–203.

30. Giannetto C, Piccione G, Giudice E. Daytime profile of the intraocular pressure and tear production in normal dog. Vet Ophthalmol 2009;12(5):302–5.

31. Hamor R, Roberts S, Severin G, et al. Evaluation of results for Schirmer tear tests conducted with and without application of a topical anesthetic in clinically normal dogs of 5 breeds. Am J Vet Res 2000;61:1422–5.

32. Berger S, King K. The Fluctuation of Tear Production in the Dog. J Am Anim Hosp Assoc 1998;34:79–83.

33. Bolzanni H, Oriá A, Raposo A, et al. Aqueous tear assessment in dogs: Impact of cephalic conformation, inter-test correlations, and test-retest repeatability. Vet Ophthalmol 2020;23:534–43.
34. Cullen C, Ihle S, Webb A, et al. Keratoconjunctival effects of diabetes mellitus in dogs. Vet Ophthalmol 2005;8(4):215–24.
35. Williams D, Pierce V, Mellor P, et al. Reduced tear production in three canine endocrinopathies. J Small Anim Pract 2007;4:252–6.
36. Chandler J, van der Woerdt A, Prittie J, et al. Preliminary evaluation of tear production in dogs hospitalized in an intensive care unit. J Vet Emerg Crit Care 2013;23(3):274–9.
37. Williams D, Burg P. Tear production and intraocular pressure in canine eyes with corneal ulceration. Open Vet J 2017;7(2):117–25.
38. Sebbag L, Uhl I, Schneider B, et al. Investigation of Schirmer tear test-1 for measurement of tear production in cats in various environmental settings and with different test durations. J Am Vet Med Assoc 2020;256:681–6.
39. Rajaei S, Faghihi H, Williams D, et al. Evaluation of tear production using the Schirmer tear test I in healthy cats; effect of age, life stage, sex, breed and neuter status. Vet Rec 2019;184(26):799–804.
40. Uhl L, Saito A, Iwashita H, et al. Clinical features of cats with aqueous tear deficiency: a retrospective case series of 10 patients (17 eyes). J Feline Med Surg 2019;21(10):944–50.
41. Lim C, Reilly C, Thomasy S, et al. Effects of feline herpesvirus type 1 on tear film break-up time, Schirmer tear test results, and conjunctival goblet cell density in experimentally infected cats. Am J Vet Res 2009;70:394–403.
42. Shinzawa M, Dogru M, Miyasaka K, et al. The Application of Strip Meniscometry to the Evaluation of Tear Volume in Mice. Invest Ophthalmol Vis Sci 2019;60(6):2088–91.
43. Oria A, Raposo A, da Silva Cardoso de Brito V, et al. Tear Meniscometry Test Wild Animals Ciênc Rural 2019;49(11):2–5.
44. Miller R, Hofmann I, Dunbar J. Comparative tests of canine tear film status using the I-strip tear test and the Schirmer tear test Conference Proceedings 48th Annual Conference of the American College of Veterinary Ophthalmologists. Baltimore (Maryland). October 11-14, 2017.
45. Miyasaka K, Kazama Y, Iwashita H, et al. A novel strip meniscometry method for measuring aqueous tear volume in dogs: Clinical correlations with the Schirmer tear and phenol red thread tests. Vet Ophthalmol 2019;22(6):864–71.
46. Rajaei A, Mood M, Asadi F, et al. Strip meniscometry in dogs, cats, and rabbits. Vet Ophthalmol 2018;21(2):210–3.
47. Gelatt KN, Peiffer RL, Erickson JL, et al. Evaluation of tear formation in the dog, using a modification of the Schirmer tear test. J Am Vet Med Assoc 1975;166:368–70.
48. Saito A, Kotani T. Estimation of lacrimal level and testing methods on normal beagles. Vet Ophthalmol 2001;4(1):7–11.
49. McLaughlin S, Brightman A, Helper L, et al. Effect of removal of lacrimal and third eyelid glands on Schirmer tear test results in cats. J Am Vet Med Assoc 1988;193(7):820–2.
50. Feenstra R, Tseng S. Comparison of fluorescein and rose bengal staining. Ophthalmol 1992;99:605–17.
51. Ferreira T, Ghignatti J, dos Santos L, et al. 2018Antimicrobial activity of topical dyes used in clinical veterinary ophthalmology. Vet Ophthalmol 2020;23:497–505.

52. Mironovichi M, Mitchell M, Lui C-C, et al. The effect of topical ophthalmic prop-aracaine, fluorescein, and tropicamide on subsequent bacterial cultures in healthy dogs. Vet Ophthalmol 2021;00:1–8.
53. Grahn B, Sisler S, Storey E. Qualitative tear film and conjunctival goblet cell assessment of cats with corneal sequestra. Vet Ophthalmol 2005;8(3):167–70.
54. Gelatt KN. Vital staining of the canine cornea and conjunctiva with rose bengal. J Am Anim Hosp Assoc 1972;8:17–22.
55. Chodosh J, Dix RD, Howell RC, et al. Staining characteristics and antiviral activ-ity of sulforhodamine b and lissamine green b. Invest Ophth Vis Sci 1994;35:1046–58.
56. Smith S, Holt E, Aguirre G. Conjunctival staining with lissamine green as a pre-dictor of tear film deficiency in dogs. Vet Ophthalmol 2020;23:624–31.
57. Kontiola A. A new electromechanical method for measuring intraocular pres-sure. Documenta Ophthalmologica 1997;93:265–76.
58. Rajaei S, Asadi F, Rajabian M, et al. Effect of body position, eyelid manipulation, and manual jugular compression on intraocular pressure in clinically normal cats. Vet Ophthalmol 2018;21(2):140–3.
59. Rodrigues B, Montiani-Ferreira F, Bortolini M, et al. Intraocular pressure mea-surements using the TONOVET® rebound tonometer: Influence of the probe-cornea distance. Vet Ophthalmol 2021;24(Suppl. 1):175–85.
60. McLellan G, Kemmerlinga J, Kiland J. Validation of the TonoVetR Rebound Tonometer in Normal and Glaucomatous Cats. Vet Ophthalmol 2013;16(2):111–8.
61. Nagata N, Yuki M, Hasegawa T. In Vitro and In Vivo Comparison of Applanation Tonometry and Rebound Tonometry in Dogs. J Vet Med Sci 2011;73(12):1585–9.
62. von Spiessen L, Karck J, Rohn K, et al. Clinical comparison of the TonoVet® rebound tonometer and the Tono-Pen Vet® applanation tonometer in dogs and cats with ocular disease: glaucoma or corneal pathology. Vet Ophthalmol 2015;18(1):20–7.
63. Tofflemire K, Wang J, Jens J, et al. Evaluation of three hand-held tonometers in normal canine eyes. Vet J 2017;224:7–10.
64. Guresh A, Horvath S, Gemensky-Metzler A, et al. The effect of central corneal thickness on intraocular pressure values using various tonometers in the dog. Vet Ophthalmol 2021;24(Suppl. 1):154–61.
65. Minella A, Kiland J, Gloe S, et al. Validation and comparison of four handheld tonometers in normal ex vivo canine eyes. Vet Ophthalmol 2021;24(Suppl. 1):162–70.
66. Ben-Shlomo G, Muirhead S. Estimation of intraocular pressure in normal canine eyes utilizing the newly introduced TonoVet Plus and TonoPen Avia, and their comparison to the established TonoVet. Vet Ophthalmol 2021;24(Suppl. 1):171–4.
67. Shim J, Kang S, Park Y, et al. Comparative intraocular pressure measurements using three different rebound tonometers through in an ex vivo analysis and clin-ical trials in canine eyes. Vet Ophthalmol 2021;24(Suppl. 1):186–93.
68. Adelman S, Shinsako D, Kilanda J, et al. The Post-Natal Development of Intra-ocular Pressure in Normal Domestic Cats (Felis catus) and in Feline Congenital Glaucoma. Exp Eye Res 2018;166:70–3.
69. Gelatt K, MacKay E. Distribution of intraocular pressure in dogs. Vet Ophthalmol 1998;1:109–14.

70. Garzon-Ariza A, Guisado A, Galan A, et al. Diurnal variations in intraocular pressure and central corneal thickness and the correlation between these factors in dogs. Vet Ophthalmol 2018;21(5):464–70.

71. Broadwater J, Schorling J, Herring I, et al. Effect of body position on intraocular pressure in dogs without glaucoma. Am J Vet Res 2008;69:527–30.

72. Pe'er O, Chiu E, Arad D, et al. Does the order of intraocular pressure measurement affect tonometry results? Vet Ophthalmol 2021;24(Suppl. 1):146–53.

73. Pauli A, Bentley E, Diehl K, et al. Effects of the Application of Neck Pressure by a Collar or Harness on Intraocular Pressure in Dogs. J Am Anim Hosp Assoc 2006;42:207–11.

74. Oliveira1 J, Montiani-Ferreira F, Williams D. The influence of the tonometer position on canine intraocular pressure measurements using the Tonovet® rebound tonometer. Open Vet J 2018;8(1):68–76.

75. Leiva M, Naranjo C, Peña M. Comparison of the rebound tonometer (ICare®) to the applanation tonometer (Tonopen XL®) in normotensive dogs. Vet Ophthalmol 2006;9(1):7–21.

76. Miller P, Pickett P, Majors L, Kurzman I. Evaluation of two applanation tonometers in cats. Am J Vet Res 1991;52:1917–21.

77. Ghaffari M, Gherekhloo A. Effect of body position on intraocular pressure in clinically normal cats. J Fel Med Surg 2018;20(8):749–51.

78. Rusanen E, Florin M, Hässig M, et al. Evaluation of a rebound tonometer (Tonovet®) in clinically normal cat eyes. Vet Ophthalmol 2010;13(1):31–6.

79. Martin C. Gonioscopy and anatomical correlations of the drainage angle of the dog. J Small Anim Pract 1969;10:171–84.

80. Bedford P. Gonioscopy in the dog. J Small Anim Pract 1977;18:615–29.

81. McLellan G, Miller P. Feline glaucoma—a comprehensive review. Vet Ophthalmol 2011;14(Suppl.1):15–29.

82. Bedford P. The aetiology of primary glaucoma in the dog. J Small Anim Pract 1975;16:217–39.

83. Pearl R, Gould D, Spiess B. Progression of pectinate ligament dysplasia over time in two populations of Flat-Coated Retrievers. Vet Ophthalmol 2015;18:6–12.

84. Oliver J, Ekiri A, Mellersh C. Pectinate ligament dysplasia in the Border Collie, Hungarian Vizsla and Golden Retriever. Vet Rec 2017;180(11):279–83.

85. Wood J, Lakhani K, Mason I, Barnett K. Relationship of the degree of goniodysgenesis and other ocular measurements to glaucoma in Great Danes. Am J Vet Res 2001;62:1493–9.

86. Trost K, Peiffer R Jr, Nell B. Goniodysgenesis associated with primary glaucoma in an adult European Short-haired cat. Vet Ophthalmol 2007;10(Suppl.1):3–7.

87. Park S, Sledge D, Colleen Monahan C, et al. Primary angle-closure glaucoma with goniodysgenesis in a Beagle dog. BMC Vet Res 2019;15(1):62–75.

88. Cynthia S, Cook L, Wilkie DA. Treatment of presumed iris melanoma in dogs by diode laser photocoagulation: 23 cases. Vet Ophthalmol 1999;2(4):217–25.

89. Featherstone H, Renwick P, Heinrich C, et al. Efficacy of lamellar resection, cryotherapy, and adjunctive grafting for the treatment of canine limbal melanoma. Vet Ophthalmol 2009;12(Suppl. 1):65–72.

90. Oliver J, Cottrell B, Newton J, et al. Gonioscopy in the dog: inter-examiner variability and the search for a grading scheme. J Small Anim Pract 2017;58:652–8.

91. Gibson TE, Roberts SM, Severin GA, et al. Comparison of gonioscopy and ultrasound biomicroscopy for evaluating the iridocorneal angle in dogs. J Am Vet Med Assoc 1998;213:635–8.

92. Hasegawa T, Kawata M, Ota M. Ultrasound biomicroscopic findings of the irido-corneal angle in live healthy and glaucomatous dogs. J Vet Med Sci 2015; 77(12):1625–31.
93. Moeller E, Blocker T, Esson D, et al. Postoperative glaucoma in the Labrador Retriever: incidence, risk factors, and visual outcome following routine phaco-emulsification. Vet Ophthalmol 2011;14(6):385–94.
94. Matusow R, Herring I, Pickett J, et al. Effects of perioperative topical dorzola-mide hydrochloride-timolol maleate administration on incidence and severity of postoperative ocular hypertension in dogs undergoing cataract extraction by phacoemulsification. J Am Vet Med Assoc 2016;249(9):1040–105.
95. Scott E, Esson D, Fritz K, et al. Major breed distribution of canine patients enucleated or eviscerated due to glaucoma following routine cataract surgery as well as common histopathologic findings within enucleated globes. Vet Oph-thalmol 2013;16(Suppl. 1):64–72.
96. Sanders M, Morton J, Kaese H, et al. Association between preoperative gonio-scopic status and postoperative glaucoma after phacoemulsification in dogs: A retrospective cohort study of 505 eyes. Vet. Ophthalmol 2021;24(Suppl.1): 39–49.
97. Zibura A, Robertson J, Westermeyer H. Gonioscopic iridocorneal angle morphology and incidence of postoperative ocular hypertension and glaucoma in dogs following cataract surgery. Vet Ophthalmol 2021;24(Suppl. 1):50–62.
98. Cochet P, Bonnet R. Corneal esthesiometery performance and practical impor-tance. Bull Soc Ophtalmol Fr 1961;6:541–50.
99. Martin X, Safran A. Corneal hypoesthesia. Surv Ophthalmol 1988;33(1):28–40.
100. Good KL, Maggs DJ, Hollingsworth SR, et al. Corneal sensitivity in dogs with diabetes mellitus. Am J Vet Res 2003;64(1):7–11.
101. Costa D, Peña M, Ríos J, et al. Evaluation of corneal anaesthesia after the appli-cation of topical 2 per cent lidocaine, 0.5 per cent bupivacaine and 1 per cent propivacaine in dogs. Vet Rec 2014;174(19):478.
102. Dorbandt D, Labelle A, Mitchell M, et al. The effects of topical diclofenac, topical flurbiprofen, and humidity on corneal sensitivity in normal dogs. Vet Ophthalmol 2017;20(2):160–70.
103. Blocker T, Hoffman A, Schaeffer D, et al. Corneal sensitivity and aqueous tear production in dogs undergoing evisceration with intraocular prosthesis place-ment. Vet Ophthalmol 2007;10(3):147–54.
104. Wieser B, Tichy A, Nell B. Correlation between corneal sensitivity and quantity of reflex tearing in cows, horses, goats, sheep, dogs, cats, rabbits, and guinea pigs. Vet Ophthalmol 2013;16(4):251–62.
105. Arnold T, Wittenburg L, Powell C. Effect of topical naltrexone 0.3% on corneal sensitivity and tear parameters in normal brachycephalic dogs. Vet Ophthalmol 2014;17(5):328–33.
106. Ledbetter E, Marfurt C, Dubielzig R. Metaherpetic corneal disease in a dog associated with partial limbal stem cell deficiency and neurotrophic keratitis. Vet Ophthalmol 2013;16(4):282–8.
107. Robin M-C, Papin Regnier A. Corneal anesthesia associated with topical appli-cation of 2% lidocaine nonophthalmic gel to healthy canine eyes. Vet Ophthal-mol 2020;23:560–6.
108. Cantarella R, de Oliveira J, Dorbandt D, et al. Effects of topical flurbiprofen so-dium, diclofenac sodium, ketorolac tromethamine and benzalkonium chloride on corneal sensitivity in normal dogs. Open Vet J 2017;7(3):254–60.

109. Telle M, Chen N, Shinsako D, et al. Relationship between corneal sensitivity, corneal thickness, corneal diameter, and intraocular pressure in normal cats and cats with congenital glaucoma. Vet Ophthalmol 2019;22(1):4–12.

110. Binder DR, Herring IP. Duration of corneal anesthesia following topical administration of 0.5%proparacaine hydrochloride solution in clinically normal cats. Am J Vet Res 2006;67:1780–2.

111. Roberts J, Meekins J, Roush J, et al. Effects of topical instillation of 0.1% diclofenac sodium, 0.5% ketorolac tromethamine, and 0.03% flurbiprofen sodium on corneal sensitivity in ophthalmologically normal cats. Am J Vet Res 2021; 82:81–7.

An Update on the Ocular Surface Bacterial Microbiota in Small Animals

Marina L. Leis, BSc, DVM, MVSc

KEYWORDS

- Ocular surface • Bacterial culture • Microbiome • Metagenomics
- Antimicrobial resistance

KEY POINTS

- Reducing contamination is imperative during sample collection for clinical investigations of diseases of the paucibacterial ocular surface.
- Clinicians will require a working knowledge of metagenomics as this technology becomes more accessible and available.
- Next-generation sequencing identifies almost all bacteria within a given sample, whereas conventional culture methods identify roughly less than 5%.
- We are reaching a turning point where antimicrobial stewardship will be critical among health-care professionals, including veterinarians, to sustain the levels of care we are able to provide to animals and humans.

INTRODUCTION

Mucosal surfaces are an interface of interaction between complex organisms and the external world. These surfaces have specific anatomic, physiologic, and immunologic functions, and act as a physical barrier to the environment. Importantly, they harbor a wide range of microorganisms. The host maintains control over this community of microorganisms, the microbiota, preventing lesions while indirectly supporting beneficial players. The ocular surface, as one of these interaction interfaces, is equipped with lysozyme and other antimicrobial molecules in tears that act as a barrier to microbial colonization and invasion. Although the ocular surface was traditionally thought to be relatively devoid of microorganisms, it is now recognized as a site hosting a unique community of microorganisms, similarly to other mucosal surfaces. However, when compared with other mucosal sites, the ocular surface hosts a low microbial biomass.[1]

This author has no commercial or financial conflicts of interest to disclose.
Western College of Veterinary Medicine, 52 Campus Drive, Saskatoon, Saskatchewan S7N 5B4, Canada
E-mail address: marina.leis@usask.ca

Knowledge of the ocular surface microbiota is integral to ophthalmic clinical practice, and it is expected that dogmas will change in the next decades as we explore it further. Bacterial culture has been the foundation for our collective understanding regarding the bacteria present in a given sample, a concept dealt with by practitioners on a near daily basis. However, in the 1980s, it was observed that a greater diversity of microbial cells was visually present in fresh samples observed microscopically, when compared with samples from agar culture plates. This is referred to as the great plate count anomaly.[2] This was an initial observation that routine bacterial culture protocols fail to support the entire microbial diversity from clinical samples. High-throughput sequencing (HTS) is a powerful technique that provides valuable insights into what microbial communities comprise a healthy versus a diseased ocular surface. Most of our understanding stems from ongoing research and the technology has yet to reach the clinic floor. Readily accessible commercial kits for the identification of the ocular surface microbiome are beginning to draw the attention of clinicians. However, great caution must be exercised in their day-to-day clinical use, as standardization of the methodology at each step (from DNA extraction to bioinformatics analysis) is required in order to produce meaningful and clinically repeatable results.

In light of these developments, this article aims to summarize the recent evidence regarding the key bacterial players of the ocular surface in dogs and cats in both healthy and diseased states.

CONTRASTING METHODOLOGIES: CULTURE VERSUS HIGH-THROUGHPUT SEQUENCING

To appreciate the clinical value and application of either culture or HTS, one must have a basic understanding of how these techniques work. One method is not better or more useful than the other, rather they are complementary techniques that yield different information.

Culture relies on the viability of bacteria harvested from a sample, and our ability to provide the required nutrients and conditions in a laboratory setting for it to replicate. This represents a potential pitfall of this method as discussed above: current diagnostic culture methods only support a fraction of the microbial diversity observed on mucosal surfaces.[3] As clinicians, we are familiar with samples often yielding negative growth, which can be explained by this limitation. Without a priori knowledge, it would be impractical, expensive, and time consuming to attempt to culture most microbes in a sample.

Conversely, HTS identifies virtually all bacteria within a given sample, not only the bacteria that can be isolated using diagnostic culture procedures (**Fig. 1**). This is achieved through a series of steps aimed at isolating the total DNA from a given sample and constructing DNA libraries that are then sequenced (**Fig. 2**). There are numerous different sequencing technologies, each with advantages and disadvantages. Comparing these techniques is beyond the scope of this study but the clinician should be aware that the bacterial microbiota of a given sample may be investigated by HTS using one of the following approaches:

- Amplicon sequencing: a specific portion of bacterial genome is amplified by targeting a barcoding gene (ie, a universal target). This is usually performed by PCR, which amplifies the gene of interest, generating an amplicon. The most common target gene is 16S rRNA (others are available, such as cpn60). This amplification step introduces bias because different PCR primers used target different regions of such genes and may artificially increase the prevalence of specific phyla.[4] A library of amplicons is then prepared and used to sequence the amplified

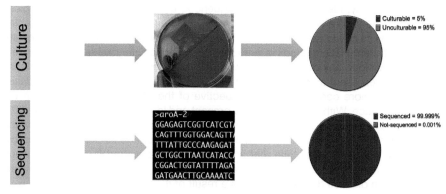

Fig. 1. Differences in the detection of bacteria from a clinical sample using routine diagnostic culture and high-throughput sequencing. Culture relies on the ability to isolate and identify a viable bacterium within a given sample, whereas next-generation sequencing is able to identify virtually all bacteria within a given sample. Data extrapolated from Venter and colleagues, 2004.

DNA. This approach is well established and due to the PCR amplification step, a lower sequencing depth (the amount of sequences generated from a given sample) is needed which helps to reduce costs.

- "Shotgun," untargeted or metagenomic sequencing: total DNA is extracted from a given sample and no further processing is performed. This results in any and all DNA of a given sample being sequenced, regardless of source (bacterial, fungal, viral, mammal). For example, detection of antimicrobial resistance (AMR) genes is a feature of shotgun sequencing, and not amplicon sequencing. Little bias is introduced using this approach when compared with the amplicon approach but a higher sequencing depth is necessary in order to obtain enough information from each sample (ie, to detect rare bacteria DNA in a sample with a large amount of dog DNA). Therefore, this approach is often more costly than amplicon sequencing.

HTS outputs several data, including text (DNA sequences) and quality control markers. Thus, algorithms developed for analysis of this type of data are used, also called the bioinformatics analyses pipelines. They facilitate the practitioner's clinical interpretation of the results by outputting meaningful metrics (discussed below). Analyses begin by removing poor-quality sequences and any other known issues (often specific to each of the sequencing technologies). Once the raw data are cleaned, elimination of contaminants from the data set (if proper controls were in place) can be

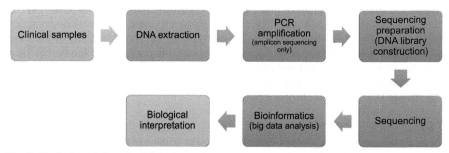

Fig. 2. Typical workflow for high-throughput sequencing from clinical specimens.

performed. Finally, identification of the sequenced DNA and estimation of biological indices can begin (**Table 1**). There is a variety of bioinformatic pipelines available, and each has its advantages and disadvantages.[5] Regardless, comparing data resulting from different HTS methods is not ideal because specific biases are introduced and this may cloud any conclusions drawn. In parallel, as discussed above, bacterial culture may represent an oversimplification of the bacterial picture in a clinical case. HTS yields a more comprehensive perspective of the bacterial players present on the ocular surface. With so many bacteria present and identified by HTS, it can be difficult to determine which ones are responsible for disease or are clinically relevant. Nonetheless, it is more realistic to envision the ocular surface as being inhabited by distinct communities of bacteria that are far more complex and fluid than we were able to appreciate with culture, and where dysbiosis of those resident communities plays a role in disease development or is a result of it.

SAMPLE COLLECTION AND GOOD DIAGNOSTIC PRACTICES IN THE ERA OF SEQUENCING

Quality control is pivotal when it comes to sampling a low microbial biomass surface such as the eye.[6] The number of microorganisms present on the ocular surface is of several orders of magnitude lower than other mucosal surfaces such as the gastrointestinal tract, skin, or oral cavity, which has implications with respect to the potential for contamination and diagnostic test analytical sensitivity. When collecting ocular surface samples for culture, only the area of interest should be touched with the swab (**Fig. 3**). In addition, gloves and a face mask should be worn and the swab should be opened to the environment for as short a time as possible.

Use of a topical anesthetic is sometimes necessary for sample collection; however, it is a known carrier of contaminants and antibacterial activity.[7,8] When possible, it is preferable to use preservative-free topical anesthetics because they are the least bactericidal.[9] However, recent clinical studies suggest that the use of topical 0.5% proparacaine before sample collection for aerobic cultures had no significant impact on growth.[10,11]

Culture

In a clinical setting, aerobic cultures of an ulcerated cornea are widely performed to rule out secondary bacterial infection. Anaerobic cultures should also routinely be performed in cases of ulcerative keratitis as bacteria were isolated in 14% of corneal ulcers in dogs and 8% of cats in one study.[12] A recent abstract presentation demonstrated that microbial samples obtained via direct sampling of a corneal ulcer with subsequent culturette submission to a laboratory did not yield significantly different culture results when compared with direct plating of the sample.[13] In addition, the use of a premoistened swab is recommended because it may significantly increase the rate of detection of gram-positive organisms, as shown in cats.[14] When directly swabbing a corneal ulcer for culture, some clinicians may have reservations about performing this when the cornea is significantly compromised (eg, in the case of a descemetocele). In these cases, sampling from the conjunctival fornix may be a suitable alternative to direct sampling of a corneal ulcer,[15] although we recommend direct sampling of the corneal ulcer because fornix cultures may identify bacteria that do not reside on the corneal surface.[1]

High-Throughput Sequencing

Standardization of methodology in metagenomics studies is the most significant limitation preventing the use of this powerful technology in both research and clinical

Table 1
Definitions for portions of the bioinformatics analysis used during high-throughput sequencing

Term	Definition
Ocular surface	Composed of the epithelial surface overlying the cornea and conjunctiva (bulbar, palpebral, and third eyelid), the margin of the eyelids, and the tears
Sequencing	Technique to establish the nucleotide sequence of DNA or RNA (through cDNA)
High-throughput sequencing ("Next" generation sequencing, Massive parallel sequencing)	A set of technologies developed since the late 1990s that yield large amounts of DNA (or cDNA) data in a single run from multiple samples simultaneously
Read/sequence	A single segment of DNA sequenced and outputted as text file by sequencing machines
Metagenome	Collection of genomes in a given sample
Ocular microbiome	Collective genetic material (genomes) belonging to microbial communities of the ocular surface
Ocular microbiota	The totality of microbes at a particular site, both commensal and pathogenic. Literally the "microbial biome (ecosystem)," which includes virus, fungi, bacteria, protozoa.
Operational Taxonomic Unit (OUT) and ASV	Groups of sequences that are similar (often >97%) to a reference sequence (eg, E coli), suggesting a read was likely obtained from a bacteria from that taxonomy. In studies of the bacterial microbiota, this is often obtained by sequencing the 16S rRNA gene
16S rRNA gene	The gene encoding the small ribosomal subunit RNA of bacteria. The nucleotide base sequence of the gene contains regions that are variable in composition. These V regions are interspersed between regions where the nucleotide base sequence is highly conserved among all bacteria. The V region sequences provide useful taxonomic information: the "signatures" of bacterial groups
Alpha diversity	Diversity of bacteria within a sample
Beta diversity	Degree of similarity between 2 (microbial) communities
Richness	Number of species in a given sample
Evenness	Abundance of each species in a given sample
Dysbiosis	Alterations in richness and community structure
Community membership	Taxa that are present in the community
Community structure	Distribution of taxa in a community

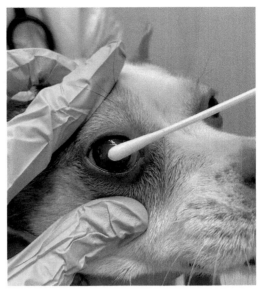

Fig. 3. Sample collection of low microbial biomass surfaces, such as the cornea and conjunctiva, requires caution. Precise targeting of the area of interest and the utilization of personal protective equipment are important in the minimization of contamination for HTS processing.

settings.[16] At each step of the analysis when dealing with a paucibacterial surface such as the cornea or conjunctiva, there is the potential for contamination that outweighs the true microbiome signal. This is particularly challenging because, different from culture, HTS does not require live cells for detection—just DNA. Therefore, it is paramount that one is rigorous about the inclusion of negative controls at each step of the analysis, beginning with clinicians who should choose to include a control swab with each submission. Recent study has evidenced that while sterile, common diagnostic swabs and even Schirmer tear strips are contaminated with bacterial DNA (**Fig. 4**).[1] The clinician should be aware that downstream processing by the diagnostic laboratory may also affect the results. Small differences in procedural techniques will end up in large differences in the results obtained. As discussed above, differences in primer pairs used for amplicon sequencing affect the results, meaning completely different conclusions could be drawn depending on which PCR primers were used.[4] This obviously puts into question the utility of metagenomics studies altogether. This shortcoming is present at each step of the analysis in microbiome studies, and it is important to keep this in mind when evaluating data. In addition to the inclusion of contaminant control samples, it is suggested to include in the diagnostic submission a sample from the contralateral, healthy eye when feasible. This increases the diagnostic value of HTS, as discussed below.

INTERPRETING SEQUENCING DATA AND DIAGNOSTIC REPORTS

To become a useful instrument in the clinician's toolbox, HTS data must be properly interpreted. As discussed previously, good-quality diagnostics begins with sample collection and the inclusion of control samples. Once results are provided by the laboratory, the clinician has the opportunity to combine these with their clinical

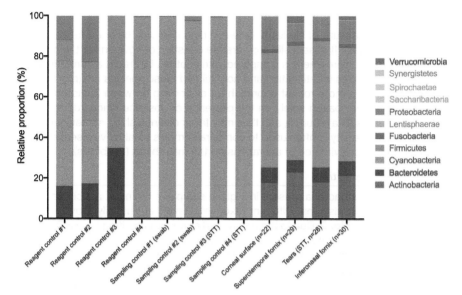

Fig. 4. Examples of sources of contamination that may affect high-throughput sequencing results. Reagent controls—no sample added, only reagents. Sampling control—Unused swab analyzed without sampling an animal. Tears/STT—Unused Schirmer tear test strip.

observation and other ancillary tests. In general, HTS data is explored based on the following metrics: alpha diversity, beta diversity, and phylogenetic composition (regardless of the method used to generate the data). Detailed descriptions of such metrics may be found in previous reviews.[17] **Table 1** provides a glossary as a quick reference guide for the clinician.

Alpha Diversity

Alpha-diversity relates to the species evenness and richness in a given sample. Richness relates to the number of species (how many microbes?) observed in a given habitat (or sample, eg, a swab). Evenness is the abundance of each species within a given habitat (do some species dominate others?). Diversity considers both richness and evenness, and is usually described as an index. During the years, multiple alpha diversity indices were developed with different goals. The most commonly used in microbial ecology are Shannon's index (estimates species richness and evenness, with more weight on richness), Simpson's index: (estimates species richness and evenness, with more weight on evenness) and Chao1 index (abundance-based estimator of richness only). In limited cases, alpha diversity may be simply reported as the number of species present in a sample (eg, operational taxonomic unit [OTU] count). The use of one of the indices mentioned above is preferred, and confers a more complete overview of the bacterial community of a sample.

In general, microbial diversity on mucosal surfaces decreases following disease onset. Thus, as recommended in "Sample collection and good diagnostic practices in the era of sequencing" section of this article, submission of paired (healthy and diseased eye) samples from the same animal are helpful for evaluation of both alpha and beta diversity. Keep in mind that species identification (phylogeny) is irrelevant for alpha-diversity analysis.

Beta-Diversity

This metric is a measure of similarity between (and can only be used for) 2 or more habitats (or samples). It essentially answers the question of how similar the microbial community in one environment is compared with another. Unifrac is a common metric that considers species identification and how related those species are (phylogenetic distance), offering a more robust approach for discerning between 2 microbial communities. Others are based solely on the presence or absence (Jaccard) or species abundance counts (Bray-Curtis), and thus may fail at distinguishing somewhat related samples. Beta-diversity is often used to compare samples (healthy vs diseased eyes), thus offering further evidence of alterations on the microbiota (dysbiosis).

Phylogenetic Composition

Identification of the bacteria present in a given sample is the most anticipated result from diagnostic submissions. Different taxonomic levels are usually provided in this report, as shown in **Fig. 5**. Due to the untargeted approach resulting from HTS, phylogenetic composition is often reported as a relative proportion of different taxa. At this point, the clinician should be familiar with 2 terms that may seem in diagnostic reports: OTU and amplicon sequence variant (ASV). Due to genomic mutations, sequences obtained from microbial communities are often not 100% similar to those deposited in the reference databases used for bacterial identification. Therefore, in simple terms, OTU and ASV are grouping strategies to cluster sequences that are somewhat similar to a known, reference sequence (eg, sequences that are 97% similar to Escherichia coli). **Fig. 4** exemplifies the relative proportion of bacterial phyla in a given sample, as this type of data is usually reported. Based on the author's experience and previously published data,[18] the clinician is advised that pathogenic bacteria may not be detected in large proportions, and yet may still be the causative insult associated with disease.

BIOGEOGRAPHY OF THE OCULAR SURFACE MICROBIOME

Similar to the gastrointestinal tract, where different anatomic sites are associated with different bacterial communities, there is evidence that different areas of the ocular surface provide specialized niches for bacteria to thrive.[19] However, due to the low biomass present on the ocular surface and the specificity of classic microbiology methods, the biogeography of the ocular surface remained unexplored until recently. The assumption that the ocular surface is colonized by one contiguous and homogenous bacterial community is no longer acceptable. The application of HTS seems to

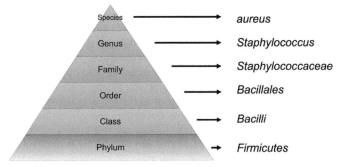

Fig. 5. Taxonomic levels for S aureus from highest (top) to lowest (bottom) resolution.

demonstrate that specific bacteria inhabit the cornea and these are distinct from the rest of the ocular surface. This was reported in a study of the ocular surface in pigs, where bacteria inhabiting the cornea were less diverse than the conjunctiva and specific to the cornea.[1] This initial evidence suggests that the cornea harbors specific bacterial taxa, distinct from the superotemporal and inferonasal fornices (**Fig. 6**). Therefore, when sampling the ocular surface, the site sampled should be the affected structure, otherwise it may not be representative of the bacteria of interest.

COMPOSITION OF THE OCULAR SURFACE MICROBIOTA

When referring to the microbiota of the ocular surface in normal, healthy animals, the conjunctiva is typically the anatomic site of interest, although this could be questioned as previously discussed. Conversely, when reporting results from animals with ulcerative keratitis, the lesion within the cornea itself represents the area of interest. Given that the epithelia from the cornea and conjunctiva are contiguous with each other, it is generally thought that the bacterial communities present would be the same across these regions. Although this is logical and clinically relevant, there is now evidence from a metagenomics perspective that distinct regions on the ocular surface are associated with distinct bacterial communities (see "Biogeography of the ocular surface microbiome" section). The core conjunctival microbiome likely plays an important role in the maintenance of health and protection from opportunistic infections, however also represents a source of potential pathogens.

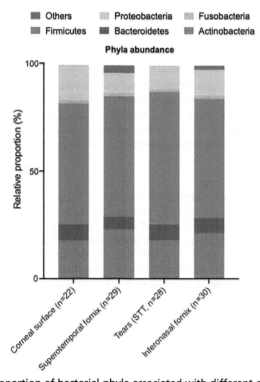

Fig. 6. Relative proportion of bacterial phyla associated with different ocular surface structures from pigs. STT—Schirmer tear test strip.

Healthy Canine Microbiota

Culture

Ever since the twentieth century, there is general consensus from a culture perspective that gram-positive bacteria predominate on the ocular surface in both health and disease.[20–22] In healthy dogs, gram-positive bacteria predominate over gram-negative bacteria and *Staphylococcus*, *Bacillus*, *Neisseria*, and *Corynebacterium* spp are among the most frequently isolated genera[23–25] (**Table 2**).

High-throughput sequencing

Exploration of the canine ocular microbiota by HTS is in its infancy. Pioneering studies have demonstrated that the bacteria frequently recovered by culture of the normal canine conjunctiva over time have largely been overrepresented[26–28] (**Table 3**). Recent studies evidenced that *Staphylococcus*, *Bacillus*, *Neisseria*, and *Corynebacterium* spp isolated by culture represented a small proportion of the total bacterial load on the ocular surface. Genera such as *Bifidobacterium* and *Acinetobacter* were found to represent a larger proportion of the bacterial community found in ocular surface samples[26,28] and went largely undetected with culture-dependent methods likely due to limitations of the techniques used. It was also shown that the ocular surface bacterial microbiome in normal dogs was stable over 7 days and did not change significantly following daily topical neomycin-polymyxin-bacitracin therapy.[27]

This finding, and similar findings across veterinary and human medicine, put into question what we knew and understood regarding the normal ocular surface bacterial microflora. Suddenly, a new and overwhelming world of data became available for discovery. Although sequencing studies generate and continue to generate large volumes of data, resolution to the species level does not easily occur.

Healthy Feline Microbiota

Culture

The predominance of gram-positive bacteria over gram-negative bacteria isolated from the normal conjunctiva is much the same in cats as it is in dogs.[20–22] In clinically normal cats, culture of the conjunctiva revealed a wide-ranging positivity rate (4% to 67%) where primarily *Staphylococcus*, *Streptococcus*, *Enterococcus*, and *Moraxella* were isolated.[14,29–31] Similarly, the most commonly isolated conjunctival bacteria in Persian cats were *Staphylococcus*, *Streptococcus*, *Corynebacterium*, and *Escherichia*[32,33] (see **Table 2**).

High-throughput sequencing

HTS studies have uncovered largely ignored bacteria that undoubtedly fulfill a role as part of the normal ocular surface microflora, such as *Acinetobacter*, *Psychrobacter*, *Bacteroides*, and other genera[34,35] (see **Table 3**). In addition, the bacterial ocular surface microbiome in clinically normal cats before and after treatment with topical erythromycin did not change significantly and was stable during 1 week.[36] However, the environment seems to play an important role in seeding the ocular microbiota. Cats introduced to a feline shelter undergo significant changes in the bacterial communities (both membership and structure) after 1 week, including a potential shift toward known feline ocular surface pathogens.[34]

CLINICAL RELEVANCE OF THE OCULAR SURFACE MICROBIOTA

Keratoconjunctivitis Sicca in Dogs

The ocular surface microbiota of dogs with keratoconjunctivitis sicca, or dry eye, has not been thought to play a role in disease development. However, there is increasing

Table 2
Bacterial microflora of the ocular surface in the dog and cat as determined by aerobic and anaerobic culture

Family	Isolates	Disease	Source
Canine	*Staphylococcus, Bacillus, Corynebacterium, Clostridium*	Healthy	McDonald *et al*, 1976
Canine	*Staphylococcus, Streptococcus, Bacillus, E coli, Proteus*	Conjunctivitis, blepharitis, dacryocystitis, or corneal ulceration	Murphy *et al*, 1978
Canine	*Staphylococcus, Streptococcus, Pseudomonas*	External ocular disease	Gerding et al, 1988
Canine	*Staphylococcus, Streptococcus, Corynebacterium, Enterobacter, Escherichia, Klebsiella, Acinetobacter Staphylococcus, Streptococcus, Corynebacterium, Enterobacter, Escherichia, Pseudomonas, Proteus*	Healthy Corneal ulcerations	Prado *et al*, 2005
Canine	*Staphylococcus, Streptococcus, Pseudomonas*	Bacterial keratitis	Tolar *et al*, 2006
Canine	*Staphylococcus, Streptococcus, Micrococcus, Stomatococcus, Neisseria, Corynebacterium, Rhodococcus, Acinetobacter, Pseudomonas, Moraxella, Enterobacteriaceae, Salmonella, Proteus Staphylococcus, Streptococcus, Micrococcus, Stomatococcus, Neisseria, Corynebacterium, Rhodococcus, Acinetobacter, Pseudomonas, Moraxella, Enterobacteriaceae*	Healthy Corneal ulcerations	Wang *et al*, 2008
Canine	*Clostridium, Peptostreptococcus, Actinomyces, Fusobacterium, Bacteroides*	Ulcerative keratitis	Ledbetter *et al*, 2008
Canine	*Streptococcus, Staphylococcus, Pseudomonas*	Bacterial keratitis	Hindley *et al*, 2016
Feline	*Staphylococcus, Streptococcus Staphylococcus, Streptococcus, Chlamydophila, Mycoplasma*	Healthy Conjunctivitis	Shewen *et al*, 1980
Feline	*Peptostreptococcus, Fusobacterium, Bacteroides*	Ulcerative keratitis	Ledbetter *et al*, 2008
Feline	*Staphylococcus, Streptococcus, Chlamydophila, Micrococcus, Mycoplasma, Corynebacterium, Pseudomonas, Enterobacteriaceae*	Conjunctivitis and upper respiratory disease	Hartmann *et al*, 2010

(*continued on next page*)

Table 2 (continued)			
Family	Isolates	Disease	Source
Feline	Staphylococcus, Micrococcus, Streptococcus, Moraxella, Bacillus, Acinetobacter, Pseudomonas, Pantoea, Pasteurella, Escherichia, Neisseria	Healthy	Buttner et al, 2019
Feline	Staphylococcus, Streptococcus, Corynebacterium, Escherichia	Healthy Persian cats	Aftab et al, 2019 Arteaga et al, 2021

evidence that human patients with dry eye harbor a distinct ocular microbiome compared with healthy controls where microbial diversity was lower and the relative abundance of several genera was reduced.[37,38] Interplay between inflammation, a lack of aqueous tears, and microbial dysbiosis may contribute to disease pathogenesis. In dogs with dry eye, the ocular surface microbiota is not well described. One study demonstrated a reduced rate of bacterial isolation from the conjunctiva of dogs with keratoconjunctivitis sicca following response to topical cyclosporine treatment.[39] However, among eyes that did not respond to treatment, a significant change over time in prevalence or type of bacteria isolated was not found.[39] Currently, it remains unclear whether changes in the ocular microbiota of dogs affected by dry eye is a cause or a consequence of the disease. Further research in this field is required to help clarify this.

Contact Lens Wear

Bandage contact lenses are often applied to the cornea by ophthalmologists because they facilitate a multifaceted treatment of canine indolent corneal ulcers (otherwise known as superficial chronic corneal epithelial defect). The bacterial microflora as determined by culture was not found to be altered during bandage contact lens wear in dogs with 2 types of commercially available lenses, and the most common bacterial organisms isolated before and following bandage contact lens placement for 14 days were, as expected, Staphylococcus, Streptococcus, and Bacillus spp.[40] Similarly, there were no differences in in vivo bacterial adhesion between 2 types of contact lenses worn by dogs for 24 hours.[41] Metagenomics studies in humans have demonstrated that contact lens wear significantly alters the structure of the conjunctival microbiota, rendering it more similar to the skin microbiota, and possibly increasing the risk of keratitis.[7,42] To this point, no data is yet available from small animal patients.

Ulcerative Keratitis

The ocular surface condition in veterinary medicine that has received the most attention with respect to investigations of bacteria is ulcerative keratitis. This is a condition where the corneal epithelium is ulcerated, and where there is potential for bacterial infection (bacterial keratitis) by commensals and pathogens. When corneal ulceration progresses to involve deeper portions of the corneal stroma, vision, and the integrity of the globe are threatened. Empiric use of antimicrobials is essential in the multilayered management of corneal ulceration and bacterial keratitis, while awaiting aerobic and anaerobic culture and antimicrobial susceptibility results. Special attention to isolates

Table 3

Bacterial microflora of the ocular surface in the dog and cat as determined by next-generation sequencing (genera contributing to 5% or more of the total DNA present within a sample)

Family	Disease	Genera	Source
Canine	Healthy conjunctiva	Bifidobacterium, Acinetobacter, Corynebacterium	Leis et al, 2019
Canine	Healthy conjunctiva	Unclassified Micrococcaceae, unclassified Pasteurellaceae, unclassified Pseudomonadaceae	Rogers et al, 2020
Canine	Healthy conjunctiva	Acinetobacter, unclassified Moraxellaceae	Banks et al, 2020
Feline	Healthy FIV	Staphylococcus, Pseudomonas, Acinetobacter, unclassified Clostridiales, Psychrobacter, Aerococcus Staphylococcus, Pseudomonas, unclassified Enterobacteriaceae, Sporosarcina	Weese et al, 2015
Feline	Healthy	Unclassified Helicobacteraceae, Corynebacterium	Darden et al, 2019
Feline	Healthy Cats with upper respiratory disease	Bacteroides, Fusobacterium Bacteroides	Lucyshyn et al, 2021

demonstrating AMR and judicious use of antimicrobials is paramount in these cases (see "Antimicrobial resistance" section).

Factors predisposing dogs to corneal ulceration and infection are trauma, being a brachycephalic breed, previous ocular surgery, prior or concurrent use of a topical corticosteroid, aqueous tear deficiency (tear production <10 mm/min), and concurrent ocular surface disease.[43–45]

Staphylococcus, Streptococcus, Pseudomonas, Corynebacterium, Escherichia spp were the most commonly isolated bacteria in culture studies of ulcerative keratitis and bacterial keratitis.[15,23,25,43–49]

Bacterial infections are not thought to play a large role in indolent corneal ulcer formation, and one study demonstrated that healing rates were not significantly different between indolent ulcers where bacteria were isolated (most commonly *Staphylococcus* and *Streptococcus*) from indolent ulcers where bacteria were not isolated.[50]

Although metagenomics studies in veterinary ophthalmology are currently lacking, the microbiome was found to be altered in humans with ulcerative keratitis, where *Pseudomonas* was present at a greater relative abundance, the abundance of potential pathogens was increased, and the abundance of commensals was reduced.[51,52] This corroborates previous data from dogs/cats, suggesting that *Pseudomonas* spp may play a role in ulcerative keratitis development regardless of the host species.

Feline Diseases

Cats are more frequently affected by primary viral and bacterial infectious conjunctivitis. In cats with clinical signs of conjunctivitis, bacteria detected by culture included *Streptococcus, Staphylococcus, Mycoplasma, Micrococcus*, and *Chlamydophila*.[29,53] The performance of culture is sometimes of limited diagnostic value because these organisms can be present both in health and disease, and positive bacterial cultures occur in cats with and without clinical signs of conjunctivitis.[31] In cats with ulcerative keratitis, the most commonly isolated gram-positive bacteria were *Staphylococcus* species while *Pseudomonas aeruginosa* was the most common Gram-negative bacteria.[54] This further supports the findings discussed above for human and canine subjects.

One study using HTS did demonstrate that the conjunctival microbiome community membership and structure in cats with systemic feline immunodeficiency virus (FIV) infection was significantly different from FIV-uninfected controls, with differences in community membership.[35] Metagenomics studies regarding ocular surface disease in cats are lacking but we expect that they will become more prevalent with time.

ANTIMICROBIAL RESISTANCE

Multiple public and private organizations have declared AMR to represent a major threat to human, animal, and environmental health.[55,56] The global economic cost of AMR is approximately US$3 trillion in gross domestic product losses annually.[57] In Canada, it was estimated that AMR accounted for more than 14,00 deaths in 2018 and cost the Canadian health-care system about US$1.4 billion in 2018 and could reach US$6 to US$8 billion by 2050 (https://cca-reports.ca/wp-content/uploads/2018/10/When-Antibiotics-Fail-1.pdf, accessed November 23, 2021). Similar to the Canadian data, it was estimated that 2.8 million infections and more than 35,000 deaths from antimicrobial resistant bacteria occur annually in the United States (https://www.cdc.gov/drugresistance/biggest-threats.html, accessed November 23, 2021).

There is wide consensus that a coordinated One Health approach is urgently needed in order to even begin to combat this global public health emergency, and veterinarians have a major role in mitigation of AMR through judicious use of antimicrobials and good antimicrobial stewardship.[58]

The interpretation of in vitro antimicrobial susceptibility and resistance testing is a challenge with respect to infections of the ocular surface as they are based on blood and tissue levels of the drug. However, it is currently the information clinicians have available and, although imperfect, is the cornerstone of decisions regarding antimicrobial therapy particularly in cases of infected corneal ulcers.

Staphylococcus spp

Staphylococcus aureus and *Staphylococcus pseudintermedius* are associated with the emergence of methicillin resistance, which represents an important problem not only in the disease management of a particular patient, but are significant concerns for animal and public health.[59]

In a study investigating canine external eye disease, *Staphylococcus* was isolated in 59% of cases, where *Staphylococcus intermedius* was the most frequent species, followed by *S aureus* and the coagulase-negative species *Staphylococcus epidermidis*, and *S simulans*. Of great concern was that resistance to at least one drug was observed in 92.5% of the isolates, and multidrug resistance in 72.5% of isolates. The most effective antimicrobials in this study were ceftiofur and cefalexin.[60] Another study of ulcerative keratitis in dogs revealed that more than 50% of the *S intermedius* isolates were resistant to erythromycin, gentamicin, neomycin, and polymyxin B.

Following cataract surgery, dogs treated with ofloxacin 4 times daily for 3 weeks had a higher bacterial load and a higher proportion of *Staphylococcus* spp that were resistant to ofloxacin at the 3 week mark, demonstrating the intentional selection of resistant bacteria in day-to-day clinical practice.[61]

The ocular surface is a potential source of Methicillin-resistant *S pseudintermedius* (MRSP), a pathogenic and zoonotic bacterium of great clinical significance, and the prevalence was found to be less than 1% in the conjunctival sac of healthy dogs.[62] However, cross-contamination of MRSP from dogs and cats affected by ophthalmic disease to the environment,[63] as well as bacterial contamination of slit lamps[64] was demonstrated in a veterinary ophthalmology setting, and represents a concerning source of nosocomial infections and zoonoses. In another study, ophthalmic cases yielded a 40% positivity rate for *S pseudintermedius* in dogs and cats, where the prevalence of MRSP was 3% (dogs only).[65] Therefore, appropriate infection control precautions such as cleaning are paramount in preventing transfer of these pathogens to other animals and humans.

STREPTOCOCCUS SPP

Beta-hemolytic *Streptococcus* is another concerning pathogen with growing AMR in ocular surface disease, including ulcerative keratitis in dogs where more than 80% of beta-hemolytic *Streptococcus* spp isolates were resistant to neomycin, polymyxin B, and tobramycin.[44] Another study in dogs with ulcerative keratitis and in vitro antimicrobial susceptibility patterns demonstrated that monotherapy with ciprofloxacin was ineffective in ulcers caused by β-hemolytic *Streptococcus* spp but it remained susceptible to chloramphenicol and cephalexin.[43] *Streptococcus* was also found to be resistant to ciprofloxacin in a study regarding ulcerative keratitis in dogs.[49]

PSEUDOMONAS SPP

In dogs with ulcerative keratitis, *P aeruginosa* isolates were resistant to chloramphenicol, cephalexin, and fusidic acid; however, greater than 90% were susceptible to ciprofloxacin, polymyxin B, and gentamicin.[43] Further research in animals with ocular surface infections with *Pseudomonas* demonstrated increasing resistance to tobramycin.[66] Yet another study in dogs reported more than 50% of *Pseudomonas* isolates were resistant to 11 of the 15 antibiotics tested, and that amikacin and ciprofloxacin were active against the greatest proportion of isolates.[49] In contrast, most of the bacteria (*Staphylococcus*, *Streptococcus*, and *Pseudomonas*) isolated from feline eyes with ulcerative keratitis demonstrated less resistance, and ciprofloxacin and gentamicin were found to be highly effective against most of the isolates.[54]

SUMMARY

HTS techniques have revolutionized the way we understand microbial communities in both research and clinical settings and are elucidating what organisms contribute to a healthy ocular surface and a diseased one. As more diagnostic laboratories incorporate HTS into their technique repertoire, and as the methodology is refined and normalized, practitioners can expect this technology to become increasingly accessible for clinical practice, potentially becoming the new standard in the future.

AMR is a global public health threat where veterinarians have a large and urgent role to play. In addition to profiling the microbiota, the detection of AMR genes using shotgun sequencing will become a powerful tool for mitigation of AMR.

CLINICS CARE POINTS

- Donning appropriate personal protective equipment such as gloves and a mask prior to sample collection may help to reduce contamination when investigating the low microbial biomass of the ocular surface using HTS
- The inclusion of environmental controls (swabs open to ambient air but not in contact with the ocular surface) is imperative to remove contaminant sequences
- Considerable work remains in order to make high-throughput sequencing applicable and accessible to a clinical setting

REFERENCES

1. Leis ML, Madruga GM, Costa MO. The porcine corneal surface bacterial microbiome: A distinctive niche within the ocular surface. PLoS One 2021;16(2): e0247392.
2. Staley JT, Konopka A. Measurement of in situ activities of nonphotosynthetic microorganisms in aquatic and terrestrial habitats. Annu Rev Microbiol 1985;39: 321–46.
3. Lagkouvardos I, Overmann J, Clavel T. Cultured microbes represent a substantial fraction of the human and mouse gut microbiota. Gut Microbes 2017;8(5): 493–503.
4. Brooks JP, Edwards DJ, Harwich DHJ, et al. The truth about metagenomics: quantifying and counteracting bias in 16S rRNA studies. BMC Microbiol 2015; 15:66.
5. Siegwald L, Touzet H, Lemoine Y, et al. Assessment of Common and Emerging Bioinformatics Pipelines for Targeted Metagenomics. PLoS One 2017;12(1): e0169563.

6. Doan T, Akileswaran L, Andersen D, et al. Paucibacterial Microbiome and Resident DNA Virome of the Healthy Conjunctiva. Invest Ophthalmol Vis Sci 2016; 57(13):5116–26.
7. Shin H, Price K, Albert L, et al. Changes in the Eye Microbiota Associated with Contact Lens Wearing. mBio 2016;7(2):e00198.
8. Onerci Celebi O, Celebi ARC. The Effect of Topical Ocular Anesthetic Proparacaine on Conjunctival and Nasal Mucosal Flora in Dry Eye Disease Patients. J Clin Med 2018;7(4).
9. Pelosini L, Treffene S, Hollick EJ. Antibacterial activity of preservative-free topical anesthetic drops in current use in ophthalmology departments. Cornea 2009; 28(1):58–61.
10. Fentiman KE, Rankin AJ, Meekins JM, et al. Effects of topical ophthalmic application of 0.5% proparacaine hydrochloride on aerobic bacterial culture results for naturally occurring infected corneal ulcers in dogs. J Am Vet Med Assoc 2018; 253(9):1140–5.
11. Edwards SG, Maggs DJ, Byrne BA, et al. Effect of topical application of 0.5% proparacaine on corneal culture results from 33 dogs, 12 cats, and 19 horses with spontaneously arising ulcerative keratitis. Vet Ophthalmol 2019;22(4): 415–22.
12. Ledbetter EC, Scarlett JM. Isolation of obligate anaerobic bacteria from ulcerative keratitis in domestic animals. Vet Ophthalmol 2008;11(2):114–22.
13. Abstracts: The 52nd Annual Scientific Meeting of the American College of Veterinary Ophthalmologists, Indianapolis, IN Sept 29-Oct 2, 2020. Vet Ophthalmol, 2021.
14. Buttner JN, Schneider M, Jaqueline C, et al. Microbiota of the conjunctival sac of 120 healthy cats. Vet Ophthalmol 2019;22(3):328–36.
15. Auten CR, Urbanz JL, Dees DD. Comparison of bacterial culture results collected via direct corneal ulcer vs conjunctival fornix sampling in canine eyes with presumed bacterial ulcerative keratitis. Vet Ophthalmol 2020;23(1):135–40.
16. Scott EM, Lewin AC, Leis ML. Current ocular microbiome investigations limit reproducibility and reliability: Critical review and opportunities. Vet Ophthalmol 2021;24(1):4–11.
17. Lucas R, Groeneveld J, Harms H, et al. A critical evaluation of ecological indices for the comparative analysis of microbial communities based on molecular datasets. FEMS Microbiol Ecol 2017;93(1).
18. Kuroda M, Sekizuka T, Shinya F, et al. Detection of a possible bioterrorism agent, Francisella sp., in a clinical specimen by use of next-generation direct DNA sequencing. J Clin Microbiol 2012;50(5):1810–2.
19. Ozkan J, Wilcox M, Wemheuer B, et al. Biogeography of the human ocular microbiota. Ocul Surf 2019;17(1):111–8.
20. Gaskin JM. Microbiology of the canine and feline eye. Vet Clin North Am Small Anim Pract 1980;10(2):303–16.
21. Gerding PA Jr, Kakoma I. Microbiology of the canine and feline eye. Vet Clin North Am Small Anim Pract 1990;20(3):615–25.
22. Whitley RD. Canine and feline primary ocular bacterial infections. Vet Clin North Am Small Anim Pract 2000;30(5):1151–67.
23. Prado MR, Rocha MFG, Brito EHS, et al. Survey of bacterial microorganisms in the conjunctival sac of clinically normal dogs and dogs with ulcerative keratitis in Fortaleza, Ceara, Brazil. Vet Ophthalmol 2005;8(1):33–7.
24. McDonald PJ, Watson DJ. Microbial flora of normal canine conjunctivae. J Small Anim Pract 1976;17(12):809–12.

25. Wang L, Pan Q, Zhang L, et al. Investigation of bacterial microorganisms in the conjunctival sac of clinically normal dogs and dogs with ulcerative keratitis in Beijing, China. Vet Ophthalmol 2008;11(3):145–9.

26. Leis ML, Costa MO. Initial description of the core ocular surface microbiome in dogs: Bacterial community diversity and composition in a defined canine population. Vet Ophthalmol 2019;22(3):337–44.

27. Rogers CM, Scott EM, Sarawichitr B, et al. Evaluation of the bacterial ocular surface microbiome in ophthalmologically normal dogs prior to and following treatment with topical neomycin-polymyxin-bacitracin. PLoS One 2020;15(6): e0234313.

28. Banks KC, Giuliano EA, Busi SB, et al. Evaluation of Healthy Canine Conjunctival, Periocular Haired Skin, and Nasal Microbiota Compared to Conjunctival Culture. Front Vet Sci 2020;7:558.

29. Shewen PE, Povey RC, Wilson MR. A survey of the conjunctival flora of clinically normal cats and cats with conjunctivitis. Can Vet J 1980;21(8):231–3.

30. Espinola MB, Lilenbaum W. Prevalence of bacteria in the conjunctival sac and on the eyelid margin of clinically normal cats. J Small Anim Pract 1996;37(8):364–6.

31. Kielbowicz Z, Ploneczka-Janeczko JB, Bania J, et al. Characteristics of the bacterial flora in the conjunctival sac of cats from Poland. J Small Anim Pract 2015; 56(3):203–6.

32. Aftab G, Rajaei SM, Pot SA, et al. Seasonal Effects on the Corneoconjunctival Microflora in a Population of Persian Cats in Iran. Top Companion Anim Med 2019;34:30–2.

33. Arteaga K, Aftab G, Rajaei SM, et al. Comparison of conjunctival microbiota of clinically normal Persian cats with and without nasolacrimal duct obstruction. Vet Ophthalmol 2021;24(5):455–9.

34. Lucyshyn DR, Maggs DJ, Cooper AE, et al. Feline conjunctival microbiota in a shelter: effects of time, upper respiratory disease and famciclovir administration. J Feline Med Surg 2021;23(4):316–30.

35. Weese SJ, Nichols J, Jalali M, et al. The oral and conjunctival microbiotas in cats with and without feline immunodeficiency virus infection. Vet Res 2015;46:21.

36. Darden JE, Scott EM, Arnold C, et al. Evaluation of the bacterial ocular surface microbiome in clinically normal cats before and after treatment with topical erythromycin. PLoS One 2019;14(10):e0223859.

37. Willis KA, Postnikoff CK, Freeman A, et al. The closed eye harbours a unique microbiome in dry eye disease. Sci Rep 2020;10(1):12035.

38. Andersson J, Vogt JK, Dalgaard MD, et al. Ocular surface microbiota in patients with aqueous tear-deficient dry eye. Ocul Surf 2021;19:210–7.

39. Salisbury MAR, Kaswan RL, Brown J. Microorganisms isolated from the corneal surface before and during topical cyclosporine treatment in dogs with keratoconjunctivitis sicca. Am J Vet Res 1995;56(7):880–4.

40. Braus BK, Riedler D, Tichy A, et al. The effects of two different types of bandage contact lenses on the healthy canine eye. Vet Ophthalmol 2018;21(5):477–86.

41. Kita M, Kanai K, Ono HK, et al. Retention, Bacterial Adhesion, and Biofilm Formation between Anionic and Zwitterionic Bandage Contact Lenses in Healthy Dogs: A Pilot Study. Vet Sci 2021;8(10).

42. Retuerto MA, Szczotka-Flynn L, Mukherjee PK, et al. Diversity of Ocular Surface Bacterial Microbiome Adherent to Worn Contact Lenses and Bacterial Communities Associated With Care Solution Use. Eye Contact Lens 2019;45(5):331–9.

43. Hindley KE, Groth AD, King M, et al. Bacterial isolates, antimicrobial susceptibility, and clinical characteristics of bacterial keratitis in dogs presenting to referral practice in Australia. Vet Ophthalmol 2016;19(5):418–26.

44. Tolar EL, Hendrix DVH, Rohrbach BW, et al. Evaluation of clinical characteristics and bacterial isolates in dogs with bacterial keratitis: 97 cases (1993-2003). J Am Vet Med Assoc 2006;228(1):80–5.

45. Suter A, Voelter K, Hartnack S, et al. Septic keratitis in dogs, cats, and horses in Switzerland: associated bacteria and antibiotic susceptibility. Vet Ophthalmol 2018;21(1):66–75.

46. Gerding PA Jr, McLaughlin SA, Troop MW. Pathogenic bacteria and fungi associated with external ocular diseases in dogs: 131 cases (1981-1986). J Am Vet Med Assoc 1988;193(2):242–4.

47. Murphy JM, Lavach JD, Severin GA. Survey of conjunctival flora in dogs with clinical signs of external eye disease. J Am Vet Med Assoc 1978;172(1):66–8.

48. Ollivier FJ. Bacterial corneal diseases in dogs and cats. Clin Tech Small Anim Pract 2003;18(3):193–8.

49. Lin CT, Petersen-Jones SM. Antibiotic susceptibility of bacterial isolates from corneal ulcers of dogs in Taiwan. In: Journal of small animal practice. 2007. p. 271–4.

50. Levitt S, Osinchuk SC, Bauer B, et al. Bacterial isolates of indolent ulcers in 43 dogs. Vet Ophthalmol 2020;23(6):1009–13.

51. Kang Y, Zhang H, Hu M, et al. Alterations in the Ocular Surface Microbiome in Traumatic Corneal Ulcer Patients. Invest Ophthalmol Vis Sci 2020;61(6):35.

52. Cavuoto KM, Galor A, Banerjee S. Ocular Surface Microbiome Alterations Are Found in Both Eyes of Individuals With Unilateral Infectious Keratitis. Transl Vis Sci Technol 2021;10(2):19.

53. Hartmann AD, Hawley J, Werckenthin C, et al. Detection of bacterial and viral organisms from the conjunctiva of cats with conjunctivitis and upper respiratory tract disease. J Feline Med Surg 2010;12(10):775–82.

54. Lin CT, Petersen-Jones SM. Antibiotic susceptibility of bacteria isolated from cats with ulcerative keratitis in Taiwan. J Small Anim Pract 2008;49(2):80–3.

55. McCubbin KD, Anholt RM, de Jong E, et al. Knowledge Gaps in the Understanding of Antimicrobial Resistance in Canada. Front Public Health 2021;9:726484.

56. Watkins RR, Bonomo RA. Overview: The Ongoing Threat of Antimicrobial Resistance. Infect Dis Clin North Am 2020;34(4):649–58.

57. Naylor NR, Atun R, Zhu N, et al. Estimating the burden of antimicrobial resistance: a systematic literature review. Antimicrob Resist Infect Control 2018;7:58.

58. Lloyd DH, Page SW. Antimicrobial Stewardship in Veterinary Medicine. Microbiol Spectr 2018;6(3).

59. Weese JS, van Duijkeren E. Methicillin-resistant Staphylococcus aureus and Staphylococcus pseudintermedius in veterinary medicine. Vet Microbiol 2010; 140(3–4):418–29.

60. Varges R, Penna B, Martins G, et al. Antimicrobial susceptibility of Staphylococci isolated from naturally occurring canine external ocular diseases. Vet Ophthalmol 2009;12(4):216–20.

61. Sandmeyer LS, Bauer BS, Poor SMM, et al. Alterations in conjunctival bacteria and antimicrobial susceptibility during topical administration of ofloxacin after cataract surgery in dogs. Am J Vet Res 2017;78(2):207–14.

62. Mouney MC, Stiles J, Townsend WM, et al. Prevalence of methicillin-resistant Staphylococcus spp. in the conjunctival sac of healthy dogs. Vet Ophthalmol 2015;18(2):123–6.

63. Gentile D, Allbaugh RA, Adiguzel MC, et al. Bacterial Cross-Contamination in a Veterinary Ophthalmology Setting. Front Vet Sci 2020;7:571503.
64. Casola C, Winter-Kempf E, Voelter K. Bacterial contamination of slit lamps in veterinary ophthalmology. Vet Ophthalmol 2019;22(6):828–33.
65. Soimala T, Lubke-Becker A, Hanke D, et al. Molecular and phenotypic characterization of methicillin-resistant Staphylococcus pseudintermedius from ocular surfaces of dogs and cats suffering from ophthalmological diseases. Vet Microbiol 2020;244:108687.
66. Leigue L, Montiani-Ferreira F, Moore BA. Antimicrobial susceptibility and minimal inhibitory concentration of Pseudomonas aeruginosa isolated from septic ocular surface disease in different animal species. Open Vet J 2016;6(3):215–22.

Optical Coherence Tomography

A Review of Current Applications in Veterinary Ophthalmology

Maria Vanore, DMV, MSc, DECVO[a],*,
Marie-Odile Benoit-Biancamano, DMV, PhD, FIATP, DACVP, DECVP[b]

KEYWORDS

- Animals • Eye • In vivo microscopy • OCT • Ophthalmology

KEY POINTS

- Optical coherence tomography (OCT) systems allow high-resolution imaging of the anterior segment (cornea and iridocorneal angle), the retina, and the optic nerve. In human and veterinary ophthalmology, OCT has become an important tool, with a near-histological resolution, that greatly facilitates clinical and research applications.
- OCT images are representations of biologic tissue structure based on the optical backscattered intensity, which is highly dependent on the optical properties of the tissue structure.
- OCT has the potential to detect and diagnose early stages of diseases before physical symptoms and irreversible vision loss can occur. OCT allows visualization of corneal and retinal lesions at the cellular level and evaluation of their evolution after systemic or topical treatments and after surgical procedures.

INTRODUCTION

Optical coherence tomography (OCT) is a powerful, no-contact biomedical imaging that uses low-coherence light sources to obtain in-depth scans of biological tissues. OCT provides cross-sectional images of structures below the tissue surface in detail that are analogous to histologic examination (**Fig. 1**).[1] Axial resolution of 10 to 15 μm can be achieved by standard-resolution OCT. However, recently, ultrahigh-resolution

The authors have nothing to disclose.
[a] Ophthalmology Service, Veterinary Teaching Hospital, Université de Montréal, 3200 Rue Sicotte, Quebec, Canada; [b] Department of Pathology and Microbiology, Groupe de Recherche sur les Maladies Infectieuses en Production Animale (GREMIP), Faculté de Médecine Vétérinaire, Université de Montréal, 3200 Rue Sicotte, Quebec, Canada
* Corresponding author.
E-mail address: maria.vanore@umontreal.ca

Vet Clin Small Anim 53 (2023) 319–338
https://doi.org/10.1016/j.cvsm.2022.10.003
0195-5616/23/Published by Elsevier Inc.
vetsmall.theclinics.com

imaging with axial resolutions as fine as 1 to 2 μm has been obtained.[1] The image resolution of OCT is 10 to 100 times finer than ultrasound imaging, magnetic resonance imaging, or computed tomography. The maximum imaging depth in most opaque tissues is limited to approximately 2 to 3 mm due to optical attenuation and scattering, as opposed to the eye, where whole-depth images can be taken thanks to the transparency of the matrices.[1]

OCT also allows high-resolution imaging of the anterior segment (cornea and iridocorneal angle), the retina, and the optic nerve in human and veterinary ophthalmology and has become an important diagnostic tool used in clinical and research applications.

TECHNOLOGY

The principle of OCT imaging is analogous to that of ultrasound B-mode imaging, except that OCT uses light rather than acoustic waves.[1] OCT permits high-resolution, cross-sectional, tomographic imaging of biologic microstructures by directing a focused beam of light into the biologic tissue and measuring the delay time (echo delay) for the backscattered light to return to the instrument. Light that is backscattered or reflected from a biologic tissue at varying depths will yield longitudinal (depth) information on tissue structures.[2] The optical detection method used in OCT is highly sensitive and known as low-coherence interferometry. The measurement system consists of a low-coherent, super-luminescent diode 840-nm light source used with an optic fiber, the Michelson interferometer.[2] As OCT images are representations based on the optical backscattered intensity, they are highly dependent on the optical properties of the tissue structure.[2]

Different technologies have been developed for OCT devices: time domain-OCT (TD-OCT),[3] spectral domain-OCT (SD-OCT),[4] and Fourier domain-OCT (FD-OCT). For TD-

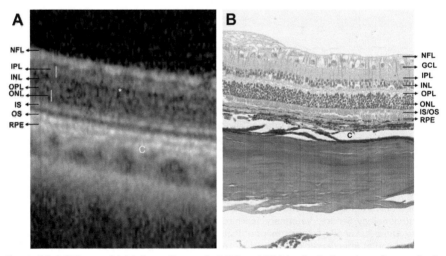

Fig. 1. (A) OCT image (Heidelberg Spectralis OCT) and (B) histological section of normal rabbit central retina. The layers of the retina can be identified: nerve fiber layer (NFL), ganglion cell layer (GCL), inner plexiform layer (IPL), inner nuclear layer (INL), outer plexiform layer (OPL), outer nuclear layer (ONL), Inner and outer segment of photoreceptors (IS/OS), retinal pigment epithelium (RPE), choroid (C). OCT image shows all the retinal layers (arrows) and INL (arrow and asterisk).

OCT technology, in which the position of the reference mirror is changed, signals reflected from the sample are detected at different depths, sequentially as a function of "time of flight." As the reported signals are time encoded, this system is called the time domain. Newer systems use broadband light sources and collect all backscattered frequencies simultaneously, using a spectrometer, as the reference mirror which remains stationary.[5] The signal is then analyzed using Fourier analysis, a mathematical transformation in which spatial frequencies are isolated from the individual components of the compound waveforms. This method allows the recognition of patterns and the mapping of object shapes, essentially expressing the data in the form of a frequency spectrum, where each frequency corresponds to a different depth of tissue. These systems are called spectral domain (SD-OCT) or Fourier domain (FD-OCT).[6]

FD-OCT is characterized by a rapid scan speed and higher resolution as compared with TD-OCT. The scan speed of TD-OCT systems depends on the mechanical cycle time of the moving reference mirror driver, whereas in FD-OCT, the reference mirror is fixed, which assists in sampling multiple points from the ocular structures simultaneously. Thus, relatively high acquisition speed (up to 26,000 A-scans per second), so FD_OCT images are ~100 times faster than TD-OCT. The resulting high scan speed with FD-OCT distinctly improves resolution, significantly reduces motion artifacts, and increases the signal-to-noise ratio.[7,8] In contrast, TD-OCT can penetrate deeper into the sclera, iris, and cornea than FD-OCT, due to the longer wavelength of its detector.[9,10]

CHALLENGES IN IMAGES ACQUISITION

Performing a good OCT scan and obtaining high image resolution of biological tissues is more difficult in veterinary ophthalmology than in human ophthalmology. This is due to a few characteristics specific to animals, such as different head and pupil sizes, and patients that are uncooperative and unable to fixate a target. Adapting the OCT standard scanning method is essential to remedy these problems.[6]

Anesthesia-Sedation

The standard method for OCT scanning in humans requires the patient to be seated in front of the scanner with the face on a chin rest and the eyes level with the scanning beam (like the position used for routine biomicroscopic examination) and the patient fixates on a target. In veterinary ophthalmology, several modifications are needed to perform an OCT. These include appropriate patient positioning and general anesthesia, similar to uncooperative adults and children, to obtain all necessary alignments that will be acquired by the examiner.[11] In veterinary medicine, clinical patients may be old and have a systemic illness, and the choices of anesthetic agents and/or sedative medications are important for the individual patient's safety,[6] and the protocol will depend on the species, the general health and the time needed to perform the OCT scan.

A horse can be placed in stocks and sedated with detomidine hydrochloride administered at a dose range between 10 and 15 mcg/kg IV.[12] A palpebral nerve blocks using lidocaine HCl 2% are administered to horses to facilitate the manipulation of the eyelids and facilitate the use of eyelid speculums.[12]

For experimental animals including primates and monkeys, ketamine and isoflurane have been used in combination, or simply ketamine alone, delivered by intramuscular injection of 20 mg/kg, followed by repeated injections of 10 mg/kg, as needed.[13,14] Cats may also be successfully anesthetized with ketamine 5 mg/kg and medetomidine

0.2 mg/kg and angiography OCT completed to evaluate retinal and choriocapillaris blood flow.[15]

Anesthesia and sedation immobilize the animal and allow for the OCT scan, but it is also necessary to dilate the pupils. Mydriasis allows a complete retinal examination with OCT. However, evaluation of the cornea, the iridocorneal angle, does not require mydriasis. To obtain a maximal mydriasis, several pharmaceuticals have been shown to induce mydriasis and extinguish pupillary light reflexes including mydriacyl or atropine given topically during pre-anesthetic induction as well as muscle relaxants pancuronium and vecuronium which are given to paralyze the extraocular muscles and maintain a central pupil to facilitate the OCT.[16] The pupillary reflex dilation is known to reflect the level of analgesia in response to a painful procedure or to a calibrated noxious stimulus.[17] Butorphanol can be used for mild to moderate sedation, however, it will slightly delay (not prevent) the onset of tropicamide-induced mydriasis, in dogs.[18] Medetomidine, an alpha-2-adrenoceptor agonist, will not antagonize mydriasis when it is combined in dogs with topical 0.5% Tropicamide.[19]

Pupil Dilation

Depending on the species, an iris dilation of short duration is best achieved using 0.5% tropicamide ophthalmic solution[20] or 1% cyclopentolate, in horses, in cats, rabbits, dogs and monkeys.[12,21–24] The pupil of primates can also be dilated with 1 drop each of 1% tropicamide, 2.5% phenylephrine hydrochloride, and 2% cyclopentolate hydrochloride.[13] For longer surgical procedures that follow OCT topical atropine may be provided before induction of general anesthesia.

Eye Position and Movements

To have full retinal exposure to the OCT scan and to obtain the best image resolution, the globe must stay in an axial position and globe movements avoided. Under sedation or general anesthesia, the globe will rotate ventrally, and this precludes retinal and optic nerve examination by OCT. The episcleral and conjunctival tissues can be held with Colibri forceps or by suture fixation to facilitate a central pupil. Similarly, pancuronium or vecuronium will paralyze the extraocular muscles and facilitate a central pupil provided that a ventilator is used during general anesthesia. An alternative retrobulbar block consisting of 0.5 mL of 2% lidocaine will reduce eye movements in most species including monkeys.[14]

Corneal Hydration

Maintaining the transparency of the cornea is crucial to obtain the best image resolution of the retina. If the cornea is dehydrated and hazy due to exposure during the OCT scan, the image resolution of the OCT scan will be poor. Variations in corneal hydration due to the use of topical anesthetics or of other diagnostic tools, such as the tonometer or corneal topographer, can affect the accuracy of the OCT image. A constant corneal hydration is therefore essential to maintain of its transparency. An edematous cornea will often preclude a thorough OCT evaluation of the posterior segment as the refractive index fluctuations scatter light.[25]

Interestingly, the OCT can be helpful in monitoring quantitatively the dynamics of the corneal response and assessing the corneal function based on the detection of changes in the optical properties and morphology of the cornea after topical application of dehydrating agents.[26]

Head Size

Depending on the type of OCT and the supporting equipment and the size and shape of the animal 's head, the acquisition of an OCT can be challenging. A dual-display handheld OCT system is available commercially for retina and optic-nerve-papilla. This particular OCT is portable and easily movable OCT with a handheld probe and computer. The probe can be fixed to the benchtop cradle and the images can be displayed in real time on the computer monitor or recorded with the handheld probe.[27]

The animal's head must be appropriately aligned and supported, whereas sedation or general anesthesia is provided (**Fig. 2**).

Image Data and Different Optical Coherence Tomography Instruments

The OCT appearance of image data is highly dependent on details of the OCT instrument, scan protocols, signal processing, and methods used to generate OCT information. The algorithms and display methods can greatly vary between different instrument manufacturers. Therefore, special care is required when comparing results between different instruments.[28] Furthermore, software designed for human ocular structures does not always provide accurate quantitative values in different species of animals.[6]

AVAILABLE SPECTRAL-DOMAIN OPTICAL COHERENCE TOMOGRAPHY SYSTEMS, CHARACTERISTICS, AND SPECIFIC ADVANTAGES

With time, OCT systems have become more sophisticated, efficient, and accurate, to aid in the diagnosis and management of a wide range of ocular diseases. Several OCT machines have been developed, with different characteristics. The different commercially available OCT instruments are listed in **Table 1**.

Spectralis OCT offers several Module System Options. The Glaucoma Module Premium Edition includes tools to assess the optic nerve head (ONH), the retinal nerve fiber layer (NFL), and the macular ganglion cell layer in glaucoma patients. The MultiColor Module uses three laser wavelengths simultaneously to provide diagnostic images that show distinct structures and pathologies at different depths within the retina not visible on ophthalmoscopy and fundus photography. The OCT system has an eye tracking system, a wide-angle views will allow fluorescein and indocyanine green angiography assessments, and also follow the dynamic movement of dye

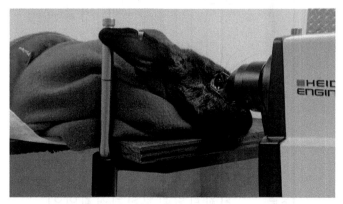

Fig. 2. OCT examination in a rabbit under sedation. A wood support for the head and body allows an appropriate ocular alignment.

Table 1
Different commercially available optical coherence tomography instruments

Device	Manufacturer	Axial Resolution (μm)	A Scan Acquisition Rate (Scans/s)
Spectralis HRA + OCT	Heidelberg Engineering, Heidelberg, Germany	3.5	40,000
Cirrus HD-OCT 6000	Carl Zeiss Meditec, Dublin, CA, USA	5	100,000
Envisu SDOIS series	Leica, Microsystems Durham, NC 27703, USA	1 to 3	34,000
EnFocus intraoperative OCT	Leica, Durham, NC 27703, USA	2.4 to 4	> 36,000
iVue80 & iFusion80	Optovue, Fremont, USA	5	80,000
RTVue 100	Optovue, Fremont, USA	5	26,000
3D-OCT 2000	Topcon, Tokyo, Japan	5 to 6	27,000
SL Scan-1	Topcon, Tokyo, Japan	8 to 9	5000
Spectral OCT/SLO	(OPKO/OTI, Miami, Florida, USA	5	27,000
SOCT Copernicus REVO	Optopol, Zawierce, Poland	2.5 to 5	80,000 to 27,000
SOCT-HR Copernicus	Optopol, Zawierce, Poland	3	52,000

through the vessels using the scanning laser angiography. The OCT 2 Module is the next generation of OCT technology, offering enhanced image quality from the vitreous to the choroid, with a fast-scanning speed of 85,000 Hz. The Anterior Segment Module allows assessment of the cornea, anterior chamber angle, and sclera. The Flex Module is conceived for patients in supine position; however, this option is not available in all countries.

Cirrus HD-OCT 6000 is the next-generation OCT from ZEISS. It delivers high-speed image capture with HD imaging detail using 100,000 A-scans/sec and a wider field of view. It provides a guided progression analysis for glaucoma, eye tracking, and anterior segment OCT imaging options. AngioPlex Metrix allows clinicians to objectively assess and track progressive eye diseases such as diabetic retinopathy and glaucoma with quantification tools such as Vessel Density, Perfusion Density, and Foveal Avascular Zone (FAZ) for the macula, and Capillary Flux Index for the ONH.

Envisu OCT R-class is designed for pre-clinical research. It offers a full set of species-specific imaging lenses, allowing examination of a large variety of animal species: mouse retina lens (50-degree field of view), rat retina (40-degree field of view), rabbit lens (70-degree field of view) and anterior imaging lens (from 10 to 20 mm field of view).

Envisu OCT C-class is most suitable for clinical use, specifically Envisu C2300, which is handheld and suitable even for premature infants. The intention of this instrument is to provide flexibility to image from the operating to the clinic examination rooms. Envisu OCT C class is approved for use in Europe, Australia, and Canada; it includes a Doppler flow, the enhanced-depth imaging (EDI) to reveal the structural details of the choroid and provides options for rodents.

EnFocus intraoperative OCT confirms in real time how ocular tissues are reacting intraoperatively to surgical maneuvers for cornea, glaucoma and retina.

iVue80 OCT system can be paired with the new high-resolution iCam12 fundus camera (high-resolution fundus and external photography) to create *iVue80&iFusion80*, a space-saving, all-in-one imaging system. iVue 80 is a high-speed OCT, three times faster than the original iVue OCT. This instrument was developed for clinical use and generates high-resolution, cross-sectional, and three-dimensional (3D) images of the retina, optic disk, and anterior segment. This system uses advanced software to provide extensive analysis of NFL thickness, ganglion cell, and nerve fiber thickness, and a range of parameters on the optic disc in simple, and it provides easy-to-read reports. It allows the anterior segment scan to visualize cross sections of the cornea, to observe and measure corneal angles, to track corneal thickness over multiple visits, and to calculate intraocular lens (IOL) powers in post-refractive surgery of humans.

RTVue 100 is a next-generation Fourier-Domain OCT, providing analysis for retina, glaucoma, and anterior segment.

3D OCT-2000 is a new generation machine that has a high resolution with the addition of noise-reducing algorithms and IR/3D tracking technology. It includes an integrated retinal photography function. The High-resolution B-scan changes the reference mirror position to the choroidal mode, hence the border between choroid and sclera can be visualized due to enhanced depth imaging. The 3D OCT-2000 has an 8.2 × 3 mm wide view area scans, allowing even the smallest area of pathology to be captured during the initial scan. It includes a combination of autofluorescence, fluorescein and indocyanine green angiography to aid the diagnosis of retinal, RPE, and choroidal diseases. It also allows for iridocorneal angle and corneal curvature and thickness measurements with automatic calculations.

SL Scan-1 system, which is marketed by Opticon includes a slit lamp adapted for anterior and posterior OCT.

Spectral OCT SLO is a combination of OCT and confocal SLO designed to image vitreous, retinal, and choroidal structures. It is indicated for *in vivo* viewing, axial, cross-sectional, and three-dimensional imaging, and measurement of posterior ocular structures including the retina, macula, retina NFL, and optic disk. Retinal maps can be viewed as a 3D volume cube, and sectional cuts can be extracted to identify structures and pathologic features below the retinal surface. A unique feature of this system is the ability to perform microperimetry, providing quantifiable measurements and difference mapping of a patients' visual functions correlated with inner retina pathologic features. An optional lens attachment allows high-resolution anterior segment imaging, corneal pachymetry, corneal topography, as well as the measurement of the anterior chamber angle to be calculated. In addition, the system can image the cornea, sclera, and conjunctiva by changing the focal position.

SOCT Copernicus REVO has real-time hardware eye-tracking functions, which compensate for blinks, loss of fixation, and involuntary eye movements during scanning. It has a 12 mm × 12 mm wide field, allowing a full range scan of the posterior segment. The system has comprehensive glaucoma analysis tools for quantification of NFL, ganglion layer, ONH for glaucoma monitoring over time. A single 3D Retina scan performs both Retina and Glaucoma analysis. The software automatically recognizes 8 retinal layers, which assists with precise diagnosis and mapping of any changes in the patient's condition. SOCT Copernicus REVO provides a complete set of biometry parameters: axial length, central cornea thickness, anterior chamber depth, and lens thickness. It supplies the anterior segment scan, angiography OCT and angiography mosaic option. It can calculate the power of an IOL implant. The REVO FC Fundus Camera is fully automated and the advanced optical system ensures high-quality imaging at a viewing angle as wide as 45°.

SOCT-HR Copernicus in addition to the macular grid, radial line, and 3D volume scans for retinal visualization, NFL and ONH analysis, and a multilingual user interface, this system also incorporates A retinal tracking system, and Doppler analysis, providing a readout indicating relative retinal blood vessel flow velocities. It provides the anterior segment scan and pachymetry. The SOCT Copernicus Glaucoma Module (SOCT-REVO and SOCT-RH) are useful for the detection and management of glaucoma.

LONGITUDINAL STUDIES

In the longitudinal study by Schuman, OCT data were also obtained in primates with experimentally induced glaucoma, which revealed inner retinal and optic nerve damage that was correlated with intraocular pressure (IOP) and histopathology. Longitudinal quantitative assessment of NFL thickness and optic papilla axon density provides an excellent indication of glaucomatous damage.[14]

In longitudinal studies, the effect of age on quantitative measurements (thickness values) needs to be taken into account. In humans, the thickness of the retinal NFL, especially in the lower and upper quadrants, and the macular thickness, except for the central fovea area, significantly decreases with age.[29]

It is also important to remember that, in longitudinal studies, retinal measurements performed with different OCT apparatus are not interchangeable, as internal OCT calibrations and algorithms are different between manufacturers.[30] This creates challenges when comparing different studies with different OCT machines.

In four species of normal diurnal birds of prey, normative OCT data for the *fovea* have been reported.[31] The retinal thickness (RT) of the perifoveal region of the central fovea was slightly increased just before the foveal depression. In all birds, the depression of the *central fovea* (where the highest visual acuity and, monocular vision is attained with sideways assessment of distant objects), was found to be deeper (median depth of 264 ± 29 µm) than the *temporal fovea* (median depth of 120 ± 52 µm) (where binocular and close visual acuity are achieved). The distance between the pecten and both *foveae* were calculated and the *central fovea* was 30% less between the pecten and the *temporal fovea*.[31]

Potential aging effect should also be taken into account when conducting long-term longitudinal animal studies. In the study by Occelli and colleagues,[32] the OCT was used to assess the thickness of the retina during maturation in healthy Beagle crossbreed dogs aged 4 to 52 weeks. In the *area centralis*, there was a thickening of the photoreceptor (PR) layer due to the predominance of cone PR. There was also a thinning of the retina on either side of the ONH, both vertically and horizontally. The superior retina was thicker than the inferior retina. Most of the RT changes peripheral to the optic nerve were due to variations in the thickness of the inner retinal layers. The outer retinal layers have a more constant thickness, especially horizontally and dorsally at the ONH.[32]

DETECTING RETINAL AND CORNEAL DAMAGE WITH OPTICAL COHERENCE TOMOGRAPHY

OCT has been widely adopted for the qualitative assessment of many human ocular pathologies, and this imaging technique will detect early stages of disease before physical symptoms and irreversible vision loss develops. Furthermore, OCT allows visualizing lesions in such detail in the cornea or retina, that ophthalmologists can now assess the effects of systemic and topical treatments, and the response to surgical procedures.

In animals, OCT scans will often identify retinal lesions presented without ophthalmoscopically detectable lesions and without clinically detectable vision impairment. Detailed OCT examination of the retinal layers allows precise characterization and diagnosis (**Fig. 3**). Both eyes should be examined to allow comparison and confirmation of unilateral versus bilateral disease (**Figs. 4** and **5**),

Corneal OCT can also be used to assess all corneal layers and review healing after ulceration and or surgical procedures completed to repair corneal disease or for the evaluation of progressive and non-progressive non-ulcerative keratopathies (**Figs. 6** and **7**). The evolution of the bullous keratopathy can be also evaluated by OCT in order

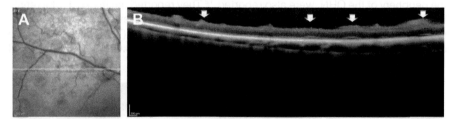

Fig. 3. (A) Image of the ocular fundus as obtained by optical coherence tomography (OCT). (B) OCT transversal image at the level of the green line in (A) demonstrating multifocal areas of nerve fiber layer (NFL) thickening and photoreceptors layer separation from the RPE, corresponding to multifocal retinal detachments (arrows) that can be related to multifocal retinopathy, in a 2-year-old dog Doodle dog (Heidelberg Spectralis OCT). The absence of rosettes excludes the diagnosis of multifocal retinal dysplasia, although indirect ophthalmoscope examination revealed the lesions were similar to retinal dysplasia lesions.

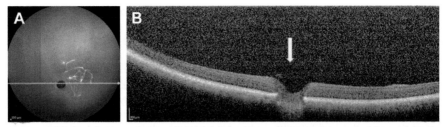

Fig. 4. (A) Image of the ocular fundus as obtained by OCT.(B) OCT transversal image at the level of the green line in (A) showing a physiologically normal optic nerve head (arrow) in a healthy, 3-year-old cat (Heidelberg Spectralis OCT). The optic nerve head appears cupped due to the absence of myelin. The ophthalmic examination of this cat did not identify any abnormalities.

to have the best understanding of the corneal condition, before considering any medical treatment or surgery (**Fig.8**).

ANIMAL STUDIES
Normative and Standards for Healthy Eye Structures

Several studies have been reported including those by Hernandez-Merino and coleagues.[33] to establish standards for the thickness of NFL, PR, and the outer nuclear layers (ONLs) in 12 healthy adult female Beagle dogs. They assessed the thickness of RT, PR, and ONL by linear scanning OCT of the dorsotemporal quadrant relative to the optic nerve (superior or tapetal retina) and the ventro-temporal quadrant (non-tapetal or inferior). They reported the thickness of RT, PR, and NFL was greater in the superior to in the inferior retina. Statistical differences were not detected for ONL thickness in the superior or inferior retina. However, the thickness of the peripapillary NFL of the superior retina was significantly greater than that of the inferior retina (**Table 2**).[33]

Other standards for normal ocular anatomy have been reported in various species. Pinto and colleagues[12] reported the OCT parameters of cornea, retina, and ONH in vivo in normal standing horses that were sedated, and under sedation. The data included descriptions of the corneal layers, as well as the total thickness of the cornea at its axial, superior, inferior, nasal, and temporal regions (**Table 3**).[12] Measurements of total RT in four quadrants (superior, inferior, nasal, and temporal) 1 and 5 mm from the periphery of the OHN, were also reported.[12] They reported the thickest total retinal layer and NFL (mean ± standard deviaiton [SD]), at the ONH level, in the nasal quadrant, followed by the temporal, superior, and inferior quadrants (**Tables 4** and **5**).[12] The dimensions of ONH and optic cup (OC) (mean ± SD) were 3.682 ± 0.276 mm and

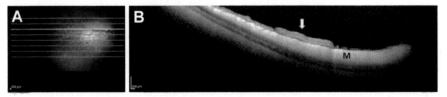

Fig. 5. (A) Image of the peripapillary area as obtained by OCT (B) Transversal image at the level of the thick green line in (A) showing a retinal vessel (arrow) and thick layer of myelin (M), in a healthy, 1-year-old rabbit (Heidelberg Spectralis OCT).

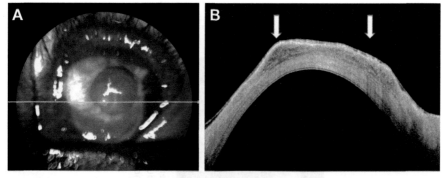

Fig. 6. (A) Image of the central cornea as obtained by OCT (B) Transversal image at the level of the green line in (A) showing a heterogenic stromal healing due to the corneal Acell Vet integration (arrows), 1 month after the surgical procedure, in a 14-year-old dog (Heidelberg Spectralis OCT).

2.175 mm ± 0.502 mm, respectively, in the horizontal axis; 3.012 ± 0.278 mm and 2.035 ± 0.488 mm in the vertical axis.[12]

Normative RTs have been established in commonly used laboratory animal models. Carpenter reported variations in RT with SD-OCT.[34] In this study, 4 adult animal models with normal eyes (5 rats, 5 rabbits, 5 dogs, and 5 mini pigs) were evaluated. Manual measurements were carried out to monitor the normal variation in RT using the Heidelberg Spectralis SD-OCT. They reported internal and external RT at fixed distances from the ONH based on mm from there (1 to 6 mm). Depending on the animal model, the total internal and external RT, measured at specific distances from the ONH, were significantly different. As expected, total RT decreases significantly with increasing distance from ONH in canine, mini-pig, and rabbit. However, the internal RT significantly decreases in dogs, pigs, and rabbits, whereas the external RT decreases significantly only in the canine model. Significant differences between the total, internal and external RT retinas of normal dog, pig, rabbit, and rat retinas were confirmed with SD-OCT, which provides a normative baseline and a standardized method for assessing RT and these serve as standards for the evaluation of future studies of many retinal disorders.[34]

Gomes' and colleagues reported the morphology of the optic nerve and the peripapillary retina in cats, using an SD-OCT Spectralis machine. The area of the optic disc, the depth of the OC (also known as the optic pit or central physiological depression of ONH), the thickness of the peripapillary retina (RT), and the thickness of the retinal NFL, were measured.[35] The NFL: RT ratio in the upper peripapillary, nasal, temporal, and inferior region, were calculated. The superior RT and NFL were the thickest, whereas the inferior RT was significantly thinner than the nasal and temporal part of the retina. The NFL: RT ratio was significantly higher in the superior retina (**Table 6**). The area of the optical disc was 1.39 ± 0.26 mm². The depth of the OC was 168.36 ± 67.74 μm. Bergmeister's papilla (remnant of the hyaloid artery located on the optic papilla) was detectable in most of these OCT images.[35]

Optical Coherence Tomography Investigations of Ocular Disorders

Grahn and colleagues[36] used OCT to investigate a multifocal retinopathy in Coton de Tulear dogs. This is the first reported OCT study in dogs with a clinical disease. The OCT images confirmed multiple focal retinal detachments with progressive development from a few weeks of age in affected puppies till they were mature at

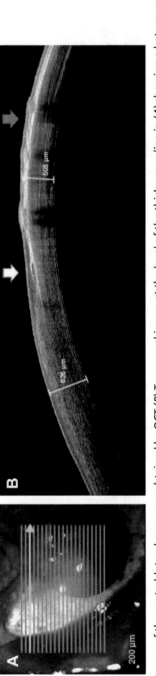

Fig. 7. (A) Image of the central-lateral cornea as obtained by OCT (B) Transversal image at the level of the thick green line in (A) showing a heterogenic superficial stromal healing due to a corneo-conjonctival transposition (arrows), 7 months after the surgical procedure, in a 14-year-old dog. The dark superficial corneal area (white arrow) is characterized by an absence of the bulbar conjunctiva compared with the white corneal superficial section, where the conjunctiva was transposed (blue arrow) (Heidelberg Spectralis OCT).

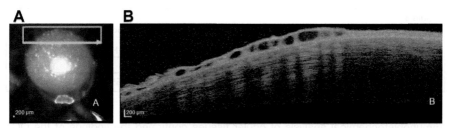

Fig. 8. (*A*) Image of the cornea of a dog obtained by OCT. (*B*) OCT transversal image at the level of the green line in (*A*) showing multiple hypoechoic round spaces in the corneal epithelium corresponding to a bullous keratopathy (Heidelberg Spectralis OCT) secondary to a corneal endothelial degeneration, in an 11-year-old dog. The OCT image of the corneal was similar to a histological image.

approximately one year of age when further development was not detected. This research confirmed that multifocal retinopathy of Coton de Tulear dogs is an inherited as an autosomal recessive disease manifested by multifocal serous detachments of the retina in homozygous puppies between 3 and 4 months old. OCT and ultrasound confirmed multifocal serous detachments of the retina. Serial fundic photographs documented the progression of lesions slightly beyond 1 year of age. Electroretinography identified a decrease in scotopic and photopic b-wave amplitude; however, only the flicker responses showed significant differences between affected Coton de Tulear dogs and control dogs of the same age. Fluorescein angiography revealed that blood-retinal barriers were intact during repeated angiograms before, during, and after the development of the retinopathy. Focal retinal thinning was detected with OCT over the focal retinal detachments and the serous content of some of the multifocal detachments decreased after several years, leaving focal areas of hyperreflectivity consistent with retinal scarring.[36]

In Rauscher's study, 45 wild and domestic birds were investigated by OCT.[37] The OCT examination revealed structural changes in retinal and choroidal tissues and these were compared with direct ophthalmoscopy findings of retinal and choroidal degeneration, retinal detachment, retinal schisis, and drusen, and histologic and

Table 2
Retinal thickness (mean ± SD) of the different retinal layers; whole retinal thickness, photoreceptor layer, nerve fiber layer, outer nuclear layer, peripapillary nerve fiber layer, in tapetal and nontapetal retina in the superior and inferior retina, in dogs

	Retinal Thickness (μm) (Mean ± SD, *P*-value), in Normal Dogs		
	Superior Retina (Tapetal)	Inferior Retina (Nontapetal)	*P*-value
WRT	198.7 ± 9.6	164.4 ± 6.4	*P*<.0001
PR	95.5 ± 6.5	78.8 ± 7.4	*P*<.0001
NFL	26.4 ± 1.6	25.0 ± 1.9	*P* = .0236
ONL	50.1 ± 6.4	44.3 ± 3.6	*P* = .0578
NLF C	91.26 ± 7.0	76.42 ± 9.2	*P*<.001

Abbreviations: NFL, nerve fiber layer; ONL, outer nuclear layer; PL, photoreceptor layer; WRT, whole retinal thickness.

Table 3				
Total corneal thickness in the axial, superior, inferior, nasal, and temporal area				
Total Corneal Thickness (μm) (Mean ± SD), in Normal Horses				
Axial	Superior	Inferior	Nasal	Temporal
800 ± 50	937 ± 61	956 ± 61	912 ± 65	884 ± 68

immunohistochemical analysis of ocular tissues confirmed the findings of the OCT examinations.[38]

Somma and colleagues[39] reported OCT examinations of progressive retinal atrophy (PRA) in Whippet dogs with clinical photographs and OCT images, and electroretinograms (ERG) and pedigree analysis. All dogs received an ophthalmic screening for hereditary eye disease, including visual tests such as the obstacle course test under scotopic (in attenuated light) and photopic (in bright light) conditions, as well as the cotton ball test, dazzle reflexes, and fundus assessment by indirect ophthalmoscopy and accompanied fundus photographs. ERG and OCT were performed in 24 dogs of which 16 were diagnosed with PRA. A visual deficit in low light associated with nystagmus was detected in the young dogs. Indirect ophthalmoscopy revealed multifocal retinal vesicle bubbles from the age of 6 months. Thinning of the retina appeared later when the vesicles were no longer detectable. OCT examination of selected young dogs revealed that the retinal vesicles were focal retinal detachments where the PR and the retinal pigment epithelium were separated. In dogs presenting a more advanced disease, OCT confirmed the development of progressive outer retinal thinning with loss of outer segments and the outer nuclear layer (ONL). The ERG recordings were expected to be diminished; however, they were not detectable in affected young Whippet dogs where the b-wave was not detectable in the scotopic and photopic recordings, which is consistent with a loss of outer segments of the rods and cones. With the progression of the disease, the ERG b-waves remained absent, consistent with a lack of functional PR. Analysis of the pedigree suggested an autosomal recessive mode of inheritance and PRA in Whippet dogs is a unique phenotype, characterized by the initial presence of retinal vesicles, absence of the ERG b-wave, and generalized progressive retinal degeneration.[39]

Grozdanic and colleagues[40] reported OCT evaluation of sudden acquired retinal degeneration (SARD). They reported 29 dogs with SARDS that were assessed using a pupil chromatic reflex (cPLR) test, a complete ophthalmologic examination, ERG, retinal photography, and OCT. Histological and immunohistochemical analysis was performed in 2 eyes with SARD, and microarray analysis was performed in 5 retinas from eyes with SARD. OCT confirmed focal retinal detachments less than 1 mm in width (RD) in 11/29 dogs which could not be detected by funduscopy or by

Table 4					
Retinal thickness in the dorsal, ventral, nasal, and temporal area of the ocular *fundus*					
Retinal Thickness (μm) (Mean ± SD), in Normal Horses					
	ONH	1 mm	2 mm	3 mm	4 mm
Dorsal	336 ± 90	239 ± 15	205 ± 16	187 ± 14	176 ± 11
Ventral	231 ± 58	133 ± 14	121 ± 15	116 ± 13	111 ± 3
Nasal	459 ± 115	276_41	216 ± 19	185 ± 18	164 ± 13
Temporal	449 ± 115	263 ± 30	213 ± 20	171 ± 21	165 ± 17

Table 5
Nerve fiber layers thickness in the dorsal, ventral, nasal, and temporal area of the ocular *fundus*

	Nerve Fiber Layers Thickness (μm) (Mean ± SD), in Normal Horses				
	ONH	1 mm	2 mm	3 mm	4 mm
Dorsal	229 ± 81	126 ± 18	91 ± 13	85 ± 14	78 ± 10
Ventral	128 ± 53	69 ± 10	59 ± 15	54 ± 17	44 _± 12
Nasal	377 ± 116	193 ± 40	142 ± 20	111 ± 19	91 ± 13
Temporal	357 ± 117	176 ± 30	132 ± 16	97 ± 19	84 ± 18

examination of retinal photographs and based on limited data they suggested that SARD may be an immune-mediated retinopathy.[38]

SARD-affected dogs were also examined with OCT by Osinchuk and colleagues.[37] They reported retinal changes detected by OCT in 10 dogs. The OCT analysis data were retrieved from four retinal quadrants (the dorsal and the ventral nasal, as well as the dorsal and the ventral temporal), and around the optic nerve. Measurements of the PR layer, ONL, outer retina, inner retina, and the full thickness of the retina in all quadrants and measurements of the ONL and outer retina were significantly reduced in all SARDS-affected dogs. OCT images of the inner and outer layer of PR revealed marked degeneration in all SARD dogs, compared with the control group. Dogs with SARD had a significant decrease in the thickness of the external retina, ONL, and the temporal global retina compared with the control dogs. These findings are consistent with previous histological reports describing diffuse ONL thinning attributed to apoptosis where pycnotic nuclei are lost.[37]

Optical Coherence Tomography Future Clinical Use in Veterinary Ophthalmology

OCT findings will offer new information to facilitate in the near future the understanding of the management of glaucoma, corneal and retinal diseases in animals.

Prognosis of Glaucoma Therapies

Glaucoma is a retinal and optic neuropathy characterized by retinal ganglion cell (RGC) loss and retinal nerve fiber layer (RNFL) atrophy that results in functional and morphological changes.[41] Dysfunction and/or loss of RGC is the primary determinant of visual loss and endpoints used in current research on experimental therapies.[42] OCT can measure the RNFL and ganglion cell complex (GCC) thicknesses.[41] Anterior segment OCT (AS-OCT) can be a useful tool to investigate glaucoma pathophysiology in several species and document therapeutic responses. In canine eyes with angle

Table 6
Retinal thickness, nerve fiber layer thickness, and ratio between RT and NFL in the superior, inferior, nasal and temporal area of the ocular *fundus*

	Retinal and Nerve Fiber Layer Thickness (μm) (Mean ± SD), in Normal Cats			
	Superior	Inferior	Nasal	Temporal
RT	264.7 ± 13.95	222.44 ± 9.63	229.92 ± 11.01	237.96 ± 11.22
NFL	70.22 ± 11.78	44.12 ± 7.51	39.19 ± 10.38	41.31 ± 14.54
NFL: RT	0.27 ± 0.04	0.2 ± 0.03	0.17 ± 0.04	0.17 ± 0.05

Abbreviaitons: NFL, nerve fiber layer; RT, Retinal thickness.

closure glaucoma (PACG), Tell and al. revealed that distal aqueous outflow channels are not identifiable by aqueous angiography (AA), despite normalization of their IOP, and intra-scleral vascular profiles are collapsed on OCT and histologic examinations. These findings indicate that severely affected PACG eyes have a combination of scleral vascular lumen abnormalities in distal outflow pathways (eg, structure, function, perfusion, lumen size, collapsibility) that could be contributing to a reduced aqueous outflow.[43]

Prognosis of Anterior Segment and Corneal Conditions

AS-OCT images can precisely evaluate the corneal tissues and will become a precedent to many corneal surgeries, and they will allow non-invasive evaluation of corneal healing after medical and surgical therapies for many corneal diseases (eg, ulcerative and non-ulcerative keratitis). In humans with granular corneal dystrophy requiring removal to decrease stromal haze, spectral domain OCT is a useful means of determining keratectomy depth.[44,45] AS-OCT will be used to evaluate the depth of corneal opacities, verify infectious agents, to choose the appropriate surgical techniques for keratopathies in most animals.[46] Serial AS-OCT evaluation with measurement of infiltration thickness and corneal thickness can be a tool for monitoring response to treatment.[46]

Shousha and colleagues[47] reported patients with Fuchs' endothelium corneal dystrophy (FECD), AS-OCT quantification of Descemet's membrane thickness had an excellent correlation with that of light microscopy.[47] Canine corneal endothelium dystrophy (CED) in Boston Terrier (BT), has the potential to be a valuable spontaneous in vivo model for FECD, as reported by Thomasy and colleagues.[48] They assessed corneal morphology using in vivo confocal microscopy (IVCM) and Fourier-domain optical coherence tomography (FD-OCT) in BT with and without CED.[48] AS-OCT could be a useful tool to investigate Descemet detachment and numerous infectious keratopathies in horses hence giving a better diagnosis and prognosis, and thereby improving vision.

Prognosticating Retinal Recoveries After Detachment

In veterinary ophthalmology, it is difficult to evaluate visual impairment during stationary or progressive retinal diseases, especially when only one eye is affected. In humans, structural changes in OCT have been correlated with different levels of visual function in rhegmathogenous retinal detachment (RRD) and central serous chorioretinopathy (CSC).[49] CSC is a human idiopathic serous retinal detachment, characterized by a fluid leakage into the subretinal space from the retinal pigment epithelium (RPE). Normal RPE prevents diffusion of fluid into the subretinal space; however, in eyes with CSC, the RPE might be dysfunctional because of abnormalities of the choroidal circulation beneath it, which results in serous retinal detachment. OCT analysis of RRD was able to show intraretinal cyst formation, intraretinal separation, and undulation of the outer detached retina, whereas CSC eyes showed none of these changes[49] Although the duration of symptoms was longer in CSC than in RRD, a more rapid visual loss was found in RRD.[49] Fujimoto and al. used FD OCT to show pigment epithelial detachment (PED) with a protruding or irregular RPE layer in CSC patients.[50] Fibrinous exudate (SFR) in the subretinal space was seen above the leakage sites and the smooth posterior detached retina became granular in the presence of residual SRF. OCT findings in the retina of CSC eyes can be compared with an inflammatory serous, and inherited multifocal retinal detachment in animals.[36,50] OCT findings may offer additional information to facilitate the differential diagnosis between an RRD and an inflammatory serous retinal detachment, giving a better prognosis on vision function in animals presenting a retinal detachment.

SUMMARY

OCT improves the diagnostic accuracy of corneal and retinal/choroidal diseases and provides images with near to histologic resolution, which allows the ophthalmologist to accurately identify lesions within ocular tissues non-invasively and follow their evolution over time. This enables the assessment of therapeutic responses of the corneal, optic nerve, or retinal disease in animals. OCT is applicable and useful and should be considered as an essential diagnostic tool in veterinary ophthalmology. It can improve the quality of the diagnostic ophthalmologic toolbox in multiple animal species and enable better characterization of disease prognosis by repeated OCT assessments over time.

CLINICS CARE POINTS

- Future developments include refinement of assessing vascular networks for the anterior segment and retina, in vivo ultra-high resolution anterior segment optical coherence tomography with histology-like detail, en-face image with 3-dimensional reconstruction as well as functional extensions of the technique.

REFERENCES

1. Fujimoto JG. Optical coherence tomography for ultrahigh resolution in vivo imaging. Nat Biotechnol 2003;21(11):1361–7.
2. Toth CA, Birngruber R, Boppart SA, et al. Argon laser retinal lesions evaluated in vivo by optical coherence tomography. Am J Ophthalmol 1997;123(2):188–98.
3. Aumann S, Donner S, Fischer J, et al. Optical Coherence Tomography (OCT): principle and technical realization. In: Bille JF, editor. High resolution imaging in microscopy and ophthalmology: new frontiers in biomedical optics. Springer Copyright 2019. The Author(s); 2019. p. 59–85.
4. Kiernan DF, Mieler WF, Hariprasad SM. Spectral-domain optical coherence tomography: a comparison of modern high-resolution retinal imaging systems. Am J Ophthalmol 2010;149(1):18–31.
5. Wojtkowski M, Leitgeb R, Kowalczyk A, et al. In vivo human retinal imaging by Fourier domain optical coherence tomography. J Biomed Opt 2002;7(3):457–63.
6. McLellan GJ, Rasmussen CA. Optical coherence tomography for the evaluation of retinal and optic nerve morphology in animal subjects: practical considerations. Vet Ophthalmol 2012;15(Suppl 2):13–28.
7. Chen TC, Cense B, Pierce MC, et al. Spectral domain optical coherence tomography: ultra-high speed, ultra-high resolution ophthalmic imaging. Arch Ophthalmol 2005;123(12):1715–20.
8. de Boer JF, Cense B, Park BH, et al. Improved signal-to-noise ratio in spectral-domain compared with time-domain optical coherence tomography. Opt Lett 2003;28(21):2067–9.
9. Zhou SY, Wang CX, Cai XY, et al. Optical coherence tomography and ultrasound biomicroscopy imaging of opaque corneas. Cornea 2013;32(4):e25–30.
10. Ramos JL, Li Y, Huang D. Clinical and research applications of anterior segment optical coherence tomography - a review. Clin Exp Ophthalmol 2009;37(1):81–9.

11. Patel CK, Chen SDM, Farmery AD. Optical coherence tomography under general anesthesia in a child with nystagmus. Am J Ophthalmol 2004;137(6):1127–9.

12. Pinto NI, Gilger BC. Spectral-domain optical coherence tomography evaluation of the cornea, retina, and optic nerve in normal horses. Vet Ophthalmol 2014; 17(Suppl 1):140–8.

13. Strouthidis NG, Grimm J, Williams GA, et al. A comparison of optic nerve head morphology viewed by spectral domain optical coherence tomography and by serial histology. Invest Ophthalmol Vis Sci 2010;51(3):1464–74.

14. Schuman JS, Pedut-Kloizman T, Pakter H, et al. Optical coherence tomography and histologic measurements of nerve fiber layer thickness in normal and glaucomatous monkey eyes. Invest Ophthalmol Vis Sci 2007;48(8):3645–54.

15. Wada T, Song Y, Oomae T, et al. Longitudinal Changes in Retinal Blood Flow in a Feline Retinal Vein Occlusion Model as Measured by Doppler Optical Coherence Tomography and Optical Coherence Tomography Angiography. Invest Ophthalmol Vis Sci 2020;61(2):34.

16. Gray AT, Krejci ST, Larson MD. Neuromuscular blocking drugs do not alter the pupillary light reflex of anesthetized humans. Arch Neurol 1997;54(5):579–84.

17. Payen JF, Isnardon S, Lavolaine J, et al. [Pupillometry in anesthesia and critical care]. Ann Fr Anesth Reanim 2012;31(6):e155–9. La pupillométrie en anesthésie-réanimation.

18. Jugant S, Grillot AE, Lyarzhri F, et al. Changes in pupil size and intraocular pressure after topical application of 0.5% tropicamide to the eyes of dogs sedated with butorphanol. Am J Vet Res 2019;80(1):95–101.

19. Wallin-Håkanson N, Wallin-Håkanson B. The effects of topical tropicamide and systemic medetomidine, followed by atipamezole reversal, on pupil size and intraocular pressure in normal dogs. Vet Ophthalmol 2001;4(1):3–6.

20. Rubin LF, Wolfes RL. Mydriatics for canine ophthalmoscopy. J Am Vet Med Assoc 1962;140:137–41.

21. Bessonnat A, Vanore M. Effect of topical cyclopentolate alone or combined with phenylephrine in healthy horses. Vet Ophthalmol 2021. https://doi.org/10.1111/vop.12896.

22. Costa D, Leiva M, Coyo N, et al. Effect of topical 1% cyclopentolate hydrochloride on tear production, pupil size, and intraocular pressure in healthy Beagles. Vet Ophthalmol 2016;19(6):449–53.

23. Kovalcuka L, Nikolajenko M. Changes in intraocular pressure, horizontal pupil diameter, and tear production during the use of topical 1% cyclopentolate in cats and rabbits. Open Vet J 2020;10(1):59–67.

24. Hussein KH, Elmeligy E, Khalphallah A, et al. Effect of Topical Cyclopentolate 1% on Ocular Ultrasonographic Features, Intraocular Pressure, Tear Production, and Pupil Size in Normal Donkeys (Equus Asinus). J Equine Vet Sci 2021;104:103700.

25. Kim YL, Walsh JT Jr, Goldstick TK, et al. Variation of corneal refractive index with hydration. Phys Med Biol 2004;49(5):859–68.

26. Hosseini K, Kholodnykh AI, Petrova IY, et al. Monitoring of rabbit cornea response to dehydration stress by optical coherence tomography. Invest Ophthalmol Vis Sci 2004;45(8):2555–62.

27. Cho NH, Park K, Wijesinghe RE, et al. Development of real-time dual-display handheld and bench-top hybrid-mode SD-OCTs. Sensors (Basel) 2014;14(2): 2171–81.

28. Spaide RF, Fujimoto JG, Waheed NK, et al. Optical coherence tomography angiography. Prog Retin Eye Res 2018;64:1–55.

29. Sung KR, Wollstein G, Bilonick RA, et al. Effects of age on optical coherence tomography measurements of healthy retinal nerve fiber layer, macula, and optic nerve head. Ophthalmology 2009;116(6):1119–24.

30. Brandao LM, Ledolter AA, Schötzau A, et al. Comparison of Two Different OCT Systems: Retina Layer Segmentation and Impact on Structure-Function Analysis in Glaucoma. J Ophthalmol 2016;2016:8307639.

31. Espinheira Gomes F, Abou-Madi N, Ledbetter EC, et al. Spectral-domain optical coherence tomography imaging of normal foveae: A pilot study in 17 diurnal birds of prey. Vet Ophthalmol 2020;23(2):347–57.

32. Occelli LM, Pasmanter N, Ayoub EE, et al. Changes in retinal layer thickness with maturation in the dog: an in vivo spectral domain - optical coherence tomography imaging study. BMC Vet Res 2020;16(1):225.

33. Hernandez-Merino E, Kecova H, Jacobson SJ, et al. Spectral domain optical coherence tomography (SD-OCT) assessment of the healthy female canine retina and optic nerve. Vet Ophthalmol 2011;14(6):400–5.

34. Carpenter CL, Kim AY, Kashani AH. Normative Retinal Thicknesses in Common Animal Models of Eye Disease Using Spectral Domain Optical Coherence Tomography. Adv Exp Med Biol 2018;1074:157–66.

35. Espinheira Gomes F, Parry S, Ledbetter E. Spectral domain optical coherence tomography evaluation of the feline optic nerve and peripapillary retina. Vet Ophthalmol 2019;22(5):623–32.

36. Grahn BH, Sandmeyer LL, Breaux C. Retinopathy of Coton de Tulear dogs: clinical manifestations, electroretinographic, ultrasonographic, fluorescein and indocyanine green angiographic, and optical coherence tomographic findings. Vet Ophthalmol 2008;11(4):242–9.

37. Osinchuk SC, Leis ML, Salpeter EM, et al. Evaluation of retinal morphology of canine sudden acquired retinal degeneration syndrome using optical coherence tomography and fluorescein angiography. Vet Ophthalmol 2019;22(4):398–406.

38. Rauscher FG, Azmanis P, Körber N, et al. Optical coherence tomography as a diagnostic tool for retinal pathologies in avian ophthalmology. Invest Ophthalmol Vis Sci 2013;54(13):8259–69.

39. Somma AT, Moreno JCD, Sato MT, et al. Characterization of a novel form of progressive retinal atrophy in Whippet dogs: a clinical, electroretinographic, and breeding study. Vet Ophthalmol 2017;20(5):450–9.

40. Grozdanic SD, Lazic T, Kecova H, et al. Optical coherence tomography and molecular analysis of sudden acquired retinal degeneration syndrome (SARDS) eyes suggests the immune-mediated nature of retinal damage. Vet Ophthalmol 2019;22(3):305–27.

41. Distante P, Lombardo S, Verticchio Vercellin AC, et al. Structure/Function relationship and retinal ganglion cells counts to discriminate glaucomatous damages. BMC Ophthalmol 2015;15:185.

42. Mead B, Tomarev S. Evaluating retinal ganglion cell loss and dysfunction. Exp Eye Res 2016;151:96–106.

43. Telle MR, Snyder KC, Oikawa K, et al. Development and validation of methods to visualize conventional aqueous outflow pathways in canine primary angle closure glaucoma. Vet Ophthalmol 2021. https://doi.org/10.1111/vop.12943.

44. Kim TI, Hong JP, Ha BJ, et al. Determination of treatment strategies for granular corneal dystrophy type 2 using Fourier-domain optical coherence tomography. Br J Ophthalmol 2010;94(3):341–5.

45. Jung SH, Han KE, Stulting RD, et al. Phototherapeutic keratectomy in diffuse stromal haze in granular corneal dystrophy type 2. Cornea 2013;32(3):296–300.

46. Konstantopoulos A, Kuo J, Anderson D, et al. Assessment of the use of anterior segment optical coherence tomography in microbial keratitis. Am J Ophthalmol 2008;146(4):534–42.

47. Shousha MA, Perez VL, Wang J, et al. Use of ultra-high-resolution optical coherence tomography to detect in vivo characteristics of Descemet's membrane in Fuchs' dystrophy. Ophthalmology 2010;117(6):1220–7.

48. Thomasy SM, Cortes DE, Hoehn AL, et al. In Vivo Imaging of Corneal Endothelial Dystrophy in Boston Terriers: A Spontaneous, Canine Model for Fuchs' Endothelial Corneal Dystrophy. Invest Ophthalmol Vis Sci 2016;57(9):495–503.

49. Lee SY, Joe SG, Kim J-G, et al. Optical Coherence Tomography Evaluation of Detached Macula from Rhegmatogenous Retinal Detachment and Central Serous Chorioretinopathy. Am J Ophthalmol 2008;145(6):1071–6.e2.

50. Fujimoto H, Gomi F, Wakabayashi T, et al. Morphologic Changes in Acute Central Serous Chorioretinopathy Evaluated by Fourier-Domain Optical Coherence Tomography. Ophthalmology 2008;115(9):1494–500.e2.

Diagnosing Corneal Pigmentation in Small Animals

Amber Labelle, DVM, MS[a],*, Philippe Labelle, DVM[b]

KEYWORDS

- Cornea • Pigmentation • Pigmentary keratitis • Brachycephalic • Small animal
- Pigment • Melanin

KEY POINTS

- Brown opacities of the cornea can be corneal epithelial pigment, melanocytomas, or other, nonmelanin-containing lesions including sequestrum or foreign bodies.
- Corneal pigmentation is a nonspecific response associated with a variety of keratopathies.
- A complete ophthalmic examination is critical to making an accurate diagnosis.
- Pigmentary keratitis is a unique disease of pugs and other brachycephalic breeds of dogs that presents as pigment extending from the nasal cornea toward the axial cornea.
- No reliably effective medical treatment of reversing corneal pigmentation is available. Appropriate and accurate surgical correction of euryblepharon, lagophthalmos, and medial canthal entropion facilitates resolution of corneal pigmentation.

REVIEW OF CORNEAL ANATOMY

Understanding the normal anatomy and physiology of the cornea is critical to understanding corneal pathologic condition and response to disease (**Boxes 1** and **2**). The cornea and sclera make up the tough and protective fibrous tunic of the eye. The cornea can be described as a "fat-water-fat" sandwich; the epithelium and endothelium/Descemet's membrane are hydrophobic, whereas the stroma is very hydrophilic.

Precorneal Tear Film

The epithelium of the cornea is protected and nourished by the precorneal tear film. The tear film is composed of 3 layers listed from inner to outer: (1) mucus layer derived

The authors have nothing to disclose.
[a] Practice Owner, Bright Light Veterinary Eye Care, Ottawa, Ontario, Canada; [b] Antech Diagnostics, 7555 Danbro Crescent, Mississauga, Ontario L5N 6P9, Canada
* Corresponding author. 1445 Merivale Road, Nepean, Ontario K2E 5N9, Canada
E-mail address: hello@brightlightvet.ca
Twitter: @brightlightvet (A.L.)

Vet Clin Small Anim 53 (2023) 339–352
https://doi.org/10.1016/j.cvsm.2022.11.001
0195-5616/23/© 2022 Elsevier Inc. All rights reserved.

vetsmall.theclinics.com

Box 1
Layers of the cornea

5 layers of the cornea:

Precorneal tear film

Epithelium

Stroma

Descemet's membrane

Endothelium

---

primarily from the goblet cells of the conjunctiva, (2) watery layer produced by the orbital lacrimal gland and gland of the third eyelid, and (3) oily layer produced by the meibomian glands. The tear film has numerous functions, including lubrication, germicidal properties (lysozymes and some IgA), nutrition for the cornea, removal of debris, and general maintenance of optical clarity. A normal, healthy tear film is critical for the maintenance of corneal clarity.

Corneal Epithelium

The epithelium of the cornea is an extension of the conjunctival epithelium, with some modifications. The normal corneal epithelium is approximately 5 to 7 cells thick and is hydrophobic. The epithelium is transparent, and very firmly adherent to the underlying corneal stroma through hemidesmosomes. It is highly mitotically active with a fast regeneration rate. Corneal epithelial cells can migrate at a rate of ~1 mm/d. The epithelium has an important physical barrier function in preventing the invasion of microorganisms and the seepage of the precorneal tear film into the corneal stroma.

Corneal Stroma

The stroma comprises approximately 90% of the corneal thickness. It is composed of well-organized, parallel layers of mainly collagen fibrils with few keratocytes. Thin collagen fibrils are uniformly positioned to allow light to enter the eye without scatter. Collagen fibrils, gycosaminoglycans (keratan sulfate, chondroitin sulfate, and dermatan sulfate) and glycoproteins make up 15% to 25% of the stroma. The cornea is

---

Box 2
Differential diagnoses for brown lesions on the ocular surface beyond corneal pigmentation

Neoplasia

Sequestrum

Iris prolapse

Foreign body

Dermoid

Fungal keratitis

Pigmentary keratitis

Keratoconjunctivitis sicca

Pannus (chronic superficial keratitis)

Chronic keratitis

---

relatively dehydrated compared with other body tissues and contains only 75% to 80% water. The collagen matrix of the stroma is hydrophilic.

Descemet Membrane

Descemet's membrane is the basement membrane (10–15 μm thick) of the corneal endothelium. It thickens with age and it is hydrophobic.

Corneal Endothelium

The endothelium of the cornea is a single layer of cells lining the inner surface of Descemet's membrane. The endothelial cell layer is very active metabolically and plays the major role in maintaining corneal transparency. Pumps on the endothelial cells help to actively transport water out of the cornea in order to maintain its relatively dehydrated state. Endothelial cells are nonregenerative and cannot be replaced when lost.

Physiology of Corneal Transparency

The cornea is the clear window at the front of the eye that allows the transmission of light from the outside world into the globe. Maintaining the transparency of the cornea is critical to its role in transmitting light and the facilitation of normal vision. How does the cornea maintain transparency? What makes skin a tough, fibrous tunic that protects the body, and how does the cornea, which also has a protective function, differ?
   The cornea

- Has no pigment.
- Has no blood vessels.
- Has no epithelial cell keratinization.
- Has precise arrangement of collagen lamellae.
- Is relatively dehydrated.

Because the sclera and cornea are both made of collagen, why is the cornea transparent and the sclera white? The cornea is composed of precisely arranged parallel layers, also called lamellae. Transparency depends on this precise arrangement of fibrils and fibril diameter. Conversely, the sclera is composed of interwoven collagen without precise lattice arrangement of the fibrils, rendering it opaque.
   All diseases of the cornea can be categorized as one (or both) of the following: a loss of thickness or a loss of transparency. The *first key* to correctly diagnosing and treating corneal disease lies in the ability of the clinician to recognize which pattern is occurring. The cornea has a relatively limited repertoire of responses to a wide variety of stimuli. The cornea can ulcerate, melt (collagenolysis), vascularize, pigment, scar (fibrosis), or become edematous. Recognizing these patterns of response is the *second key* to correctly diagnosing and treating corneal disease. This review will focus on pigmented lesions that can be identified on the ocular surface of small animal patients and how to differentiate them and make an accurate diagnosis.

DIFFERENTIAL DIAGNOSES FOR BROWN LESIONS ON THE OCULAR SURFACE BEYOND CORNEAL PIGMENTATION

Pigment is brown, and the identification of a brown lesion on the ocular surface (conjunctiva and cornea) should prompt the question: what kind of pigmented lesion is this? Not all brown lesions on the ocular surface are the result of corneal pigmentation. Corneal pigmentation is the accumulation of melanin and often melanocytes or occasionally melanophages in and under the corneal epithelium, which must be differentiated from other brown-colored lesions on the ocular surface. As always, a complete and thorough ophthalmic examination is indicated but having a ready set of differential diagnoses to rule out can assist the veterinarian with making an accurate diagnosis.

Neoplasia

Ocular surface neoplasia is rare in dogs, and primary corneal melanocytoma is rare, with only a single reported canine case report.[1] Limbal melanocytomas are the most common neoplasms.[2,3] Uveal melanomas/melanocytomas can erode through the sclera and can be visible subconjunctivally.[4] Limbal melanocytomas are located at the limbus, typically dorsotemporally in an outward fan shape, and extend into the deep corneal stroma as a second dark fan shape (**Fig. 1**). This unique growth pattern results from their origin from melanocytes that are located at the limbus adjacent to Descemet's membrane. The location, dark pigmentation, and growth patterns are the 3 identifying features that allow for a clinical diagnosis of limbal melanocytoma. Golden and Labrador retrievers are overrepresented, and there seems to be a bimodal age distribution of young (age 3–4 years) and older (age 9–10 years) dogs.[2] Referral to an ophthalmologist or consultation with an ophthalmologist is recommended for these patients.[5,6]

Corneal Sequestrum

This is a condition unique to cats that results in a devitalized, discolored corneal lesion, typically in the axial cornea[7] (**Fig. 2**). Dogs are only rarely affected but brachycephalic cats are disproportionately represented.[8–10] Despite multiple laboratory investigations, the cause of feline corneal sequestrum and the reason the cornea becomes discolored remains unknown, and melanin is not the cause of the brown discoloration.[7–11] A variety of surgical interventions has been described, and a recent report summarizes the existing techniques and their outcomes.[12] Medical therapy is not recommended, and referral to or consultation with a veterinary ophthalmologist is indicated.

Corneal Foreign Body

Both superficial and penetrating foreign bodies often seem as brown opacities on or in the cornea (**Figs. 3** and **4**). Organic and nonorganic debris can adhere itself to

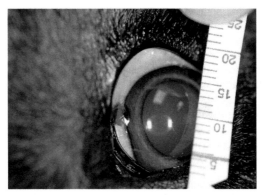

Fig. 1. The left eye of a 3-year-old M Labrador retriever. A 3 mm diameter, black slightly raised limbal melanoma/melanocytoma is visible at the dorsonasal limbus. This is a less common location for a limbal melanoma/melanocytoma. Extension into the cornea is also visible.

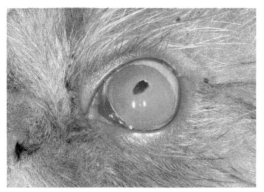

Fig. 2. The left eye of a 4-year-old FS Persian cat. A 4-mm darkly pigmented, oblong-shaped corneal sequestrum is present in the axial cornea.

the epithelial surface and be associated with corneal ulceration[13] (**Fig. 5**). Foreign bodies can be either full thickness (perforating) or partial thickness (penetrating)[14] (**Fig. 6**). Superficial corneal foreign bodies can be differentiated from other brown corneal lesions based on their location, irregular shape, and the ability to remove the foreign body from the cornea with saline hydropulsion. Other clues that the brown opacity may be a superficial corneal foreign body are blepharospasm, conjunctival hyperemia, and corneal vascularization. Penetrating foreign bodies are typically associated with blepharospasm and conjunctival hyperemia, and with perforating projectiles, there will be significant uveitis with clinical manifestations that may include hyphema, hypopyon, and aqueous flare. Although superficial foreign bodies can sometimes be removed in primary care practice, deep penetrating and perforating foreign bodies should be referred to a veterinary ophthalmologist when possible.[13,14]

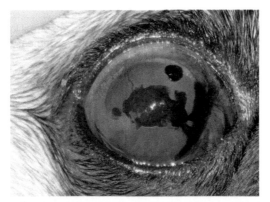

Fig. 3. The right eye of an 8-year-old FS pug. This patient previously had a conjunctival graft to repair a deep corneal ulcer in the axial cornea. The pigmentation in the axial (central) cornea is the pigmented remnants of a conjunctival graft. A prominent blood vessel extends from the dorsal limbus to the graft site at axial cornea. There is a 3 mm, dark brown lesion at the dorsal limbus at 1 to 2 o'clock. The location and shape of this brown opacity is highly unusual; limbal melanomas are usually well circumscribed and nearly black. Corneal pigmentation does not typically occur in a clump at the limbus. Close examination revealed this lesion to be an organic foreign body, likely a seedpod, that adhered itself to the cornea.

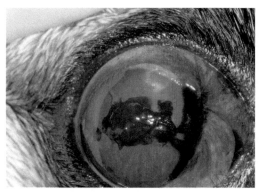

Fig. 4. The right eye of an 8-year-old FS pug. The corneal foreign body has been removed with saline hydropulsion (forceful lavage using a directed stream of sterile saline) and fluorescein has been applied to the cornea. A fluorescein-positive ulceration is present under the area where the foreign body was adhered to the cornea. The patient was treated with topical antibiotics and anticollagenases, and the ulcer resolved within a week.

Iris Prolapse

When the cornea perforates, the iris usually forms a mechanical plug to seal the wound. Acute iris prolapse can be seen as brown tissue protruding into or from the corneal or limbal surface (**Fig. 7**). If the iris prolapse has formed a good seal, the anterior chamber will be formed and no aqueous humor will be leaking from the wound. Great care should be taken to not disturb a sealed iris prolapse, which will further destabilize the globe. Poorly sealed iris prolapses are often accompanied by a shallow anterior chamber, active leakage of aqueous humor, fibrin in the wound, and hyphema. Treatment options include referral for surgical grafting of the cornea and replacement of the iris into the anterior chamber, medical management with oral and topical antibiotics, and pain-relieving medications or enucleation.[15–19]

Dermoid

Dermoids are a form of choristoma: a normal tissue in an abnormal location (**Fig. 8**). Dermoids of the ocular surface can be found on the conjunctiva, cornea, and limbus. They are

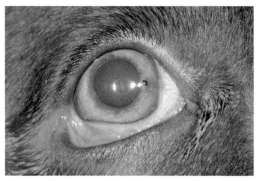

Fig. 5. The right eye of a 2-year-old MC mixed breed dog. A brown, 1.5-mm superficial corneal foreign body is present in the medial paraxial cornea. Superficial corneal vascularization extends from the limbus to the foreign body, indicating chronicity. Corneal pigmentation is rarely an isolated, circular lesion as seen here in this foreign body, which should raise the index of suspicion for a superficial corneal foreign body.

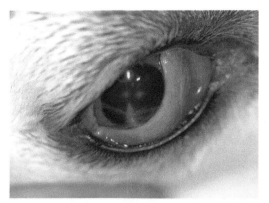

Fig. 6. The right eye of a 7-year-old mixed breed dog. A tan colored penetrating corneal foreign body is present in the temporal paraxial cornea. Removal of penetrating foreign bodies is complex and best performed using microsurgical instrumentation and techniques.

often pigmented but may vary in their level of pigmentation. They frequently have long hairs growing from their surface that can be a source of ocular irritation and excess tearing. Surgical excision is the treatment of choice and most are referred to an ophthalmologist.[20]

Fungal Keratitis

Fungal keratitis is rare in small animal patients.[13,21–25] Even more rare is fungal keratitis with pigmented dematiaceous fungus.[26] Fungal keratitis is a differential diagnosis for pigmented, ulcerative lesions of the corneal surface (**Fig. 9**). Cytology, PCR, and fungal culture may all aid in making an accurate diagnosis, and these ulcerative lesions should also be referred to an ophthalmologist for appropriate therapy.

DIFFERENTIAL DIAGNOSES OF CORNEAL PIGMENTATION
Histologic Manifestations of Corneal Pigmentation

Melanocytes located within the corneal limbus epithelium have multiple roles and are an essential component of the corneal epithelial stem cell niche. Their main function is

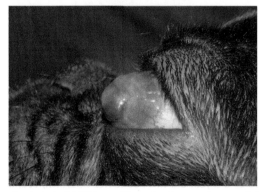

Fig. 7. The left eye of a 4-year-old MC pug. There is a large rupture of the axial cornea with prolapse of pigmented iris material. There is marked deformation of the corneal surface; rather than being smooth and curved, it is eruptive and bulbous. This patient did not have a dazzle or a consensual PLR to the fellow eye, and enucleation was elected for the patient's comfort and well-being.

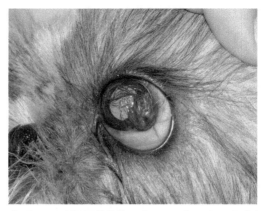

Fig. 8. The left eye of a 1-year-old MC Shih Tzu. A corneal-conjunctival dermoid is present at the temporal limbus, with long hairs originating from the dermoid and cascading across the cornea.

understood to be the transfer of melanin-containing melanosomes to adjacent limbal epithelial stem/progenitor cells to protect them from ultraviolet light damage. Limbal melanocytes also show immunomodulatory effects interpreted to protect limbal epithelial stem/progenitor cells from inflammatory injury and oxidative stress as well as preventing premature differentiation. Limbal melanocytes may also contribute to the avascular nature of the cornea by secreting antiangiogenic factors.[27,28] Normal canine limbal melanocytes can be visualized by immunohistochemistry.[29]

Limbal melanocytes may migrate in the corneal epithelium during corneal wound healing as well as a component of pathological processes. During wound healing, limbal melanocytes will accompany undifferentiated limbal epithelial stem/progenitor cells migrating onto the cornea and influence their proliferation, migration, and terminal differentiation during reepithelialization.[30]

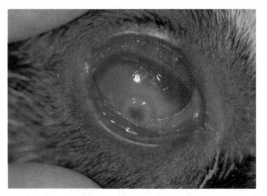

Fig. 9. The right eye of a 3-year-old MC Rat terrier. A brown, round, raised plaque surrounded by stromal loss and corneal edema is present in the axial cornea. Very dense, deep, active stromal vascularization extends 5 mm from the dorsal limbus toward the axial cornea. After keratectomy, this patient was diagnosed with a dematiaceous fungal keratitis. Dematiaceous funguses are pigmented, which makes the corneal lesion associated with this lesion pigmented as well.

In dogs, the pathogenesis and specific triggers of corneal pigmentation have not been completely established. The lesion commonly represents an adaptive response to a variety of repeated or persistent corneal injuries. Corneal pigmentation results from centripetal migration of limbal melanocytes in the epithelium and melanin accumulation within the corneal epithelial cells. The accumulation of pigment within the corneal epithelium is a histologic feature of chronic keratitis along with hyperplasia of the epithelium and, in some cases, keratinization (nonspecific chronic keratitis; **Fig. 10**). These changes result in a corneal epithelium that mimics the skin's epidermis and the changes have been termed epidermalization or "cutaneous metaplasia." Melanin pigment may also accumulate in the corneal stroma secondary to leakage of melanin from the epithelial basal cells with phagocytosis by macrophages (pigmentary incontinence). The corneal stromal lesions are typically seen with nonspecific chronic keratitis include fibrosis and neovascularization and, in some cases, the infiltration of leukocytes, typically lymphocytes and plasma cells. These adaptive changes represent an attempt to maintain corneal integrity and avoid progressive corneal ulceration even though the consequence is loss of corneal transparency.[30]

Pigmentary keratitis of brachycephalic breeds shares morphologic features with nonspecific chronic keratitis. The findings include corneal pigmentation as well as the presence of leukocytes and neovascularization of the corneal stroma. The underlying pathogenesis of pigmentary keratitis of brachycephalic breeds remains speculative (see "Pigmentary Keratitis of Pugs and Other Brachycephalic Dogs" section).[31]

Clinical Implications of Corneal Pigmentation

As discussed at the beginning of this article, the essential function of the cornea is clarity to allow the transmission of light from the outside world to the retina. Corneal pigmentation interferes with light transmission and therefore impairs vision. Unlike other forms of corneal opacity, which can resolve spontaneously or with therapy, such as vascularization or corneal infiltrate, corneal pigmentation is very difficult to reverse.[32] Therefore, early and accurate diagnosis of corneal pigmentation and its associated ocular disease is critical to preserving vision. We will now shift to focusing on individual keratopathies associated with corneal pigmentation.

Pigmentary Keratitis of Pugs and Other Brachycephalic Dogs

Pugs have been recognized in multiple studies as being disproportionately affected by corneal pigmentation.[31,33–36] The unique pattern of corneal pigmentation seen is pugs is termed pigmentary keratitis[31] (**Fig. 11**). Prevalence estimates range from 70% to

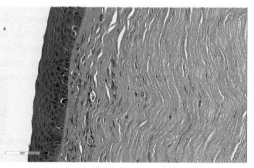

Fig. 10. Histopathology of nonspecific chronic keratitis with corneal melanosis in a dog. The corneal epithelium is hyperplastic and many cells contain melanin pigment. The underlying corneal stroma is fibrotic with neovascularization. HE staining, 400×.

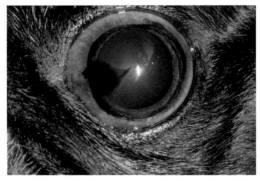

Fig. 11. The left eye of a 6-year-old FS pug. Corneal pigment is visible extending from the nasal limbus toward the axial cornea consistent with mild pigmentary keratitis.

90% of the pug population. No significant difference is detected between "pet" pugs and AKC-registered pugs who compete in conformation shows.[34] Pigmentary keratitis begins at the medial limbus and extends across the cornea toward the temporal limbus. In severe cases, the pigment can completely cover the corneal surface, causing blindness, although the majority of cases are mild. Although corneal pigmentation is recognized in other brachycephalic breeds, the severity and frequency of pigmentary keratitis is unique to pugs.[31,33,37] There is conflicting data regarding the role of eyelid conformation in the pathogenesis of pigmentary keratitis. Lagophthalmos and exposure are probably the most significant factors in the pathogenesis of this disorder. Although entropion at the medial canthus may play a role, the pathogenesis is likely multifactorial and likely has a genetic component.[34–36] Concurrent ocular disease, including corneal trauma and keratoconjunctivitis sicca (KCS), likely exacerbate the severity of pigmentary keratitis.[35,36]

Because the pathogenesis of pigmentary keratitis is not well understood, treatment strategies are similarly not straightforward or based on controlled clinical trials. Medical therapy with topical corticosteroids(prednisolone acetate 1%, dexamethasone sodium phosphate 0.1%) and immunomodulators (cyclosporine A 0.02%–2%, tacrolimus 0.02%–0.03%) have been a long mainstay of medical therapy, although there have not been long-term studies evaluating the efficacy of these therapies.[34] Cryotherapy has been evaluated as a therapeutic technique for reducing corneal pigmentation in dogs with corneal pigmentation; however, it induces significant inflammation and additional stromal scarring, and the long-term efficacy has not been evaluated.[32] Surgical canthoplasty has been reported as a therapy in textbooks and for treatment of the 2 critical eyelid issues (lagophthalmos and medial ventral entropion). Although anecdotal evidence suggests that surgery can hasten or facilitate complete pigment resolution, peer-reviewed data is not available.[38,39] Further investigation is needed into the etiopathogenesis of pigmentary keratitis in order to develop more effective treatment strategies.

Keratoconjunctivitis Sicca

KCS is a quantitative deficiency of the aqueous tear film. Because the normal cornea critically depends on a robust and healthy tear film for nutrition, immune-protection, and waste removal, tear film deficiencies lead to poor corneal health. KCS is far more common in canine patients than in feline patients, with strong breed predilections in canine patients.[33,37,40,41] Brachycephalic and spaniel breeds are overrepresented, including Shih Tzus, Lhasa Apsos, Pugs, Bulldogs, West Highland white terriers, and American cocker spaniels. Knowing the commonly affected breeds will help raise the index of suspicion for KCS in patients with early or mild clinical signs. The most common cause of KCS in canine patients is immune-mediated destruction of the lacrimal tissue.

The early clinical signs of KCS may be limited to mucoid ocular discharge, with time, the cornea responds by opacifying. Corneal pigmentation is associated with chronic KCS and may be accompanied by vascularization and fibrosis. A Schirmer tear test (STT) is required to diagnose KCS. Although most textbooks state that STT of 0 is absolute KCS, less than 5 mm is severe KCS, and 5 to 10 mm is moderate KCS, and finally 14 mm/min is early or potential KCS, the STT must be interpreted in light of the patient's clinical signs. A patient with mucoid ocular discharge, superficial corneal vascularization, corneal pigmentation and a STT of 16 mm/min has KCS, even though the STT is "normal" may require a combination of lacrimostimulants and supplemental lubrication.

Chronic Superficial Keratitis or "Pannus"

Chronic superficial keratitis, also known as pannus, is typically a bilateral, non–ulcerative keratopathy of many large breeds of dogs and the German Shepherds, Bouvier des Flandres and sighthounds are the most commonly affected breeds.[42] The lesion is characterized by superficial neovascularization and pigmentation of the cornea, typically starting from the lateral limbus and extending toward the axial cornea, opposite to what is seen in pigmentary keratitis[43,44] (**Fig. 12**). Pannus is likely immune mediated and may have a genetic component.[45,46] Exposure to high levels of UV radiation, seem to make the disease more refractory to therapy.[47] Diagnosis is made primarily by the classic appearance of the lesion and patient signalment rather than by cytology or biopsy. Treatment is aimed at limiting excessive exposure to intense UV light and topical immunosuppressives.[48]

Chronic Keratitis

Any chronic keratitis can be associated with corneal pigmentation. Corneal pigmentation may occur as part of a wound healing response after ulceration. Any mechanical abrasion of the cornea such as occurs with entropion or an eyelid mass may result in corneal pigmentation. Chronic corneal edema can also be associated with pigmentation. It is critical to remember that corneal pigmentation is a nonspecific clinical sign

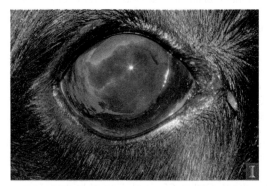

Fig. 12. The right eye of an 8-year-old FS German Shepherd. Diffuse corneal pigmentation and vascularization consistent with chronic, severe pannus (chronic superficial keratitis) is present.

that must be interpreted alongside signalment and the rest of the ocular examination in order to make an accurate diagnosis.

CLINICS CARE POINTS

- Signalment and ophthalmic examination findings are both critical to accurately diagnosing brown corneal opacities.
- Location and pattern of pigment should be considered in the making of an accurate diagnosis.
- Additional testing beyond a complete ophthalmic examination, including schirmer tear test, cytology, culture, and biopsy may be indicated.

REFERENCES

1. Bauer B, Leis ML, Sayi S. Primary corneal melanocytoma in a Collie. Vet Ophthalmol 2015;18(5):429–32.
2. Donaldson D, Sansom J, Scase T, et al. Canine limbal melanoma: 30 cases (1992-2004). Part 1. Signalment, clinical and histological features and pedigree analysis. Vet Ophthalmol 2006;9(2):115–9.
3. Wang AL, Kern T. Melanocytic ophthalmic neoplasms of the domestic veterinary species: a review. Top Companion Anim Med 2015;30(4):148–57.
4. Grahn BH, Sandmeyer LS, Bauer B. Diagnostic ophthalmology. extrascleral extension of an uveal melanoma. Can Vet J Rev Veterinaire Can 2008;49(7): 723–4.
5. Andreani V, Guandalini A, D'Anna N, et al. The combined use of surgical debulking and diode laser photocoagulation for limbal melanoma treatment: a retrospective study of 21 dogs. Vet Ophthalmol 2017;20(2):147–54.
6. Donaldson D, Sansom J, Adams V. Canine limbal melanoma: 30 cases (1992-2004). Part 2. Treatment with lamellar resection and adjunctive strontium-90beta plesiotherapy–efficacy and morbidity. Vet Ophthalmol 2006;9(3):179–85.
7. Cullen CL, Wadowska DW, Singh A, et al. Ultrastructural findings in feline corneal sequestra. Vet Ophthalmol 2005;8(5):295–303.
8. Davidson HJ, Gerlach JA, Bull RW. Determination of protein concentrations and their molecular weight in tears from cats with normal corneas and cats with corneal sequestrum. Am J Vet Res 1992;53(10):1756–9.
9. Featherstone HJ, Franklin VJ, Sansom J. Feline corneal sequestrum: laboratory analysis of ocular samples from 12 cats. Vet Ophthalmol 2004;7(4):229–38.
10. Grahn BH, Sisler S, Storey E. Qualitative tear film and conjunctival goblet cell assessment of cats with corneal sequestra. Vet Ophthalmol 2005;8(3):167–70.
11. Nasisse MP, Glover TL, Moore CP, et al. Detection of feline herpesvirus 1 DNA in corneas of cats with eosinophilic keratitis or corneal sequestration. Am J Vet Res 1998;59(7):856–8.
12. Michel J, Vigan M, Douet JY. Autologous lamellar keratoplasty for the treatment of feline corneal sequestrum: A retrospective study of 35 eyes (2012-2020). Vet Ophthalmol 2021;24(5):491–502.
13. Labelle AL, Psutka K, Collins SP, et al. Use of hydropulsion for the treatment of superficial corneal foreign bodies: 15 cases (1999-2013). J Am Vet Med Assoc 2014;244(4):476–9.

14. Tetas Pont R, Matas Riera M, Newton R, et al. Corneal and anterior segment foreign body trauma in dogs: a review of 218 cases. Vet Ophthalmol 2016; 19(5):386–97.
15. Mezzadri V, Crotti A, Nardi S, et al. Surgical treatment of canine and feline descemetoceles, deep and perforated corneal ulcers with autologous buccal mucous membrane grafts. Vet Ophthalmol 2021;24(6):599–609.
16. Thajunnisa AS, Sainulabdeen A, Dileepkumar KM, et al. Comparative evaluation of decellularized bovine omentum alone and in combination with mitomycin-C in the management of corneal injuries in dogs. Vet World 2020;13(11):2401–10.
17. Gogova S, Leiva M, Ortillés Á, et al. Corneoconjunctival transposition for the treatment of deep stromal to full-thickness corneal defects in dogs: A multicentric retrospective study of 100 cases (2012-2018). Vet Ophthalmol 2020;23(3):450–9.
18. Bussieres M, Krohne SG, Stiles J, et al. The use of porcine small intestinal submucosa for the repair of full-thickness corneal defects in dogs, cats and horses. Vet Ophthalmol 2004;7(5):352–9.
19. Paulsen ME, Kass PH. Traumatic corneal laceration with associated lens capsule disruption: a retrospective study of 77 clinical cases from 1999 to 2009. Vet Ophthalmol 2012;15(6):355–68.
20. Badanes Z, Ledbetter EC. Ocular dermoids in dogs: A retrospective study. Vet Ophthalmol 2019;22(6):760–6.
21. Ledbetter EC, Norman ML, Starr JK. In vivo confocal microscopy for the detection of canine fungal keratitis and monitoring of therapeutic response. Vet Ophthalmol 2016;19(3):220–9.
22. Scott EM, Carter RT. Canine keratomycosis in 11 dogs: a case series (2000-2011). J Am Anim Hosp Assoc 2014;50(2):112–8.
23. Grundon RA, O'Reilly A, Muhlnickel C, et al. Keratomycosis in a dog treated with topical 1% voriconazole solution. Vet Ophthalmol 2010;13(5):331–5.
24. Binder DR, Sugrue JE, Herring IP. Acremonium keratomycosis in a cat. Vet Ophthalmol 2011;14(Suppl 1):111–6.
25. Nevile JC, Hurn SD, Turner AG. Keratomycosis in five dogs. Vet Ophthalmol 2016; 19(5):432–8.
26. Pucket JD, Allbaugh RA, Rankin AJ. Treatment of dematiaceous fungal keratitis in a dog. J Am Vet Med Assoc 2012;240(9):1104–8.
27. Higa K, Shimmura S, Miyashita H, et al. Melanocytes in the corneal limbus interact with K19-positive basal epithelial cells. Exp Eye Res 2005;81(2):218–23.
28. Polisetti N, Gießl A, Zenkel M, et al. Melanocytes as emerging key players in niche regulation of limbal epithelial stem cells. Ocul Surf 2021;22:172–89.
29. Labelle P, Reilly CM, Naydan DK, et al. Immunohistochemical characteristics of normal canine eyes. Vet Pathol 2012;49(5):860–9.
30. Labelle P. The eye. In: Zachary JF, editor. Pathologic basis of veterinary disease. 7th edition. St. Louis, MO: Elsevier; 2022. p. 1431–2.
31. Vallone LV, Enders AM, Mohammed HO, et al. In vivo confocal microscopy of brachycephalic dogs with and without superficial corneal pigment. Vet Ophthalmol 2017;20(4):294–303.
32. Azoulay T. Adjunctive cryotherapy for pigmentary keratitis in dogs: a study of 16 corneas. Vet Ophthalmol 2014;17(4):241–9.
33. Costa J, Steinmetz A, Delgado E. Clinical signs of brachycephalic ocular syndrome in 93 dogs. Ir Vet J 2021;74(1):3.
34. Labelle AL, Dresser CB, Hamor RE, et al. Characteristics of, prevalence of, and risk factors for corneal pigmentation (pigmentary keratopathy) in Pugs. J Am Vet Med Assoc 2013;243(5):667–74.

35. Krecny M, Tichy A, Rushton J, et al. A retrospective survey of ocular abnormalities in pugs: 130 cases. J Small Anim Pract 2015;56(2):96–102.
36. Maini S, Everson R, Dawson C, et al. Pigmentary keratitis in pugs in the United Kingdom: prevalence and associated features. BMC Vet Res 2019;15:384.
37. Palmer SV, Gomes FE, McArt JAA. Ophthalmic disorders in a referral population of seven breeds of brachycephalic dogs: 970 cases (2008–2017). J Am Vet Med Assoc 2021;259(11):1318–24.
38. Allgoewer I, Sahr S, Neumann K. Abstracts: American College of Veterinary Ophthalmologists, Monterey, CA October 26–29, 2016 Abstract 75: Results of the evaluation of the long-term effect of different therapies on pigmentary keratitis (PK) of the Pug. Vet Ophthalmol 2016;19(6):E21–43.
39. Yi NY, Park SA, Jeong MB, et al. Medial canthoplasty for epiphora in dogs: a retrospective study of 23 cases. J Am Anim Hosp Assoc 2006;42(6):435–9.
40. Uhl LK, Saito A, Iwashita H, et al. Clinical features of cats with aqueous tear deficiency: a retrospective case series of 10 patients (17 eyes). J Feline Med Surg 2019;21(10):944–50.
41. O'Neill DG, Brodbelt DC, Keddy A, et al. Keratoconjunctivitis sicca in dogs under primary veterinary care in the UK: an epidemiological study. J Small Anim Pract 2021;62(8):636–45.
42. Bedford PG, Longstaffe JA. Corneal pannus (chronic superficial keratitis) in the German shepherd dog. J Small Anim Pract 1979;20(1):41–56.
43. Williams D, Scarff D. Chronic superficial keratitis in German shepherd dogs. Vet Rec 1992;130(20):456.
44. Drahovska Z, Balicki I, Trbolova A, et al. A retrospective study of the occurrence of chronic superficial keratitis in 308 German Shepherd dogs: 1999-2010. Pol J Vet Sci 2014;17(3):543–6.
45. Barrientos LS, Zapata G, Crespi JA, et al. A study of the association between chronic superficial keratitis and polymorphisms in the upstream regulatory regions of DLA-DRB1, DLA-DQB1 and DLA-DQA1. Vet Immunol Immunopathol 2013;156(3–4):205–10.
46. Jokinen P, Rusanen EM, Kennedy LJ, et al. MHC class II risk haplotype associated with canine chronic superficial keratitis in German Shepherd dogs. Vet Immunol Immunopathol 2011;140(1–2):37–41.
47. Chavkin MJ, Roberts SM, Salman MD, et al. Risk factors for development of chronic superficial keratitis in dogs. J Am Vet Med Assoc 1994;204(10):1630–4.
48. Balicki I, Szadkowski M, Balicka A, et al. Clinical study on the application of dexamethasone and cyclosporine/dimethyl sulfoxide combination eye drops in the initial therapy of chronic superficial keratitis in dogs. Pol J Vet Sci 2021;24(3): 415–23.

Eosinophilic Keratoconjunctivitis in Cats

Amber Labelle, DVM, MS[a],*, Philippe Labelle, DVM[b]

KEYWORDS

- Cornea • Eosinophilic • Conjunctivitis • Keratitis • Keratoconjunctivitis • Cat
- Feline • Eosinophil

KEY POINTS

- Eosinophilic keratitis is a disease of the feline cornea characterized by white to pink plaques on the corneal surface and vascularization of the cornea.
- Cytology of the affected cornea is usually diagnostic for eosinophilic keratitis.
- Immunosuppressive therapy, either topical or systemic, is the key to successful treatment.
- Eosinophilic keratitis can recrudesce after successful therapy.

INTRODUCTION

Eosinophilic keratoconjunctivitis (EK) is a disease of the feline ocular surface. Although corneal involvement with secondary conjunctivitis is the most commonly recognized manifestation, a form of primary eosinophilic conjunctivitis has been reported that does not include corneal involvement.[1] Although EK has been reported in the veterinary scientific literature for over 40 years, there is much yet to be learned about the pathophysiology of this disease.[2] A form of EK is also recognized in horses, but it remains unknown if there is shared etiopathogenesis between the disease in both species.[3–5]

CLINICAL FINDINGS

The mean affected age is approximately 5 years, and no breed predilection has been reported.[6–8] EK is most commonly unilateral but may be bilateral. Most cats present with some degree of ocular discomfort that manifests as blepharospasm. Ocular discharge may be serous or mucoid. The hallmark of EK is white to pink irregularly shaped raised plaques on the corneal surface accompanied by corneal

The authors have nothing to disclose.
[a] Bright Light Veterinary Eye Care, Ottawa, Ontario, Canada; [b] Antech Diagnostics, 7555 Danbro Crescent, Mississauga, Ontario L5N 6P9, Canada
* Corresponding author. 779 Long Point Circle, Gloucester, Ontario K1T 4H5, Canada.
E-mail address: hello@brightlightvet.ca
Twitter: @brightlightvet (A.L.)

vascularization (**Fig. 1**).[9–19] This lesion tends to originate from the dorsotemporal limbus and extends towards the central cornea (**Fig. 2**). Ulceration of the adjacent corneal epithelium may be present, and the plaques themselves will stain with fluorescein (**Fig. 3**). Corneal edema may or may not be a feature of EK, but chronic cases usually have some degree of corneal degeneration, which is visible as white crystalline opacities in the corneal stroma. In severe cases, the whole corneal surface may be affected, causing vision loss. Some cases may have superficial corneal vascularization, ulceration, and only one or two small plaques in areas other than the dorsotemporal cornea (**Fig. 4**). Mild to severe conjunctival hyperemia and chemosis are often present concurrently.

Surprisingly, EK is not typically associated with a clinically detectable reflex uveitis, and the intraocular exam is normal in most patients. The neuro-ophthalmic exam is normal in most cats, with the exception of those with severe disease, where the menace response (which is unreliable in most cats) may be absent in the affected eye. Visualizing the pupil may also be difficult with severe disease, making an assessment of the pupillary light reflex challenging.

Assessing the dazzle reflex as a proxy for retinal function can be helpful in severely affected cases.[20] The dazzle reflex is assessed by shining a very bright, focal light into the eye and observing an avoidance response, typically manifested as blinking, retraction of the globe, or movement of the head away from the light source. Critical to the assessment of the dazzle reflex is the use of a sufficiently bright light source; a weak light source will not be sufficient to trigger a dazzle reflex. Assessing the dazzle in a dark room may make it easier to assess, as a patient who is dark-adapted will show a more dramatic response. The neuroanatomy of the dazzle reflex is not completely defined, but the afferent pathway is cranial nerve II (optic nerve) and the efferent pathway is cranial nerve VII, with synapses likely in the midbrain. Because the visual cortex is not part of the dazzle reflex, it is considered a subcortical response and thus cannot be considered a conclusive assessment of vision.

What is the clinical utility of the dazzle? In patients with an opaque cornea and a negative menace, the presence of a positive dazzle is confirmation that the retina is functioning, and if corneal transparency is restored, the patient will likely regain vision.

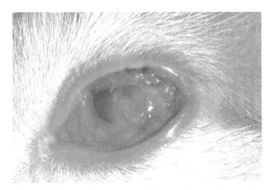

Fig. 1. Photograph of the left eye of a 4-year-old MC DSH with EK. There is mild blepharedema, severe conjunctival hyperemia, moderate-to-severe chemosis, elevation of the nictitans, and mucoid discharge. The dorsotemporal cornea has a pink-white plaque partially adhered to it surrounded by corneal vascularization. Fluorescein stain has been applied to the cornea, although there is no visible fluorescein uptake in this photograph. DLH, domestic long hair; DSH, domestic short hair; FS, female spay; MC, male castrate.

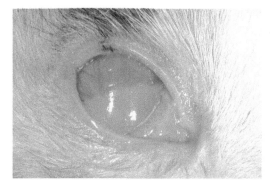

Fig. 2. Photograph of the left eye of a 6-year-old MC DLH with EK. There is moderate blepharedema, moderate-to-severe conjunctival hyperemia, moderate-to-severe chemosis, elevation and thickening of the nictitans, and serous to mucoid discharge. The dorsotemporal cornea has deep stromal vascularization extending toward the axial cornea, and thin, light pink plaque is adhered to the cornea. The pupil is mydriatic, and a yellow tapetal reflection is visible.

DIFFERENTIAL DIAGNOSES

When presented with a cat with raised white to pink corneal plaques and corneal vascularization, EK should be the top differential diagnosis. Corneal stromal abscess, foreign body, or fungal granuloma are considered the most appropriate differential diagnoses.[7,21] Because cats are frequently affected with squamous cell carcinoma (SCC) of the periocular skin, ears, and nasal planum, some clinicians may consider including SCC on their differential list.[22,23] Although other species, including dogs, horses, and cows, are more often affected by corneal SCC, there is only a single case report in the scientific literature of a corneal SCC in a cat.[24] Therefore, SCC is not an important differential diagnosis. Corneal lymphoma has not been reported in cats. Because EK has such a characteristic clinical appearance, it is important to be mindful that it is the most important differential diagnosis and to prioritize diagnostic techniques (cytology) to rule it in or out. As an anatomic pathologist working

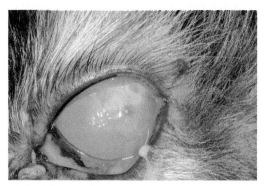

Fig. 3. Photograph of the left eye of a 4-year-old FS DSH with EK. There is mild blepharedema, moderate conjunctival hyperemia and chemosis, slight elevation of the nictitans, and mucoid discharge. The dorsotemporal cornea has a fluorescein positive plaque adhered to it, and deep stromal vessels are visible adjacent to the plaque. There is some stromal infiltrate ventral to the plaque. The pupil is mydriatic, and a yellow tapetal reflection is visible.

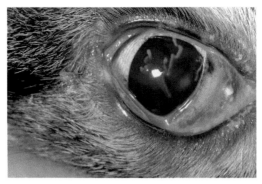

Fig. 4. Photograph of the right eye of a 6-year-old FS DSH with EK. There is very mild blepharedema, moderate conjunctival hyperemia and chemosis with elevation and thickening of the nictitans. Fluorescein has been applied to the ocular surface, and multiple linear to branching superficial corneal ulcers are visible. Multiple fluorescein positive plaques are visible on the palpebral surface of the nictitans. to the plaque. The pupil is mydriatic, and the anterior chamber and iris appear normal.

for a corporate diagnostic laboratory reports it is important to stress that I receive 1 to 2 enucleated globes with eosinophilic keratitis that are submitted yearly, and these could have been treated successfully if the diagnosis was simply confirmed before enucleation (P.L.). These cases are typically accompanied by a clinical history that includes "suspect cancer." EK is a common disease of the feline cornea whereas neoplasia of the feline cornea is rare, and therefore a clinician needs to be prepared to confirm a diagnosis of suspect EK.

Diagnostic Techniques

The diagnostic test of choice for EK is a cytologic examination of scrapings of the plaque lesions on the corneal surface.[2] To perform corneal cytology, first apply a drop of topical anesthetic to the ocular surface. Using an appropriate instrument for obtaining the cytologic sample is critical for getting a diagnostic sample.[25] Dental applicator sponges in the 2.0 mm size are an ideal cytobrush because they are small and superb at both collecting and releasing cells onto the slide (Microbrush International, Algonquin, Illinois, USA). Cotton-tipped applicators are not recommended for obtaining corneal cytology specimens, as they are ineffective at releasing cells onto the slide. A Kimura spatula is a metal blade with blunt, rounded edges that is a reusable tool that is also ideal for obtaining cytology specimens. The handle end of a scalpel blade is also an effective, disposable alternative. The specimen should be obtained from the surface of the raised plaque using a gentle but firm scraping motion across the surface (**Fig. 5**). If using a dental applicator sponge, roll the sponge surface across the slide (**Fig. 6**). If using a blade handle or Kimura spatula, gently press and wipe against the slide. The preparation of two slides is recommended. One slide can be reviewed in-house using standard Diff-Quick slide prep after air-drying, whereas the other slide can be preserved to send for evaluation by a board-certified clinical pathologist if the diagnosis is not made by the attending veterinarian.

Cytological Findings

A quality cytologic sample should be highly cellular. Eosinophils are often the dominant cell type present in eosinophilic keratitis (**Fig. 7**). Although some veterinary ophthalmologists have proposed that seeing even one eosinophil in a feline corneal cytology specimen is sufficient to make a diagnosis of EK, clinical pathologists typically describe EK as a disease where multiple eosinophils are necessary to confirm the diagnosis.[2,11,25] Neutrophils, mast cells, small lymphocytes, plasma cells, and red blood cells may all be present. Recently researchers reported the presence of a novel cell type in ocular tissue, the globule leukocyte, which was identified using a Wright-Giemsa stain.[16] The significance of the presence of this cell type remains unknown, nor has its presence in ocular tissue been reported using Diff-Quick staining.

Histopathology

The histologic diagnosis of eosinophilic keratitis is usually made in keratectomy samples (**Fig. 8**). There is almost never an indication for enucleation. The rare cases that are refractory to treatment and patients where there are at-home barriers to treatment, or noncomplaint owners are exceptions. Rarely the disease will be present in globes enucleated for other conditions. Histologically, eosinophils are always a component of corneal stromal inflammation, but may not be the predominant cell type.[2] In fact, most cases submitted for histopathologic evaluation are chronic presentations of the disease and the infiltrate is predominantly lymphoplasmacytic with variable numbers of eosinophils.[26–28] Some cases show a band of granular hypereosinophilic material near or at the epithelial basement membrane presumed to represent eosinophilic degranulation; the cause and significance of the findings is undetermined.[29] The overlying corneal epithelium is often intact with no ulceration despite significant corneal stromal infiltrates.

The cause and pathogenesis of eosinophilic keratitis have not been determined. It is plausible that some mechanisms of disease overlap with other eosinophil-rich conditions such as feline cutaneous eosinophilic granuloma complex; however, an association between these disorders has not been established.[26,27] Viral inclusions and viral cytopathic effects are not a feature of the disease and histopathologic examination provides no insight into the controversial role for feline herpesvirus 1.[26,27] Eosinophilic/allergic disease of the ocular surface in humans may offer clues that may instigate future research, but does not at this time elucidate the pathogenesis of this disease in cats.[30–33]

Treatment Strategies

The goal of treating EK is (1) to restore corneal transparency in order to restore normal vision and (2) to eliminate patient discomfort (**Figs. 9** and **10**). Topical, oral and

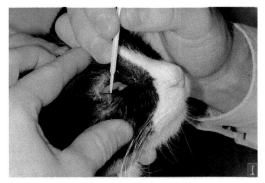

Fig. 5. In this photograph, a Microbrush is being used to obtain cytology of a corneoconjunctival lesion in a cat with suspected EK. A drop of topical anesthetic was applied to the ocular surface before obtaining the sample.

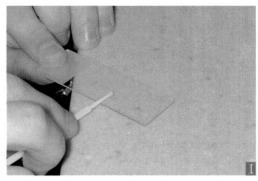

Fig. 6. In this photograph, we are demonstrating how to roll the Microbrush across a glass slide to obtain the most cellular sample possible for microscopic examination.

parenteral treatment strategies are available for EK (**Table 1**). As is generally true in veterinary medicine, when a disease has many available treatments, this generally indicates that none of the treatments are singularly effective. Factors that dictate which treatments are appropriate for the patient include:

- The presence or absence of corneal ulceration
- The ability of the caretaker to provide treatment
- The patient's temperament
- Any concurrent ocular diseases
- Any concurrent systemic diseases

Finally, by way of introduction to eosinophilic keratitis therapy, there are many successful topical and systemic medications and favored treatment regimes among ophthalmologists. However, if topical glucocorticoids have not been given, they should be given as most cases are responsive.

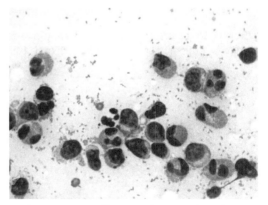

Fig. 7. Microphotograph at 100x magnification of a corneal cytology sample from a cat with EK. The sample is moderately cellular. Numerous eosinophils with rose pink granules are present, and loose granules from ruptured cells are visible scattered across the field. Small lymphocytes, plasma cells are also visible in the field with rare red blood cells and neutrophils. This is a typical cytologic specimen and it is considered strongly supportive of the diagnosis of EK.

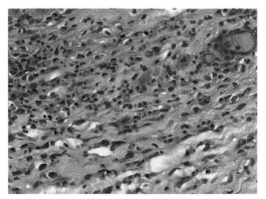

Fig. 8. Histopathology of EK in a cat. Numerous eosinophils admixed with fewer lymphocytes, plasma cells and mast cells infiltrate the corneal stroma. HE staining, 400x.

Topical corticosteroids should be avoided in cats with concurrent corneal ulceration, although this traditional dogma has been challenged.[34,35] Long-acting repositol injectable medication may be considered for fractious or difficult-to-handle cats. Systemic corticosteroids or synthetic progestins may not be the best option for obese cats or cats with diabetes.

ORAL THERAPY
Megestrol Acetate

Megestrol acetate (MgA) is a synthetic progestin that has anti-estrogen and glucocorticoid activity.[36] MgA is FDA-approved for the suppression of estrus and the treatment of false pregnancy in dogs. It has been used off-label for the treatment of feline dermatologic conditions, control of canine benign prostatic hyperplasia, and EK.[37] Oral MgA was one of the first drugs used for the treatment of EK, and although it remains highly effective, the side effects associated with its use make it a less commonly used therapy at the time of the publication of this article.[9,38,39] MgA is associated with transient

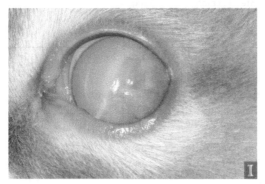

Fig. 9. Photograph of the left eye of an 11-year-old MC DSH with EK. There is very mild blepharedema. The conjunctiva of the third eyelid is mildly hyperemic. The temporal half of the cornea is covered in white to pink plaques with dense stromal vessels visible in areas with less plaque formation. The pupil is mydriatic, and a yellow tapetal reflection is visible. The iris is normal and the anterior chamber is clear.

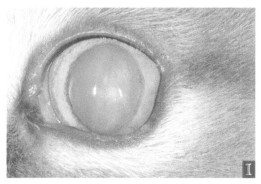

Fig. 10. Photograph of the left eye of the patient from **Fig. 9**, approximately 1 month after treatment with oral megestrol acetate for EK. The eyelids and third eyelid appear normal. There is slight serous ocular discharge. The corneal plaques have resolved, and regressing vessels are visible in the temporal one-third of the cornea. The pupil is moderately mydriatic, and the iris and anterior chamber are normal.

diabetes mellitus, endometrial hyperplasia, mammary hypertrophy, and less commonly, mammary neoplasia.[40] Avoiding use of MgA in obese or inactive patients mitigates some of the risk of the development of diabetes mellitus.[41] The efficacy of this drug and the rareness of the side effects should not warrant it's complete elimination as a treatment strategy; however, newer, more efficacious therapies may not justify the risk of sideeffects.[12,15,40]

Parenteral Therapy

Triamcinolone acetonide is a potent glucocorticoid available as an injectable suspension with a wide variety of indications.[42] Subconjunctival injection has long been

Table 1			
Medical therapy for eosinophilic keratitis			
Route	**Drug**	**Dose and Route**	**Frequency**
Oral	Megesterol acetate	5 mg PO	q24 h × 7 days, then 2.5 mg q24 h × 7 days, then 2.5 mg EOD x 7 doses
Parenteral	Triamcinolone acetonide	0.1 to 0.2 mg/kg SQ	Can repeat 7 to 15 days after first injection
	Triamcinolone acetonide	1 to 4 mg subconjunctival injection	Can repeat 4 to 6 weeks
Topical	Prednisolone acetate 1% suspension	1 drop	q4 to 8 h
	Dexamethasone 0.1% solution	1 drop	q4 to 8 h
	Cyclosporine A 0.2% to 1.5% solution	1 drop	q8 to q12 h
	Tacrolimus 0.02% to 0.5% solution	1 drop	q8 to q12 h
	Megestrol acetate 0.5% solution	1 drop	q16 to q12 h

reported, with doses of up to 4 mg injected at one site.[6,38] Recently clinical reports have shown the utility of subcutaneous injection of triamcinolone for the management of EK.[15,17] Advantages parenteral administration of triamcinolone include obviating the need for daily administration of medication and excellent immunosuppression. Systemic side effects seem to be limited, and the development of diabetes mellitus has not been reported in cats treated with triamcinolone for EK.[43]

TOPICAL THERAPY
Corticosteroids

Topical corticosteroids have long been a cornerstone of achieving ocular immunosuppression. They are generally readily available and inexpensive. Dexamethasone sodium phosphate 0.1% and prednisolone acetate 1% are the two most commonly used topical corticosteroids in veterinary medicine. Newer, more potent corticosteroids are now available for clinical use; however, there are few studies in dogs and no studies in cats evaluating their safety and efficacy.[44–46] Successful administration of eye drops requires mobility and skill on the part of the administrator and compliance on the part of the owner and cat and therefore may not be achievable for all affected cats. Conversely, topically administered corticosteroids have few systemic effects in the cat and thus may be more desirable for those with comorbidities.[47]

Megestrol Acetate Ophthalmic Solution

Recently the use of a compounded, topical formulation of MgA 0.5% has been reported for the treatment of EK.[12] The advantage of a topical formulation over systemic administration of MgA is a decreased risk of systemic side-effects associated with MgA administration. Topical MgA is reported to be safe for use in ulcerated corneas, an advantage over corticosteroids that cannot safely be used in EK-affected cats with concurrent corneal ulceration.

Immunomodulators

The lacrimostimulant calcineurin inhibitors, cyclosporine A and tacrolimus, also act as immunomodulators through their role in inhibiting T-cell activation. Although they have poor intraocular penetration, they are efficacious in the treatment of ocular surface disease. They have been reported as monotherapy treatment of EK and as part of a combination therapy.[11,17] Response to topical cyclosporine A is reported to be slower than response to corticosteroids, but given the wide safety profile of this drug, it can be an excellent treatment option for affected cats where other modalities are not effective.[11]

CONTROVERSIES
Eosinophilic Keratoconjunctivitis and Feline Herpesvirus-1

The role of feline herpesvirus-1 (FHV-1) in the etiopathogenesis of EK remains uncertain. FHV-1 DNA was recovered using polymerase chain reaction (PCR) from 76% of cytologic or keratectomy samples in one study but only 33% of samples using immunofluorescence in another.[6,48] Another study describes recovering FHV-1 DNA using PCR in 85% of corneal or conjunctival cytology samples that contain eosinophils.[49] It has been suggested that EK is either a type I hypersensitivity reaction that is mediated by IgE, mast cell degranulation, and resultant tissue damage from the degranulation of eosinophils, or a type IV reaction mediated by T lymphocytes, the production of IL-5, and tissue damage from the recruitment and degranulation of eosinophils.[2] Although the use of antivirals as part of EK treatment has been widely reported, antivirals alone

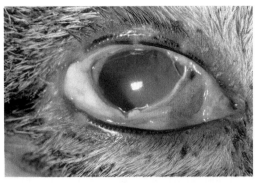

Fig. 11. Photograph of the right eye of a 9-year-old MC DSH with eosinophilic conjunctivitis. There is moderate blepharedema, severe conjunctival hyperemia, moderate-to-severe chemosis, elevation and thickening of the nictitans, with caseous white plaques visible on the conjunctival surfaces. The corneal surface appears dull. The pupil is mydriatic, the anterior chamber and iris appear normal.

are insufficient to induce regression of the disease.[6,10,15,17] It is possible that FHV-1 infection plays a role in initiating hypersensitivity responses, but further studies are necessary to test this hypothesis.

Related Syndromes

Eosinophilic conjunctivitis has been recognized as a unique clinical syndrome that is differentiated from EK by its lack of corneal involvement.[1] Affected cats have depigmentation and ulceration of the eyelid margins, conjunctival hyperemia, chemosis, ocular discharge, and blepharospasm (**Fig. 11**). Cytology of the conjunctiva is the diagnostic test of choice and shows a good correlation with histopathologic findings of conjunctival and eyelid biopsies. Treatment is similar to EK, with topical and systemic routes of immunosuppression indicated for the resolution of the disease.

CLINICS CARE POINTS

- Eosinophilic keratoconjunctivitis (EK) is an important differential diagnosis in all cases of pink/white masses or lesions of the feline cornea.
- Cytology of the affected cornea confirms the diagnosis of EK.
- Selection of treatment should consider any comorbidities, the patient's temperament, and the ability of the caretaker to administer treatment.
- EK can be chronic and recurrent and may require long-term therapy.
- Eosinophilic conjunctivitis is similar to EK but the cornea is unaffected. Treatment is similar.

REFERENCES

1. Allgoewer I, Schäffer EH, Stockhaus C, et al. Feline eosinophilic conjunctivitis. Vet Ophthalmol 2001;4(1):69–74.
2. Prasse KW. Cytology and histopathology of feline eosinophilic keratitis. Vet Comp Ophthalmol 1996;6:74–81.

3. Edwards S, Clode AB, Gilger BC. Equine eosinophilic keratitis in horses: 28 cases (2003-2013). Clin Case Rep 2015;3(12):1000–6.

4. Knickelbein KE, Luethy D, Thomasy SM, et al. Equine eosinophilic keratoconjunctivitis in California: retrospective study of 47 eyes from 29 cases (1993-2017). Vet Ophthalmol 2019;22(4):510–9.

5. Lassaline-Utter M, Miller C, Wotman KL. Eosinophilic keratitis in 46 eyes of 27 horses in the Mid-Atlantic United States (2008-2012). Vet Ophthalmol 2014; 17(5):311–20.

6. Morgan RV, Abrams KL, Kern TJ. Feline eosinophilic keratitis: a retrospective study of 54 cases: (1989–1994). Vet Comp Ophthalmol 1996;6(2):131–4.

7. Paulsen ME, Lavach JD, Severin GA, et al. Feline eosinophilic keratitis: a review of 15 clinical cases. J Am Anim Hosp Assoc 1987;23(1):63–9.

8. Dean E, Meunier V. Feline eosinophilic keratoconjunctivitis: a retrospective study of 45 cases (56 eyes). J Feline Med Surg 2013;15(8):661–6.

9. Bedford P. What is your diagnosis? Eosinophilic keratoconjunctivitis. J Small Anim Pract 1997;38(6):233–70.

10. Colitz CMH, Davidson MG, Gilger BC. Bilateral proliferative keratitis in a Domestic Long-haired cat. Vet Ophthalmol 2002;5(2):137–40.

11. Spiess AK, Sapienza JS, Mayordomo A. Treatment of proliferative feline eosinophilic keratitis with topical 1.5% cyclosporine: 35 cases. Vet Ophthalmol 2009; 12(2):132–7.

12. Stiles J, Coster M. Use of an ophthalmic formulation of megestrol acetate for the treatment of eosinophilic keratitis in cats. Vet Ophthalmol 2016;19(Suppl 1): 86–90.

13. O'Connell KE, Bruce CJ, Cazzini P. Pathology in Practice. Eosinophilic keratitis in a cat. J Am Vet Med Assoc 2017;251(2):165–7.

14. Villatoro AJ, Claros S, Fernández V, et al. Safety and efficacy of the mesenchymal stem cell in feline eosinophilic keratitis treatment. BMC Vet Res 2018;14(1):116.

15. Lucyshyn DR, Good KL, Knickelbein KE, et al. Subcutaneous administration of triamcinolone as part of the management of feline eosinophilic keratoconjunctivitis. J Feline Med Surg 2021;23(6):575–83.

16. Lucyshyn DR, Vernau W, Maggs DJ, et al. Correlations between clinical signs and corneal cytology in feline eosinophilic keratoconjunctivitis. Vet Ophthalmol 2021; 24(6):620–6.

17. Romaneck AK, Sebbag L. Case Report: Clinical remission in a cat with severe bilateral eosinophilic keratitis receiving combined immunosuppressive therapy (triamcinolone acetonide and tacrolimus). Front Vet Sci 2021;8:580396.

18. Collins BK, Swanson JF, MacWilliams PS. Eosinophilic keratitis and keratoconjunctivitis in a cat. Mod Vet Pract 1986;67(1):32–5.

19. Chisholm WH. Feline eosinophilic keratitis. Can Vet J Rev Veterinaire Can 1989; 30(5):438.

20. Gelatt KN. Visual disturbance: where do I look? J Small Anim Pract 1997;38(8): 328–35.

21. Moore PA. Feline corneal disease. Clin Tech Small Anim Pract 2005;20(2):83–93.

22. Manuali E, Forte C, Vichi G, et al. Tumours in European Shorthair cats: a retrospective study of 680 cases. J Feline Med Surg 2020;22(12):1095–102.

23. Murphy S. Cutaneous squamous cell carcinoma in the cat: current understanding and treatment approaches. J Feline Med Surg 2013;15(5):401–7.

24. Delgado EC. Topical chemotherapy with mitomycin C in a feline corneal squamous cell carcinoma. JFMS Open Rep 2020;6(1). 2055116920917833.

25. Sharkey LC, Radin MJ, Seelig D. Veterinary cytology. Wiley-Blackwell; 2021.

26. Diseases of the cornea and sclera. In: Dubielzig RR, Ketring KL, McLellan GJ, et al, editors. Veterinary ocular pathology: a comparative review. Saunders Elsevier; 2010. p. 213–6.

27. Labelle P. The eye. In: Pathologic basis of veterinary disease. 7th edition. Elsevier; 2022. p. 1431–2.

28. Diseases of the corena. In: Grahn B, Peiffer R, Wilcock B, editors. Histologic basis of ocular disease in animals. John Wiley & Sons, Ltd; 2019. p. 161.

29. Fettrelet T, Gigon L, Karaulov A, et al. The Enigma of Eosinophil Degranulation. Int J Mol Sci 2021;22(13):7091.

30. Tan C, Wandu WS, St Leger A, et al. Unlike Th1/Th17 cells, Th2/Th9 cells selectively migrate to the limbus/conjunctiva and initiate an eosinophilic infiltration process. Exp Eye Res 2018;166:116–9.

31. Nunomura S, Kitajima I, Nanri Y, et al. The FADS mouse: a novel mouse model of atopic keratoconjunctivitis. J Allergy Clin Immunol 2021;148(6):1596–602.e1.

32. Imai Y, Hosotani Y, Ishikawa H, et al. Expression of IL-33 in ocular surface epithelium induces atopic keratoconjunctivitis with activation of group 2 innate lymphoid cells in mice. Sci Rep 2017;7(1):10053.

33. Martin CL. Cornea and sclera in ophthalmic disease in veterinary medicine. Manson Publishing; 2005. p. 258–9.

34. Wu YT, Truong TN, Tam C, et al. Impact of topical corticosteroid pretreatment on susceptibility of the injured murine cornea to Pseudomonas aeruginosa colonization and infection. Exp Eye Res 2019;179:1–7.

35. Sharma B, Soni D, Mohan RR, et al. Corticosteroids in the Management of Infectious Keratitis: A Concise Review. J Ocul Pharmacol Ther Off J Assoc Ocul Pharmacol Ther 2021;37(8):452–63.

36. Romatowski J. Use of megestrol acetate in cats. J Am Vet Med Assoc 1989; 194(5):700–2.

37. Plumb DC. Megestrol. In: Plumb's Veterinary Drugs. Available at: https://app. plumbs.com/drug-monograph/qTK6MzMZTaPROD. Accessed March 12, 2022.

38. Brightman AH, Vestre WA, Helper LC. Chronic eosinophilic keratitis in the cat. Feline Pr 1979;9(3):21–3.

39. Martin CL. Feline ophthalmologic diseases. Mod Vet Pract 1982;63(2):115–22.

40. Romagnoli S. Progestins to control feline reproduction: Historical abuse of high doses and potentially safe use of low doses. J Feline Med Surg 2015;17(9): 743–52.

41. McCann TM, Simpson KE, Shaw DJ, et al. Feline diabetes mellitus in the UK: the prevalence within an insured cat population and a questionnaire-based putative risk factor analysis. J Feline Med Surg 2007;9(4):289–99.

42. Plumb DC. Triamcinolone. In: Plumb's Veterinary Drugs. https://app.plumbs.com/ drug-monograph/bxThYXphcjPROD. Accessed March 12, 2022.

43. Schaer M, Ginn PE. Iatrogenic Cushing's syndrome and steroid hepatopathy in a cat. J Am Anim Hosp Assoc 1999;35(1):48–51.

44. Allbaugh RA, Wehrman RF, Sebbag L. Comparison of topically administered 0.05% difluprednate and 1% prednisolone acetate for inhibition of aqueocentesis-induced breakdown of the blood-aqueous barrier in healthy dogs. Am J Vet Res 2020;81(3):260–6.

45. Quantz K, Anderson AL, Harman CD, et al. Localized alopecia and suppression of hypothalamic-pituitary-adrenal (HPA) axis in dogs following treatment with difluprednate 0.05% ophthalmic emulsion (Durezol®). BMC Vet Res 2021; 17(1):366.

46. OD BJS OD, Heather Whyte DeMarco. Steroid Wars: New Drugs Challenge Old Habits. Available at: https://www.reviewofoptometry.com/article/steroid-wars-new-drugs-challenge-old-habits. Accessed March 12, 2022.
47. Gosling AA, Kiland JA, Rutkowski LE, et al. Effects of topical corticosteroid administration on intraocular pressure in normal and glaucomatous cats. Vet Ophthalmol 2016;19(Suppl 1):69–76.
48. Nasisse MP, Glover TL, Moore CP, et al. Detection of feline herpesvirus 1 DNA in corneas of cats with eosinophilic keratitis or corneal sequestration. Am J Vet Res 1998;59(7):856–8.
49. Volopich S, Benetka V, Schwendenwein I, et al. Cytologic findings, and feline herpesvirus DNA and Chlamydophila felis antigen detection rates in normal cats and cats with conjunctival and corneal lesions. Vet Ophthalmol 2005;8(1): 25–32.

Feline Glaucoma

Bruce Grahn, DVM

KEYWORDS

- Feline • Glaucoma • Irido-corneal angle • Anterior segment dysgenesis • Uveitis
- Primary and metastatic intraocular neoplasia
- Feline aqueous misdirection glaucoma
- Feline secondary, congenital and primary glaucoma

KEY POINTS

- The clinical signs of feline glaucoma are subtle so always complete tonometry during ocular examinations on cats.
- All glaucomatous cats can be categorized as congenital/early onset and associated with anterior segment dysgenesis, or primary (idiopathic), or secondary based on a thorough ophthalmologic examination.
- Therapeutic decisions are best guided by the category of glaucoma and if it is acute or chronic, and if there is potential for vision.
- Feline glaucoma is challenging to treat and maintain vision long term so referral to an ophthalmologist should be prompt once the intraocular pressures are within a normal range or if that is not achieved quickly.
- End-stage, blind, glaucomatous feline eyes should be enucleated, fixed, and histologically examined by a pathologist with experience in ocular diseases to ensure that the correct category of glaucoma was diagnosed and the contralateral globe treated or monitored as required.

INTRODUCTION

To diagnose and treat glaucoma accurately in cats and generally in all species, three fundamental concepts need to be understood by all veterinarians (**Table 1**). *First*, glaucoma is not a single disease in any animal, rather there are multiple variations unique to each species and often the breed of animal affected, yet all are characterized by an elevated intraocular pressure (IOP). If the IOPs remain elevated, initially the inner retinal layers (nerve fiber, ganglion cell, inner plexiform, and inner nuclear) and the optic nerve axons will degenerate and atrophy. With chronic glaucoma, all intraocular tissues will be damaged and buphthalmos and blindness will develop in the cat.[1–3]

The author has nothing to disclose.
Western College of Veterinary Medicine, Prairie Ocular Pathology Service, Prairie Diagnostic Laboratory, University of Saskatchewan, 52 Campus Drive, Saskatoon, Saskatchewan S7N 5B4, Canada
E-mail address: bruce.grahn@usask.ca

Vet Clin Small Anim 53 (2023) 367–387
https://doi.org/10.1016/j.cvsm.2022.10.002

Table 1
Categorizing feline glaucoma

Acquired: Secondary Glaucoma	Congenital/Anterior Segment Dysgenesis Associated Glaucoma	Idiopathic/ Primary Glaucoma
Endophthalmitis due to chronic anterior uveitis and idiopathic endophthalmitis	Idiopathic anterior segment dysgenesis associated	Burmese narrow-angle glaucoma
Intraocular neoplasia Primary neoplasms include diffuse iris melanoma (most common), occasionally documented secondary to ciliary adenoma/ adenocarcinoma, post-traumatic sarcoma. Metastatic neoplasia where lymphosarcoma is by far the most common, but also secondary to occasional metastatic carcinomas and spindle cell neoplasms.	Anterior segment dysgenesis inherited as the LBT2 mutation	Idiopathic open-angle glaucoma in mixed breeds and others
Feline aqueous misdirection glaucoma		
Lens disorders (cataract lens luxation, phacoclastic uveitis)		
Orbital neoplasia and secondary glaucoma.		

Glaucoma in all species is one of the most difficult blinding conditions to treat effectively. *Second*, the diagnosis of glaucoma is based on the determination of elevated IOPs. There are two distinct conditions, ocular hypertension, and glaucoma that require differentiation. To differentiate these the IOPs need to be measured frequently and trends monitored carefully in response to treatment or lack thereof. When considering ocular hypertension and glaucoma, the veterinarian must also understand circadian rhythms (discussed later) and their daily effects on IOP. Hypertension is typically a mild elevation of, or pressures simply in the upper limit of normal (25–30 mm Hg) and there is no concurrent glaucomatous retinal and optic nerve atrophy. Ocular hypertension is often transient with or without anti-glaucoma therapy, and it is commonly diagnosed after intraocular surgery. Ocular hypertension may spontaneously recrudesce or it may progress to overt glaucoma, which is persistent and usually requires lifelong therapy to control. *Thirdly*, tonometry (the estimation of IOP), must be mastered by repeated use in all ocular examinations in animals, not just those that look like glaucoma. This allows the veterinarian to gain confidence to accurately estimate the IOP on all globes and thereby accurately diagnose hypertension, and glaucoma when they are present. To master tonometry practice is essential to develop dexterity, as well as tonometer and periocular finger placement that allows for consistent and accurate estimates of IOP. This should be easy to achieve as tonometry is required in all ocular examinations completed by veterinarians and it should be included in geriatric health and wellness examinations in cats.[4] Sadly, although stressed to veterinary students and veterinarians, tonometry is often missed during ocular examinations of cats today. This often leads to misdiagnoses and progressive glaucoma and delays in treatment and referral to the ophthalmologist. Many tonometer's effectively estimate IOP in cats. These include indentation tonometer's,[5,6] applanation tonometer's,[7,8] and rebound tonometer's.[9] There are inherent strengths and weaknesses to each type of tonometer and most ophthalmologists prefer the rebound tonometer today. However, repeated usage with most types of tonometers will give the veterinarian confidence and accuracy in their diagnosis of glaucoma.

Once those three fundamentals are understood, a review of some general clinical observations on glaucoma for all species will aid the veterinarian and the ophthalmology resident in the diagnosis, treatment, and management of all types of glaucoma. These include; glaucoma may manifest unilaterally, however it commonly affects both eyes at varied time intervals. Often the first eye affected is visually impaired or blind when the elevated IOP are initially first detected. Only a complete neuro-ophthalmic examination will detect these unilateral blind eyes. Glaucoma is always a disorder that arises from a lack of aqueous humor filtration from the globe, not an overproduction of this fluid. The lack of aqueous humor exit may be difficult to establish (for example primary glaucoma) or it may be detectable on ophthalmoscopic examination such as noted in secondary glaucoma cases (feline aqueous misdirection glaucoma or pupillary block and iris bombe, filtration angle obliteration, etc.). Therapeutic management of glaucoma is diverse and often includes initially topical medications followed by multiple medications and finally some form of surgery. However, the order of these is not necessarily pragmatic rather they are simply what we have become engrained to believe as appropriate. The transition from topical medications, to laser therapy and intraocular surgery, seems logical to most based on doing the least invasive therapy first, when in fact, it may not be so at all and future controlled studies are needed to evaluate the therapeutic approach to this blinding disease. Because glaucoma is usually progressive and challenging to treat and may affect both eyes eventually, referral and/or consultation with a veterinary ophthalmologist is essential. Blind glaucomatous globes that are non-responsive to medications and surgical therapies should be enucleated or eviscerated as there is no doubt that sustained elevations of IOP in any species are painful and analogous to a head ache described in humans with chronic uncontrolled glaucoma. Finally, all enucleated globes should be fixed promptly, examined grossly, and then histologically by a laboratory that does significant ocular pathology to warrant expertise to confirm the etiologic diagnosis in all animals. This is especially important in cats given their high numbers of secondary glaucoma that develops because of inflammatory and neoplastic conditions. Unfortunately, many of us still observe chronic glaucomatous eyes that are ignored by owners as they are deemed not painful, and then when they are enucleated the globes are not submitted for histologic examination.

This article provides the reader with a review: of the production and filtration of aqueous humor in cats, three categories of feline glaucoma, and a summary of clinical, gross, and histologic differentiation and treatment of these types of feline glaucoma.

THE PHYSIOLOGY OF AQUEOUS HUMOR PRODUCTION AND FILTRATION IN CATS

The production of aqueous humor in cats involves both active secretion and passive mechanisms (ultrafiltration, diffusion). However, the latter is not a significant contributor as very limited amounts of fluid diffuse from the ciliary body across the pigmented and non-pigmented ciliary epithelium related to its tight junctions. Only small amounts of aqueous humor will seep from within the ciliary body and drain forth through the iris, which lacks an epithelium on its anterior surface.[10]

Active production is the mainstay of aqueous humor production in all species of animals and accounts for approximately 90% of its production.[11] This occurs by secretion of NaCl into the posterior chamber, which creates an osmotic gradient that allows water to follow. This is an energy-driven cellular mechanism, provided by adenine triphosphate (ATP) and this process requires carbonic anhydrase and triphosphatase to activate the NaK pumps, which are located in the ciliary epithelium.[12] This production of aqueous humor occurs within the non-pigmented ciliary epithelium and is only affected slightly (adversely) by increasing IOPs (i.e. hypertension or glaucoma). Aqueous humor is produced in cats at a relatively constant rate of 6 to 7 µl/min.[13] Therefore, the exit of fluid is the determinant of IOPs and all cases of glaucoma are the result of alterations of movement of aqueous humor within the anterior segment or alteration of the exit of aqueous humor through the filtration angle and ciliary cleft and across the endothelium of the aqueous collecting and the choroidal veins.

There is a circadian rhythm to aqueous production which also induces a similar rhythm to daily IOPs in cats and in contrast to the dog where production of aqueous is highest in the early morning, cats aqueous production and therefore IOPs are highest in the evening and early nighttime.[14] There are probably many other factors that affect the IOP of cats including but not limited to reproductive status where queens in estrus had significantly higher IOPs compared with normal cats.[15,16]

Aqueous humor flows through the posterior chamber and pupil and circulates within the anterior chamber as it cools on the cornea it gravitates towards the ventral region and enters the filtration angle in the normal cat eye. The aqueous nourishes the lens and corneal endothelium. As the aqueous humor leaves the filtration angle, it will exit the globe through either the conventional outflow through the ciliary cleft and then across the endothelium of the aqueous collecting veins. A small amount of aqueous will leave via the non-conventional way into the choroid and out of the globe via the ciliary veins.[11,17]

The predominant (97%) exit of aqueous humor in cats is via the conventional outflow. Aqueous humor gains access to the vascular circulation by crossing the aqueous collecting vein endothelium by at least four cellular mechanisms (micro-pinocytosis, giant vacuoles, transcellular pores, and phagocytosis).[11] The scleral venous pressure of normal cats is approximately 8-12 mm Hg and the aqueous outflow C values in the cat are 0.27 -0.32 ul/min.[13] The non-conventional outflow of aqueous humor from the feline globe represents a very small portion (3%) of the total aqueous exit so we will not review it further.

CATEGORIES OF FELINE GLAUCOMA

Feline glaucoma has been categorized many different ways. It is interesting to note that non-domestic captive feline species have a very low incidence of glaucoma, and the limited cases reported document that ocular trauma and uveitis were integral in the pathogenesis in most wild feline species.[18] This is markedly different from our domestic feline breeds and hints that genetic and environmental factors may be involved in the development of glaucoma in domestic cats. Similar to the canine and equine species it is most appropriate to consider feline glaucoma as acquired, or developmental, or idiopathic. Given those parameters, feline glaucoma is most appropriately categorized as 1. Secondary glaucoma: acquired secondary to endophthalmitis or neoplasia or occasionally other primary or secondary ocular diseases. This category accounts for over 90% of all cases of feline glaucoma. Affected cats may have unilateral or bilateral glaucoma and most commonly they are middle-aged to older felids. 2. *Congenital/ASD-associated glaucoma*: this form of feline glaucoma is either present at birth or develops early in life and is usually associated with ASD, which is a congenital disorder. This may develop unilaterally or bilaterally in young cats usually less than 3 years old. 3. *Primary/idiopathic*: these forms appear to be the least common types in cats. This type of glaucoma will often manifest bilaterally or become bilateral over time in middle-aged to older cats.

CLINICAL DIAGNOSIS OF IDIOPATHIC UVEITIS AND INTRAOCULAR NEOPLASIA THAT INDUCE SECONDARY GLAUCOMA OF CATS

The most important diagnostic procedure to confirm glaucoma in the cat is a thorough ophthalmologic examination of the entire eye and documentation of an elevated IOP and/or buphthalmos in the affected eye(s).[19–22] As mentioned previously, several tonometer's accurately estimate the IOP in cats. When the IOP exceeds 30 mm Hg in cats, glaucoma is confirmed. It is critical to finish the complete ocular examination, before beginning the process of categorizing glaucoma and instituting therapy. Establishing the type of feline glaucoma will be based on all of the examination findings and consideration of the age and breed of the cat. Given that, greater than 90% of feline glaucoma is secondary to uveitis or intraocular neoplasia it is prudent to examine the cornea, iris, pupil and the filtration angle and anterior and posterior chambers and vitreous and retina and choroid, for evidence of either tumors or synechiae, and inflammatory debris. The clinical signs of uveitis and hyalitis in cats with secondary glaucoma are often quite subtle. They include mild corneal edema and vascularized keratitis, miosis or mydriasis, grey discoloration of the iris, lymphocytic nodular iritis, pre-iridal vascular membranes (rubious iridis), subcapsular cataracts, cyclitis, opaque vitreous and occasionally chorioretinitis (**Figs. 1** and **2**). Although a plethora of infectious organisms can induce uveitis/hyalitis, in most cases despite rigorous

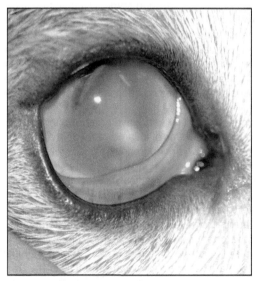

Fig. 1. These are the typical clinical manifestations of secondary glaucoma and idiopathic uveitis in the right eye of a domestic shorthaired cat. Note the anterior chamber fibrin, the miosis, grey–yellow (muddy) colored iris, and the elevated and congested third eyelid. The intraocular pressure was 40 mm Hg.

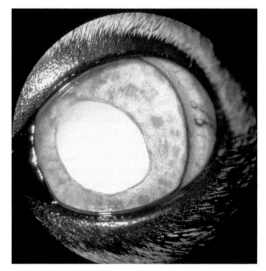

Fig. 2. This photograph reveals the much more subtle manifestations of secondary glaucoma associated with anterior iriditis, cyclitis, and hyalitis. Note the grey nodules within the iris, the congested episcleral blood vessels, and the prolapsed degenerate vitreous draped over the superior pupillary margin. The eye was blind and the intraocular pressure markedly elevated.

diagnostics, many of these cases remain idiopathic. It is assumed, that the evidence for the causative organism or injury has long dissipated or healed and what remains is a self-perpetuating immune-mediated anterior uveitis and hyalitis. It is important to remember that Felv, FIV, FIP viruses, and some systemic fungal disorders may cause unilateral or bilateral uveitis and appropriate serum tests or skin biopsies or IHC of enucleated globes should be considered to accurately diagnose these.

The filtration angle can usually be visualized by direct examination in the cat, with a focused light source such as a trans illuminator. Often the angle is open (**Fig. 3**), unless it is covered by iridal tissues that are swollen by inflammation or neoplasia. Similarly, the ciliary cleft is usually open unless diffuse inflammatory and neoplastic cells have obliterated it.

Based on our experience, many cats have anterior uveitis and have hyalitis and a few have panuveitis with collections of inflammatory debris within the folds of pars plicata and within the vitreous, and chorioretinitis. This is important as hyalitis and choroiditis dictate the consideration of systemic anti-inflammatory therapy often in conjunction with topical therapy. Hyalitis and indeed choroiditis are quite easy to overlook with miosis, fibrin clots within the anterior chamber, and lenticular opacities (see **Fig. 1**). It is important to remember that secondary glaucoma due to uveitis and hyalitis in cats can be unilateral, however, many cases are bilateral, and to complicate this further, the glaucoma often develops at different times in each inflamed eye.[23,24] Many veterinarians either forego or forget to use topical mydriatics (tropicamide), perhaps because they are reported to elevate the IOP in the treated and untreated eyes of normal cats within 90 min of application[25,26] or they simply forget to complete the posterior segment examination. We recommend pupillary dilatation of both eyes when the posterior segment cannot be examined adequately without mydriasis, to rule out posterior segment disease. It is prudent to measure the IOPs post-

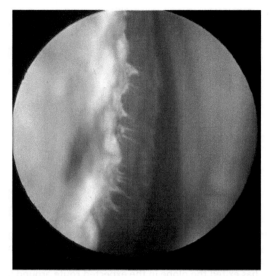

Fig. 3. This is a photograph of the filtration angle of a cat with a single brown iris patch. The filtration angle of cats is visible with a light source and direct examination with or with an ophthalmoscope or biomicroscope. Note the thin yellow pectinate fibers that span the filtration angle and the ciliary cleft behind.

dilatation. If significant increases are present then appropriate therapy is instituted promptly. It is also very important to assess vision in both eyes, and establish a likely category for glaucoma (secondary, congenital, or primary) first before selecting a therapy with anti-glaucoma medications. Finally, all cases of feline glaucoma will benefit from referral to or consultation with an ophthalmologist for appropriate additional diagnostic examinations (optical coherence tomography (OCT), ocular ultrasound, etc.) and specialized treatment options.

Some controversy exists in the literature as to whether neoplasia or uveitis is the most frequent cause of secondary feline glaucoma. Large pathology databases have described larger percentages of glaucoma secondary to neoplasia. However, veterinarians more commonly submit apparent neoplastic disorders to the pathologist. This may account for a bias. In our histologic database, the most common form of secondary glaucoma in cats is chronic idiopathic uveitis followed by intraocular neoplasia. Perhaps this is result of the enucleation of globes with an intraocular neoplasm before glaucoma develops. Suffice to say, uveitis and intraocular neoplasia account for over 90% of all feline glaucoma submissions.

It is always prudent to consider a diffuse neoplastic invasion of uveal tissues, as it induces a secondary inflammation (uveitis). As a result, feline ocular neoplasms commonly masquerade with clinical manifestations of uveitis. These neoplasms may be primary or metastatic to the eye. Diffuse iridal melanoma and ciliary adenomas and adenocarcinomas, medulloepitheliomas, and post-traumatic sarcomas are the five *primary* intraocular neoplasms reported to induce glaucoma, and the melanoma is by far the most common. Diffuse iridal melanoma is diagnosed by confirmation of progressive iridal pigmentation usually by sequential anterior segment photographs **(Fig. 4)**. Glaucoma develops later when the melanoma compromises the filtration angle and ciliary cleft (see **Fig. 4**). Primary ciliary neoplasms (adenomas, adenocarcinomas, and medulloepitheliomas) and post-traumatic sarcomas although less

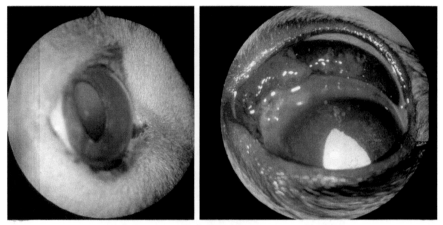

Fig. 4. Cats with chronic diffuse iris melanoma that has been progressing for years will manifest with secondary glaucoma frequently. Both of these cat eyes were blind due to chronic glaucoma and diffuse iris melanoma has effaced the anterior uvea and the filtration angle and ciliary cleft and has exited the globe in the expected route around the aqueous collecting veins and into the episcleral tissues under the bulbar conjunctiva.

common, can induce glaucoma in cats secondary to the invasion of the filtration angle and more importantly their induction of pre-iridal vascular and neoplastic membranes which cover the angle, or obstruct the flow of aqueous humor through the pupil or angle and thereby reduce aqueous humor outflow. *Metastatic* neoplasms (lymphosarcoma, carcinomas, and spindle cell neoplasms) have all been reported to induce secondary glaucoma. Lymphosarcoma is the most common cause of glaucoma secondary to metastatic neoplasia in cats. Lymphosarcoma is not readily seen during the ophthalmologic examination, as it is a diffuse uveal infiltrate. It typically invades the anterior uvea and induces uveitis and masquerades as an inflammatory disorder. The neoplasia is only confirmed when the enucleated globe is examined histologically. Diagnostic imaging including ocular OCT or US and CT may support a presumptive diagnosis of primary or metastatic intraocular neoplasia.

GROSS PATHOLOGY AND HISTOLOGIC CONFIRMATION OF SECONDARY GLAUCOMA OF CATS WITH UVEITIS AND NEOPLASIA

Examination of gross and histologic sections of feline globes will confirm the diagnosis of secondary glaucoma (**Figs. 5–9**) and rule out the important differentials of ASD-associated, primary lens luxation-associated, aqueous misdirection and primary glaucoma of cats. Given that all categories of glaucoma can develop bilaterally in cats, histologic examination of enucleated globes should be completed to confirm the type of glaucoma and help to determine the risk of developing the contralateral ocular disease. Fixation post-enucleation should be prompt, and the best ocular fixative is Davidson's solution. When using formalin, the most commonly used fixative in general practice, a ½ −1 cc injection of formalin just superior to the optic nerve through a 25-gauge needle into the vitreous greatly enhances the fixation.[27]

Gross sections will reveal the characteristic plasmoid aqueous, vitreous, and swollen uvea (see **Figs. 5** and **6**).[27] Gross examination of globes with intraocular neoplasia and secondary glaucoma will often reveal variable uvea thickness and tumors, discoloration, and a thin retina and cupped optic nerve.

Histologic examination of the retina confirms the diagnosis of glaucoma by revealing a loss of inner retinal layers including the ganglion cell, nerve fiber, inner plexiform, and inner nuclear layers[22,27,28] (see **Fig. 7**). Often, superior (tapetal) retinal tissues are less affected and this is termed tapetal or dorsal sparing. Generally, the histologic manifestations of glaucomatous retinal and optic nerve atrophy in cats are much more subtle than changes noted in dogs. The optic nerve cupping although challenging in the clinical examination room is readily detectable on images taken with optical coherence tomography or gross examination, subgross, and histologic examinations (see **Fig. 8**A–C). The most consistent histologic feature of glaucoma secondary to uveitis in cats is an anterior lymphocytic and plasmacytic anterior uveitis (see **Fig. 9**A, B)[22,27,28] and rarely an eosinophilic uveitis.[29] The lymphocytic uveitis may be diffuse or nodular and the anterior uvea and the ciliary cleft are predominantly affected (see **Fig. 9**A, B). Pre-iridal fibrovascular membranes, which are very common in the dog, are seen sometimes in the horse, and are only occasionally incremented histologically as a part of the pathogenesis of feline glaucoma when they span the filtration angle.[30] These membranes are easy to overlook in the cat with uveitis compared with those seen histologically in the dog. That is usually the result of their small stature and the covering of the iridal leaflets by inflammatory cells and debris and are therefore likely more common than suspected.

Diffuse neoplastic uveal infiltration is readily apparent histologically when it is responsible for feline secondary glaucoma (see **Fig. 9**). The pathogenesis of glaucoma secondary to primary or metastatic intraocular neoplasia usually involves obstruction of the filtration angle and ciliary cleft with neoplastic tissues and inflammatory debris.

TREATMENT OPTIONS FOR FELINE GLAUCOMA THAT IS SECONDARY TO UVEITIS OR INTRAOCULAR NEOPLASIA

Uveitis and hyalitis in cats is treated by topical and systemic immune suppression most commonly. Topical 1% prednisolone acetate or 0.1% dexamethasone given QID will suppress anterior uveitis and some cyclitis and prednisone 1-2 mg/kg of body weight will suppress hyalitis and choroiditis when they are present. If the IOP is higher than 50 mm Hg and the affected eye has the potential for vision, then

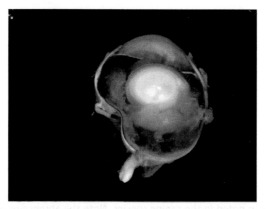

Fig. 5. This photograph reveals the gross pathology of uveitis and secondary glaucoma in a formalin fixed feline globe. Note the inflammatory debris in the anterior and posterior chamber, plasmoid vitreous with inflammatory debris coating the ciliary body and the optic nerve atrophy with degenerate vitreous extending into the atrophic optic nerve beyond the sclera.

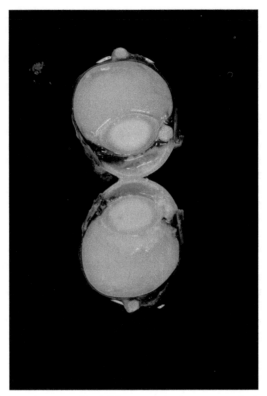

Fig. 6. This semi-bisected Buoin's fixed feline reveals the gross pathologic changes associated with endophthalmitis. Histologic examination confirmed endophthalmitis, secondary glaucoma and cat claw scleral perforation with a ciliary abscess.

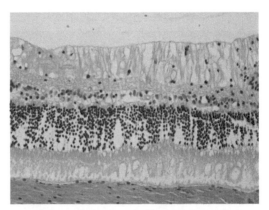

Fig. 7. Histologic manifestations of the retinal effects of chronic feline glaucoma are generally more subtle than noted in the canine species. Note the absence of ganglion cells, glial cell proliferation within the space left by the atrophic nerve fiber layer, which also exposes the linier Mueller fibers that connect to the inner limiting membrane of the retina, and the atrophy of the inner plexiform and inner nuclear layers. These inner retinal changes confirms chronic feline glaucoma.

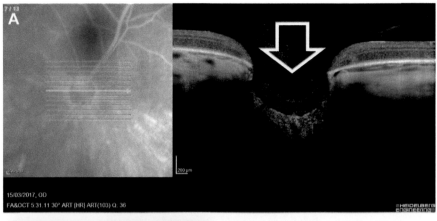

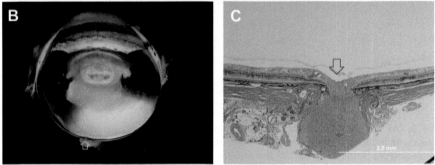

Fig. 8. (*A*). Optical coherence tomography (OCT) readily confirms optic nerve atrophy in cats. In contrast to the dog where optic nerve cupping is readily discernable on ophthalmoscopic examination, feline optic nerve atrophy is challenging to see with an ophthalmoscope due to the small size of the papilla and lack of myelin. The use of OCT has greatly enhanced the ophthalmologist's ability to evaluate and prognosticate glaucomatous retinal and optic nerve damage in cats. (*B*) Optic nerve cupping (atrophy) is readily discernable on gross sections of feline globes with chronic glaucoma. Note the prominent nodules within the iridal leaflet, which are lymphoid follicles. (*C*) Optic papillary atrophy is less dramatic in cats with chronic glaucoma than dogs but discernable.

intravenous mannitol may be administered at a dose of 1-3 gm/kg body weight in addition to appropriate topical glaucoma medications. Most secondary glaucoma due to uveitis or neoplasia will have moderate IOPs in the 30 to 40 mm Hg range. These cases are treated initially with carbonic anhydrase inhibitors (Dorzolamide 2%) at a q 8 or q 12 h. This in combination with appropriate anti-inflammatory therapy will usually reduce the IOPs to a normal range until an enucleation can be completed.[31] Topical ophthalmic carbonic anhydrase inhibitors although quite effective at lowering the IOP in cats with secondary glaucoma will necessitate systemic monitoring of K levels. Dorzolamide is reported to induce hypokalemia in cats.[32]

Combinations of Dorzolamide 2% and timolol (0.05%) will lower the IOP better than just Dorzolamide alone.[33,34] Aproclonidine although effective at reducing IOP in normal cats has significant systemic side effects that preclude it administration in this species.[35] Topical application of prostaglandins for feline glaucoma remains controversial. Topical prostaglandins are reported to reduce the IOP in normal cats significantly.[36] However, other studies report limited to no effect of bimatoprost

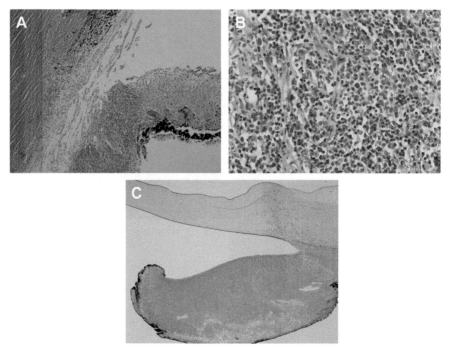

Fig. 9. (A). Lymphocytic plasmacytic anterior uveitis is commonly associated with secondary glaucoma in cats. A diffuse round cell population infiltrates the iris and filtration angle. (B) High-power photomicrograph of the anterior uvea of the cat in Fig. 10A, confirming the diffuse population of lymphocytes and occasional plasma cells. (C) Feline lymphosarcoma will induce secondary glaucoma in cats. It characteristically effaces the anterior uvea as noted in this PAS stained photomicrograph.

or Latanaprost, or unoprostone isopropyl in normal cats.[37,38] Anecdotal reports at least some short-term IOP lowering with prostaglandins including travaprost in the treatment of glaucoma in cats but peer-reviewed publications documenting responses in glaucomatous cats are lacking at this time. Uveitis and secondary glaucoma requires long-term management with frequent monitoring of IOPs and re-examination of the uvea and vitreous to ensure that endophthalmitis is controlled. When monitoring the IOPs long-term to ensure a therapeutic response, it is important to complete tonometry whenever possible at approximately the same time of the day. The normal circadian rhythm of aqueous humor production and IOP curves in cats will vary individual readings. The highest IOPs are usually recorded in the early evening.[14]

Once the inflammation is controlled, the oral and topical immune suppressive medications are reduced gradually over many months. The topical carbonic anhydrase inhibitors are maintained at a frequency that maintains an IOP of 13 to 20 mm Hg. Recrudescence of inflammation and secondary glaucoma are common in these cats. Adjusting the frequency of topical glaucoma medications and systemic therapy is warranted to maintain control of the inflammation and IOPs as long as the affected eye remains visual. Some cats with glaucoma will develop increased IOP when topical dexamethasone or prednisone are initiated, so monitoring the IOP within in a few days of onset of corticosteroids is important.[39]

The optic nerve is small in the cat and evaluation of the loss of axons is challenging even with direct ophthalmoscopy. However, the advent of OCT (see **Fig. 8**A) has greatly facilitated the staging the severity of feline glaucoma. OCT allows for accurate measurements of the inner retinal layers and the axons as they exit the optic nerve. Although this diagnostic tool requires general anesthesia it should be considered in all cats with glaucoma to ensure that therapies are effective by ruling out progressive loss of nerve fiber and ganglion cell layers over time.

Laser cytophotocoagulation with an ND: Yag or diode laser,[40,41] may be completed to reduce IOP in glaucomatous cat eyes. Complications include corneal ulceration, hyphema, post-treatment ocular hypertension, retinal detachments, and recrudescence of glaucoma and long-term IOP control is challenging. The combination of laser therapy and gonioimplants are also a feasible therapy in cats. Park and colleagues[42] reported an Ahmed implant that maintained normal IOP in a Russian Blue cat with primary glaucoma for 7 months. However, there are no published reports of implants in glaucomatous feline eyes due to uveitis. One may hypothesize that anterior chamber shunts would obstruct inflammatory debris when placed in the anterior chamber of these cats.

Once the affected eye is blind and glaucoma is present despite treatment, the most appropriate therapy is trans conjunctival or more often a trans palpebral enucleation or exenteration. The latter is used when the potential of neoplastic extension out the globe is suspected. Evisceration and intrascleral prostheses is an alternative provided when the ophthalmologist is convinced that intraocular neoplasia is not present. However, metastatic intraocular neoplasia should always be considered in cats with uveitis and secondary glaucoma so the most common therapy is enucleation. The most common metastatic neoplasm to the cat's eye (lymphosarcoma) is a frequent cause of secondary glaucoma in cats.[43] It is important to refer focal anterior uveal tumors to ophthalmologists early as small to medium-sized primary anterior uveal neoplasms can be surgically removed or laser ablated long before they would ever induce secondary glaucoma. These forms of therapy are generally widely available today, and the success rate for retention of a sighted eye without secondary glaucoma is excellent. However, uveal neoplasms that are diffuse or too large or too inflamed at presentation to justify vision-sparing surgeries, surgical enucleation remains the treatment of choice.

FELINE AQUEOUS MISDIRECTION GLAUCOMA

Aqueous misdirection glaucoma is a unique disorder in the cat where aqueous becomes misdirected into the vitreous. Misdirected aqueous humor expands the vitreous and displaces the lens and iris leaflets forward and collapses the anterior and posterior chambers, markedly narrows the filtration angle, and collapses the ciliary cleft.[44,45] This tends to be a disease of older cats (12.9 years) and most cats (5/7) are affected bilaterally.[44] The clinical diagnosis is straightforward based on an ophthalmoscopic or biomicroscopic appearance of a small or absent anterior chamber with a lens and iris displacement onto or near to the corneal endothelium (**Fig. 10**A–C). The IOPs are usually variable but often high (40 to 80 mm Hg), compared with secondary glaucoma and ASD-associated glaucoma of cats. Gross examination of sectioned feline globes with aqueous misdirection will reveal very shallow anterior chambers and collapse of the posterior chambers with the lens displaced forward and the vitreous cavity enlarged (see **Fig. 10**B). The pathogenesis is unknown. Condensation of the anterior vitreous face will usually be noted on histologic examination. The histologic confirmation of glaucoma is atrophy of the inner retinal layers and atrophy of the optic nerve.

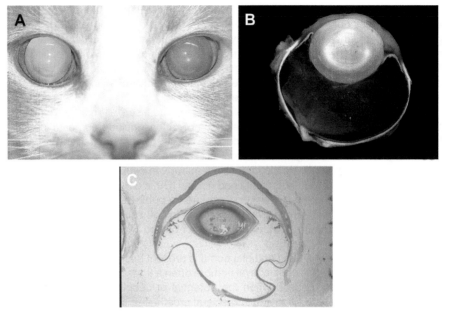

Fig. 10. (A) This cat has bilateral aqueous misdirection and both lens are being displaced forward along with the both irides. The anterior chambers were both shallow and the intraocular pressures were markedly elevated. (B) Gross sections of eyes with aqueous misdirection glaucoma will have characteristic signs including displacement of the lens and iris into the anterior chamber and condensed vitreous on the posterior lens capsule. (C) The filtration angle and ciliary cleft of the feline globe with aqueous misdirection glaucoma, may appear open and normal as this histologic section is or they may be closed and collapsed related to the forward displacement of the lens and iris leaflets. They do not however have significant anterior uveitis or endophthalmitis.

Initial medical management with topical Dorzolamide 2% ophthalmic solution is usually not successful; however, prostaglandin analogs may lower the IOP. If those fail a vitrectomy and phacoemulsification of the lens with or without lens implantation is reported as successful.[44] Reported case numbers are low as expected with such a rare condition. Most will attempt medical management before surgical therapies and the small numbers of cases have precluded long-term follow-up studies with a comparison of medical to surgical therapy.

INCIDENTAL SYSTEMIC AND PERIOCULAR CAUSES OF GLAUCOMA IN CATS

Diffuse infiltrative orbital neoplasia will occasionally induce secondary glaucoma in cats by obstructing aqueous humor drainage. Exophthalmos and high IOPs are the most common clinical signs. Sectional imaging and biopsy or exenteration, and histologic examination of exenterated globes confirm orbital neoplasia diagnosis. Lymphosarcoma is the most common metastatic neoplasm to cause this and systemic chemotherapy may be effective at reducing the tumor and allowing for effective aqueous humor movement through aqueous collecting veins with improved orbital venous drainage. Topical anti-glaucoma therapy during the clinical workup usually includes BID to TID Dorzolamide to decrease aqueous humor production and this is the initial treatment of choice. The prognosis for orbital neoplasia in cats is poor even with appropriate therapies and early diagnosis.

LENS LUXATION, CATARACTS, AND THEIR RELATIONSHIP TO SECONDARY GLAUCOMA IN CATS

Immature, mature, and hypermature cataracts do induce mild phacolytic uveitis in cats occasionally, and zonular and vitreous degeneration may develop secondary to this inflammation. This may result in a lens subluxation or luxation, which may lead to secondary glaucoma. However, this is much less frequent in the cat compared with the dog.

Primary zonular dysplasia, lens subluxation, and luxation are reported in the cat. This is a rare condition based on limited peer-reviewed reports.[46] The diagnosis is confirmed with histochemical stains (PAS, Masson's trichrome, and elastin) that allow zonular dysplasia to be documented on enucleated globes. However, unlike the dog it is not associated with ADAMTs 17 gene mutation.[46] Closely related feline who were gene mapped revealed that the FBN1 may be a candidate gene. Glaucoma secondary to the primary lens luxation was confirmed in only one of these affected cats.[46]

Most lens luxations in cats develop secondary to chronic glaucoma and buphthalmos, therefore a consequence of, not the initiating factor. Rarely, trauma will induce secondary lens luxation and vitreous prolapse into the anterior chamber and secondary glaucoma in cats.[47] Anterior lens luxation appears very similar in clinical appearance to feline aqueous misdirection and they are challenging to differentiate. Usually, lens luxation secondary to glaucoma presents with less severe IOP elevations, and the predisposing uveitis or intraocular neoplasia is evident on a thorough examination. Primary lens luxation in a visual eye is amendable to surgical lens removal and replacement with a ciliary sulcus lens so prompt referral to a qualified surgical ophthalmologist is recommended.

CLINICAL, GROSS, AND HISTOLOGIC DIAGNOSIS AND TREATMENT OF CONGENITAL/ANTERIOR SEGMENT DYSGENESIS ASSOCIATED FELINE GLAUCOMA

This disorder manifests in young cats (kittens to 3 years of age) with buphthalmos and keratitis (**Fig. 11**A). This is in contrast to the vast majority of cats with secondary glaucoma who are middle-aged to older.[48–52] The gross and histologic findings that confirm the diagnosis of anterior segment dysgenesis, which include combinations of the following, lenticular hypoplasia (small lenses) that are often round (spheropahakia) with or without abnormal shapes (lenticonus), and occasional incomplete separation of the lens from the corneal stroma, and most often there are multiple cataracts (**Fig. 11**B–D). This is usually accompanied by marked keratitis and buphthalmos (see **Fig. 11**A), uveal hypoplasia (lack of iridal, ciliary development, and minimal smooth muscle development), and elongated hypoplastic ciliary processes and atrophy of inner retinal layers and axonal atrophy and gliosis of the optic nerve. These clinical, gross, and histologic features (see **Fig. 11**A–D) of anterior segment dysgenesis are the consequence of surface ectodermal defects that occur in the early stages of ocular development or contribute to glaucoma development in utero or within the first few years of life. The filtration angle may be so severely recessed by the buphthalmos, that it precludes clinical and histologic angle assessment. The cornea is often scarred, enlarged, and vascularized and there may be striae. The ciliary cleft is typically collapsed or closed or hypoplastic. Optic nerve cupping and often complete retinal atrophy confirm the diagnosis of glaucoma. Intravitreous vascular membrane developments have been reported in 22 affected kittens under the age of one at the time of clinical diagnosis, and anterior segment dysgenesis associated glaucoma and retinal detachment and avascular retinas were confirmed histologically.[53] However, many

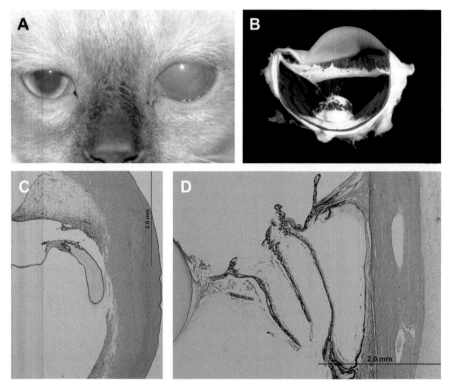

Fig. 11. (*A*). The left eye of this young cat is buphthalmic and the cornea is opaque due to edema, generalized vascularization. Histologic examination of this globe confirmed anterior segment dysgenesis associated glaucoma. (*B*) Examination of gross sections of buphthalmic feline globes such as this greatly facilitate the diagnosis of anterior segment dysgenesis and glaucoma. Note microphakia and lens luxation into the posterior segment onto the optic papilla, elongated ciliary processes, optic nerve cupping, and filtration angle recession in this feline globe with ASD associated glaucoma. (*C*) This is a PAS stained low-power histologic section of a cat with ASD and glaucoma. Note the hypoplastic filtration angle and ciliary cleft, and microphakia and abnormal lens capsule. (*D*) This PAS stained low-power histologic section of elongate ciliary process and their attachment to the lens with degenerating zonulae. Note the uveal hypoplasia. The lens was microphakic and the filtration angle and ciliary cleft are hypoplastic. The inner retina and optic nerve were atrophic.

young cats manifest with only signs of anterior segment dysgenesis and glaucoma, without avascular retinas.[27] ASD-associated glaucoma is likely under-diagnosed in general practice related to the clinical challenges of buphthalmic determination in cats, coupled with marked keratitis that precluded thorough anterior and posterior segment examinations, and finally the lack of submission of many enucleated globes with presumptive keratitis and blindness in affected kittens and young cats. In the acute stages of ASD-associated feline glaucoma, the affected eye may retain vision due to the rapid development of buphthalmos because of thin pliable sclera. As the sclera thins further due to stretching, this may facilitate aqueous humor to seep through in these young cats. This further complicates the clinical diagnosis, as the IOPs can be normal or even low in affected cats. These cases are best diagnosed by globe measurement by direct or ultra-sonographic measures with comparison to a normal contralateral globe or aged-matched control cat eye if the condition is bilateral. As a final complexity, not all cats with ASD develop glaucoma, and whether there is a need for contralateral prophylactic glaucoma therapy is unknown, and variably applied by veterinary ophthalmologists.

Topical carbonic anhydrase inhibitors will decrease the aqueous humor production and lower the IOP in cats with anterior segment dysgenesis and glaucoma,[54] at least in the short term and this is often the first topical ophthalmic medication applied in these cats. Topical ocular therapy with tropicamide has been reported to significantly increase the IOP in cats with congenital glaucoma[55] so if the pupils are being dilated to facilitate a complete ophthalmologic examination, then the post-dilatation IOPs should be monitored. Timolol maleate is reported to have minimal clinical benefit for the management of feline congenital glaucoma.[56] However, most ASD-associated glaucomatous feline eyes are blind at presentation to the general veterinarian and ophthalmologist, and the most appropriate therapy for the affected eye is enucleation. The ongoing keratitis, lens luxation, and glaucoma in these cases are very challenging to manage effectively, and the globe is best enucleated and histologically examined at a qualified laboratory.

Most ASD/congenital glaucoma seen in cats is an incidental uncommon idiopathic condition. There are exceptions to this as reported in purpose-bred cats with the LBT2 mutation and anterior segment dysgenesis. This is a simple autosomal recessive condition diagnosed initially in Siamese cats and also domestic short-hair cats and originally classified as a congenital primary condition and later changed to the more appropriate term inherited congenital glaucoma with anterior segment dysgenesis. In kittens, with this LBT2 mutation the IOP is significantly higher in affected animals at 10 weeks of age and continues to increase over 6-12 months in contrast to normal kittens where adult IOP readings are attained at 3 months of age.[57] The progressive IOP increase is accompanied by visual impairment, blindness, and buphthalmos due to the loss of ganglion cells and their axons.[58,59] The characteristic elongated ciliary processes and small lenses, which may be spherophakic, confirm this as congenital anterior segment dysgenesis. The filtration angle has been reported as mildly dysplastic and similar to goniodysgenesis. The differentiation of hypoplasia from the clinical term goniodysgenesis is yet to be reported. Both appear identical on gonioscopy examinations when corneal clarity allows for gonioscopy or direct biomicroscopic examination.

Gene therapy would seem to be a logic treatment for this inherited ASD-associated glaucoma but there are no published reports at this time. However, allogeneic transplantation of Muller-derived retinal cells has been reported, and this appears to improve retinal function in cats with ganglion cell depletion.[60]

DIAGNOSIS AND TREATMENT OF PRIMARY/IDIOPATHIC FELINE GLAUCOMA

Primary/idiopathic glaucoma is the rarest form of glaucoma in cats.[61–63] Recent anecdotal reports may reveal an upward trend in the incidence of this type of glaucoma in cats. The clinical diagnosis is based on the exclusion of all the predisposing intraocular disorders and confirmation of IOPs that are consistently greater than 30 mm Hg. Most cats are mild aged and both sexes are affected and the condition may be unilateral or bilateral. A thorough biomicroscopic anterior segment examination, and direct and indirect ophthalmoscopic examination of the posterior segment, will be normal in the acute stages and with time the inner retina and optic nerve axons will atrophy which can be documented best with OCT. Typically the IOPs are elevated but often minimally in the mid 30s to low 40s. If the disease is not diagnosed, blindness will develop. When these globes are enucleated and examined grossly and histologically primary glaucoma will be confirmed. Some of the histologically examined primary glaucoma cases have a discernable myxoid change around the aqueous collecting veins,[62] but many do not have these changes. When the globe is visual and affected by glaucoma, topical antiglaucoma therapy with Dorzolamide should be instituted. The IOPs need to be monitored repeatedly in the first month and then occasionally life-long to ensure the maintenance of the IOPs in a normal range. Usually, there is the prompt lowering of the pressure although resistant cases may require either topical prostaglandin therapy or even laser ciliary cytophotocoagulation based on unreported cases that we have managed.

SUMMARY

Glaucoma is a subtle progressive feline disease that develops most commonly as a secondary disease to idiopathic anterior uveitis and hyalitis or intraocular neoplasia. Less common forms include those associated with anterior segment dysgenesis, primary (idiopathic, which will progress to bilateral disease), and the least common aqueous misdirection associated glaucoma.

CLINICS CARE POINTS

- Glaucoma secondary to idiopathic uveitis and hyalitis is the most common category of this ocular disease in middle aged to older cats and it often involves both eyes over time
- Early onset onset glaucoma in cats is most common associated with subtle congenital anomalies and usually manifests with marked corneal disease.
- Primary (idiopathic) glaucoma of cats is the least common disorder and clinical and histologic examinations reveal no apparent predisposing disease.
- Therapeutic management of all categories of glaucoma in cats involves topical antiglaucoma medications that decrease aqueous production and often topical or systemic antiinflammatory medications while the globe is visual.Blind glaucomatous feline globes should be enucleated and submitted for histologic examination.

REFERENCES

1. Luescher M, Haessig M, Pot SA, et al. Epidemiology of feline glaucoma. Kleintier-Praxis 2013;58:393.
2. McLellan GJ, Miller PE. Feline Glaucoma-a comprehensive review. Vet Ophthalmol 2011;14:15–29.
3. McLellan GJ, Teizeira LBC. The Vet Clinics of North America. Small Anim Pract 2015;45:1307–33.
4. Kroll MM, Miller PE, Rodanl. Intraocular pressure measurements obtained as part of a comprehensive geriatric health examination for cats seven years of age or older. J Am Vet Med Assoc 2001;219:1406–10.
5. Miller PE, Pickett JP. Comparison of the human and canine Schiotz tonometry conversion tables in clinically normal cats. J Am Vet Med Assoc 1992;201:1017–20.
6. Passaglia CL, Guo X, Chen J, et al. Tono-Pen XL calibration curves for cats, cows, and sheep. Vet Ophthalmol 2004;7:261–4.
7. Andrade SF, Cremonezi T, Zachi CA, et al. Evaluation of the Perkins handheld applanation tonometer in the measurement of intraocular pressure in dogs and cats. Vet Ophthalmol 2009;12:277–84.

8. Miller PE, Pickett JP, Majors LJ, et al. Evaluation of two applanation tonometer in cats. Am J Vet Res 1991;52:1917–21.

9. Rusanen E, Florin M, Hassig M, et al. Evaluation of a rebound tonometer (tonovet) in clinically normal cat eyes. Vet Ophthalmol 2010;13:31–6.

10. Bill A. Formation and drainage of the aqueous humor in cats. Exp Eye Res 1966; 5:185–90.

11. Tripathi RC. Ultrastructure of the exit pathway of the aqueous humor of cats. Exp Eye Res 1971;12:311–4.

12. Pederson JE, Green K. Aqueous humor dynamics: experimental studies. Exp Eye Res 1973;15:77–297.

13. Hendrix DVH, Thomasy SM, Gum GG. Physiology of the eye. In: Gelatt KN, editor. Veterinary ophthalmology. 6th edition. Hoboken NJ: John Wiley & Sons; 2021. p. 142.

14. Del Sole MJ, Sande PH, Bernades JM, et al. Circadian rhythm of intraocular pressure in cats. Vet Ophthalmol 2007;10:155–61.

15. Ofri R, Shub N, Galin Z, et al. Effect of reproductive status on intraocular pressure in cats. Am J Vet Res 2002;63:159–62.

16. Oikawa d, Teixeira LBC, Keikhosravi A, et al. Microstructure and resident cell-types of the feline optic nerve head resemble that of humans. Exp Eye Res 2021;202:108315.

17. Richardson TM, Marks MS, Ausprunk DH, et al. A morphologic and morphometric analysis of the aqueous outflow system of the developing cat eye. Exp Eye Res 1985;41:31–51.

18. Nguyen L, Boorstein J, Wynn ER, et al. Prevalence and type of ocular disease in a population of aged captive nondomestic felids. Vet Ophthalmol 2022;25:31–43.

19. Blocker T, van der Woerdt A. The feline glaucoma's: 82 cases (1995-1999). Vet Ophthalmol 2001;4:81–5.

20. Ridgway MD, Brightman AH. Feline glaucoma: a retrospective study of 29 clinical cases. J Am Anim Hosp Assoc 1989;25:485–90.

21. Walde I, Rapp E. Feline glaucoma. Clinical and morphological aspects (a retrospective study of 38 cases). Euro J Comp Anim Pract 1993;4:87–105.

22. Wilcock BP, Peiffer RL Jr, Davidson MG. The causes of glaucoma in cats. Vet Path 1990;27:35–40.

23. Coop MC, Thomas JR. Bilateral glaucoma in the cat. J Am Vet Med Assoc 1958; 133:369–70.

24. Feline Glaucoma Dietrich U. Clin Tech small Anim Pract 2005;20:108–16.

25. Stadtbaumer K, Kostlin RG, Zahn KJ. Effects of topical 0.5% tropicamide on intraocular pressure in normal cats. Vet Ophthalmol 2002;5:107–12.

26. Stadtbaumer K, Frommlet F, Nell B. Effects of mydriatics on intraocular pressure and pupil size in the normal feline eye. Vet Ophthalmol 2006;9:233–7.

27. Grahn BH, Peiffer RL, Wilcock BP. Glaucoma. In: Histologic basis of ocular disease in animals. Hoboken NJ: John Wiley & Sons; 2019. p. 255–86.

28. Rapp E, Walde I. Light microscopical studies of glaucoma in the cat. Anatomia, Histologia, Embryologia. 1991;20:345–53.

29. Newbold GM, Premanandan C. An unusual case of eosinophilic uveitis in a cat. Vet Ophthalmol 2022;25:73–7.

30. Peiffer RL Jr, Wilcock BP, Yin H. The pathogenesis and significance of pre-iridal fibrovascular membranes in domestic animals. Vet Path 1990;27:41–5.

31. Maslanka T. A review of pharmacology of carbonic anhydrase inhibitors for the treatment of glaucoma in dogs and cats. Vet J 1997;203:278–84.

32. Czepiel TM, Wasserman NT. Hypokalemia associated with topical administration of Dorzolamide 2% ophthalmic solution in cats. Vet Ophthalmol 2021;24:12–9.

33. Slenter IJM, Djajadiningrat-Laanen SC, Elders DJ, et al. The effects of Dorzolamide 2% and brinzolamide 1% either alone or in combined with timolol 0.5% on intraocular pressure, pupil diameter, and heart rate in healthy cats. Vet Ophthalmol 2020;23:16–24.

34. Dietrich U. Feline glaucoma in small animal practice. Clin Tech Small Anim Pract 2005;20:108–16.

35. Maslanka T. Autonomic drugs in the treatment of canine and feline glaucoma— Part II: Medications that lower intraocular pressure by reducing aqueous humor production. Polish J Vet Sci 2014;17:753–63.

36. Bito LZ, Srinivasan BD, Baroody RA, et al. Noninvasive observations on eyes of cats after long-term maintenance of reduced intraocular pressure by topical application of prostaglandin E2. Invest Ophthalmol Vis Sci 1983;24:376–80.

37. Bartoe JT, Davidson HJ, Horton MT, et al. The effects of bimatoprost and unoprostone isopropyl on the intraocular pressure of normal cats. Vet Ophthalmol 2005; 8:247–52.

38. Studer ME, Martin CL, Stiles J. Effects of 0.005% Latanaprost solution on intraocular pressure in healthy dogs and cats. Am J Vet Res 2000;61:1220–4.

39. Gosling AA, Kiland JA, Rutkowski LE, et al. Effects of corticosteroid administration on intraocular pressure in normal and glaucomatous cats. Vet Ophthalmol 2016;19:69–76.

40. Abrams K. 2001.

41. Rosenberg et al. 1995.

42. Park S, Kim JY, Choo SW, et al. Ahmed glaucoma valve implantation with Ologen* Collagen matrix for the surgical treatment of feline glaucoma. Vet Ophthalmol 2018;21:96–100.

43. Dublielzig RR, Ketring KL, McLellan GJ, et al. The glaucomas. In: Veterinary ocular pathology (a comparative review). Toronto (Canada): Saunders Elsevier; 2010. p. 419–48.

44. Atkins RM, Armour MD, Hyman JA. Surgical outcome of cats treated for Aqueous humor misdirection syndrome: a case series. Vet Ophthalmol 2016;19:136–42.

45. Czederpiltz JM, La Croiz NC, van der Woerdt A, et al. Putative aqueous humor misdirection syndrome as a cause of glaucoma in cats: 32 cases (1997-2003). J Am Vet Med Assoc 2005;227:1434–41.

46. Payen G, Hanninen RL, Mazzucchelli S, et al. Primary lens instability in ten related cats: clinical and genetic considerations. J Small Anim Pract 2011;52:402–10.

47. Olivero DK, Riis RC, Dutton AG, et al. Feline lens displacement: a retrospective analysis of 345 cases. Prog Vet Comp Ophthalmol 1991;1:239–44.

48. Aguirre GD, Bistner SI. Microphakia with lens luxation and subluxation in cats. Vet Med Sm Anim Clin 1973;68:498–500.

49. Brown A, Munger R, Peiffer RL Jr. Congenital glaucoma and iridoschisis in a Siamese cat. Vet Comp Ophthalmol 1994;4:121–4.

50. Molleda JM, Martin E, Ginel PJ, et al. Microphakia associated with lens luxation in the cat. J Am Anim Hosp Assoc 1995;31:209–12.

51. Payen G, Hanninen RL, Mazzucchelli S, et al. Bilateral anterior segment dysgenesis with the presumed Peter's anomaly in a cat. J Vet Med Sci 2018;80:297–301.

52. Telle MR, Chen N, Shinsako D-, et al. Relationship between corneal sensitivity, corneal thickness, corneal diameter, and intraocular pressure in normal cats and cats with congenital glaucoma. Vet Ophthalmol 2019;22:4–12.

53. Beckwith-Cohen B, Hoffman A, Mclellan GJ Dubielzig R. Feline neovascular vitreoretinopathy and anterior segment dysgenesis with concurrent glaucoma in domestic cats. Vet Path 2019;56:259–68.

54. Sigle KJ, Camano-Garcia G, Carriquiry AL, et al. The effect of Dorzolamide 2% on circadian intraocular pressure in cats with primary congenital glaucoma. Vet Ophthalmol 2011;14:48–53.

55. Espinheira GF, Bentley E, Lin T_L, et al. Effects of unilateral topical administration of 0.5% tropicamide on anterior segment morphology and intraocular pressure in normal cats and cats with primary congenital glaucoma. Vet Ophthalmol 2011;14: 75–83.

56. Kiland JA, Voss AM, McLellan GJ. Effect of timolol maleate gel-forming solution on intraocular pressure, pupil diameter, and heart rate in normal and glaucomatous cats. Vet Ophthalmol 2016;19:91–6.

57. Adelman S, Shinsaka D, Kiland JA, et al. The post-natal development of intraocular pressure in normal domestic cats (*Felis catus*) and in feline congenital glaucoma. Exp Eye Res 2018;166:70–3.

58. Adelman SA, Oikawa K, Senthilkumar G, et al. Mapping retinal ganglion cell somas in a large-eyed glaucoma model. Mol Vis 2021;27:608–21.

59. Teixiera LBC, Guhr KA, Bowie O, et al. Quantifying optic nerve axons in a cat glaucoma model by semi-automated targeted counting method. Mol Vis 2014; 20:376–85.

60. Becker S, Eastlake K, Jayaram H, et al. Allogeneic transplantation of Mueller-derived retinal ganglion cells improves retinal function in feline model of ganglion cell depletion. Stem Cells Translational Med 2016;5:192–205.

61. Hampson EC, Smith RI, Bernays ME. Primary glaucoma in Burmese cats. Aust Vet J 2002;80:672–80.

62. Jacobi S, Dubielzig RR. Feline primary open angle glaucoma. Vet Ophthalmol 2008;11:162–5.

63. Trost K, Peiffer RL Jr, Nell B. Goniodysgenesis associated primary glaucoma in an adult European shorthaired cat. Vet Ophthalmol 2007;10:3–7.

The Clinical Approach to Canine Glaucoma

Lynne Sandmeyer, DVM, DVSc

KEYWORDS

- Canine • Glaucoma • Iridocorneal angle • Pectinate ligament dysplasia
- Anterior segment dysgenesis • Uveitis

KEY POINTS

- Glaucoma can be congenital, primary, or secondary, and evaluation of age, breed, and ocular changes noted clinically and pathologically will help to differentiate these categories.
- Therapeutic decisions can be guided by determining what category the glaucoma is, if it is acute or chronic, and if there is potential for vision.
- Emergency therapy is used for eyes that have potential for vision.
- Glaucoma should be considered a referral disease because differentiating the category and providing vision-preserving therapy is challenging for veterinarians.
- The long-term prognosis for all glaucoma is poor and end-stage, blind, glaucomatous eyes should be enucleated, placed in a fixative, and submitted to an appropriate laboratory for light microscopic examination and confirmation of the type of glaucoma.

INTRODUCTION

Glaucoma is a heterogeneous group of clinical syndromes that are characterized by elevated intraocular pressure (IOP) ultimately leading to optic nerve damage and blindness. Glaucoma is common in the dog and is not only blinding but also painful if the IOPs are not maintained within a normal range. Glaucoma can be a challenging disease to manage in veterinary medicine, and all cases benefit from referral to a veterinary ophthalmologist. However, the primary care veterinarian is the initial contact and thus requires a basic understanding of this disease. This article provides a simplified approach to diagnosis and clinical decision making in cases of canine glaucoma for the general practitioner. An overview of the anatomy, physiology, and pathophysiology related to canine glaucoma is provided as a foundation. Classifications of glaucoma based on cause are described as congenital, primary, and secondary, and a

The authors have nothing to disclose.
Veterinary Ophthalmology, Department of Small Animal Clinical Sciences, Western College of Veterinary Medicine, University of Saskatchewan, 52 Campus Drive, Saskatoon, Saskatchewan S7N 5B4, Canada
E-mail address: Lynne.sandmeyer@usask.ca

discussion of key clinical examination findings is provided to guide appropriate therapy and prognostication. Finally, a discussion of emergency and maintenance therapy is provided.

Anatomy and Physiology Relating to Glaucoma

The elevation of IOP that occurs in glaucoma is always secondary to a decreased exit of aqueous humor from the eye.[1] Aqueous humor is the fluid that circulates within the anterior segment of the globe. This fluid is continuously produced by the processes of diffusion, secretion, and ultrafiltration by the nonpigmented ciliary body epithelium. After formation, aqueous humor enters the posterior chamber (the space between the lens and iris) and circulates through the pupil into the anterior chamber (the space between the iris and cornea) providing nourishment and waste removal for the lens and cornea, in addition to maintaining the IOP of the globe. In the normal eye, the rate of production of aqueous humor is equal to the rate of outflow, and the IOP is maintained by this equilibrium.[2]

Aqueous humor exits the eye through 2 basic pathways: the conventional and the unconventional pathways. Approximately 85% of aqueous humor exit in the dog is via the conventional pathway in which aqueous humor exits at the iridocorneal angle (ICA) and enters the aqueous collecting veins. The ICA is the peripheral, circumferential portion of the anterior chamber where the base of the iris meets the cornea and sclera. At the face of the ICA, there are large spaces separated by thin beams of uveal tissue called pectinate ligaments, which connect the base of the iris to the peripheral cornea.[2] Aqueous humor passes between pectinate ligaments and into the ciliary cleft, which is a triangular space with a base that extends from the pectinate ligaments and apex toward the ciliary body. The ciliary cleft is filled with the uveal trabecular meshwork made up of irregular anastomosing trabecular beams separated by interlacing spaces (spaces of Fontana). The trabecular beams are lined by specialized cells (trabecular cells), which play a role in phagocytizing particles and provide a clearance mechanism for particulate debris from the aqueous humor. The aqueous humor then flows around an elaborate meshwork of veins known as the angular aqueous plexus (AAP).[3] These veins are lined by vascular endothelium and the aqueous humor bathes these collecting veins and crosses these endothelial cells by at least 4 distinct processes including direct flow through small intracellular pores, micropinocytosis, phagocytosis, and large vacuoles.[3,4] Aqueous humor then enters the vascular system via the AAP, which is a complex venous network located at the transition zone between the ICA and the ciliary cleft (**Fig. 1**). The unconventional pathway for aqueous humor exit is the uveoscleral outflow and is said to account for only 15% of total aqueous humor outflow in the dog.[5] In this exit route, aqueous humor bypasses the trabecular outflow described earlier, passively percolating through the ciliary body into the suprachoroidal space.[2] This flow is independent of IOP and is driven mainly by osmosis.[2] It is important to note that within the outflow pathways, morphologic, physiologic, and biochemical changes occur with age and with tissue remodeling. Thus, the functional anatomy associated with the maintenance of IOP within a normal range and the onset of glaucoma is dynamic and complex.[6]

Classification of Glaucoma

Grouping glaucoma into categories based on cause significantly helps the clinician and the ophthalmologist guide treatment and determine prognosis for the affected and fellow eye. Three useful basic categories for differentiating glaucoma in dogs are congenital, primary, and secondary. Deduction of the category is aided by signalment (age and breed), complete ocular examination findings, and referral to an

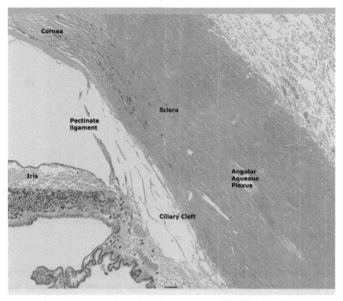

Fig. 1. Normal canine iridocorneal angle (ICA). The ICA represents the anatomic region for conventional aqueous humor outflow. The pectinate ligaments (PLs) span the opening between the base of the iris and the cornea. Aqueous humor filters between the PLs into the ciliary cleft and then enters the vascular system via the angular aqueous plexus. Hematoxylin and eosin stain, 4x magnification)

ophthalmologist for other specialized evaluations such as gonioscopy, and advanced imaging modalities such as high-frequency ultrasonography and optical coherence tomography (OCT).

Congenital Glaucoma and Those Associated with Anterior Segment Dysgenesis

Congenital glaucoma is classically described as manifesting in utero or in neonates and is associated with congenital ocular anomalies known as anterior segment dysgenesis (ASD)[7–11]; it may be unilateral or bilateral. Congenital glaucoma is the least common form of glaucoma diagnosed in the dog, and the cause is unknown. We have diagnosed glaucoma associated with ASD in dogs aged up to 3 years, because this form of glaucoma may manifest in dogs a little later in life. As a result, it is most appropriate to term these early-onset glaucomas in all species as congenital glaucoma/ASD associated. It is also important to note that not all dogs with ASD develop glaucoma. ASD is characterized by concurrent ocular anomalies of the formation of the uvea and lens, including abnormalities of the lens such as microphakia, spherophakia, aphakia, lenticonus, lens coloboma, and cataract and uveal anomalies including hypoplasia of the iris, ciliary body, elongated ciliary processes, and a hypoplastic ICA that contribute to the pathogenesis of reduced aqueous humor outflow and glaucoma.[9,10,12,] These anomalies are readily detected clinically and on gross and histologic examination of enucleated globes.

Because of the elasticity of the young dog sclera, globes often develop marked buphthalmos early in the course of disease (**Fig. 2**). Chronic buphthalmos results in corneal exposure, and keratitis resulting in ulceration, pigmentation, and scarring. Some puppies may retain vision despite buphthalmos, perhaps due to an elevation

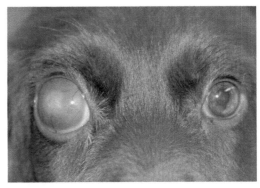

Fig. 2. Congenital glaucoma in an 8-month-old bloodhound cross dog. Note marked buph-thalmia of the left eye. Anterior segment dysgenesis was noted on clinical examination with lack of separation of the uveal tissue from the cornea. Exposure keratitis is evident with extensive corneal vascularization.

of IOP before development of the retina. The prognosis with congenital/ASD-associated glaucoma is poor because most dogs become blind and the extensive buphthalmos can lead to progressive and severe exposure keratitis.

Primary Glaucoma (Inherited and Idiopathic Glaucoma that will Affect Both Eyes)

The term primary glaucoma is used to describe inherited forms of glaucoma that are not caused by antecedent ocular disease. Primary glaucoma is described in many breeds of dogs **(Table 1)**.[1,13–38] Although there are breed-related differences in age of onset and disease progression, there are generalities that can be made about this form of glaucoma.[1] Primary glaucoma is a bilateral condition that typically mani-fests in middle- to older-aged dogs. The disease typically presents unilaterally initially, with the fellow eye developing glaucoma months to years later. The 2 basic clinical forms of primary glaucoma described in the literature are primary glaucoma associ-ated with goniodysgenesis and primary open-angle glaucoma (POAG). Goniodysgenesis-related glaucoma (GDRG) is the most common form of primary glaucoma in the dog. This form is associated with a bilateral congenital anatomic ab-normality of the ICA in which there is a failure of rarefaction of the mesoderm within the ICA. Thus, normal pectinate ligaments and spaces between them fail to form[1,15–18]; this is called pectinate ligament dysplasia (PLD). Goniodysgenesis and PLD are often used interchangeably when discussing canine glaucoma. This anatomic anomaly is only a marker for primary glaucoma, rather than the cause, because its presence does not ensure development glaucoma later in life, because only some of the dogs with goniodysgenesis will develop glaucoma.[1,17] This form of glaucoma is also frequently called primary angle closure glaucoma (PACG) in the literature. Although this is a common term used clinically, it creates diagnostic confusion with secondary glaucoma disorders in which peripheral anterior synechiae cause physical closure of the ICA, which is challenging to differentiate from goniodysgenesis clinically, but is readily apparent histologically.[12,39] The authors, therefore, prefer to avoid the use of PACG, and simply describe this as primary glaucoma associated with goniodysgene-sis. It is important to stress that goniodysgenesis is a congenital anomaly and it does not progress as such. The appearance of the ICA will change with collection of pigment and other cellular debris, which is common in globes with GDRG.[29] In addi-tion, growth of the lens throughout life and the subtle effects of glaucomatous

Table 1
Common canine breed predisposed to primary glaucoma

Primary Glaucoma/ Pectinate Ligament Dysplasia –Associated	Primary Open Angle Glaucoma
American Cocker Spaniel[15]	Beagle[30]
Basset hound[15]	Basset hound[32]
Border Collie[16]	Basset Fauve de Bretagne[32]
Bouvier des Flandres[17]	Chinese Shar-Pei[33]
Chow Chow[18]	Norwegian elkhound[34]
Dandie Dinmont Terrier[19]	Petit Basset Griffon Vandeen[35]
English Cocker Spaniel[15]	
English Springer Spaniel[20]	
Flat-coated Retriever[21]	
Golden retriever[16]	
Welsh springer Spaniel[22]	
Great Dane[23]	
Miniature and Toy Poodle[24]	
Leonberger[25]	
Norwegian elkhound[26]	
Samoyed[27]	
Shiba Inu[28]	
Shih Tzu[28]	
Siberian husky[29]	
Vizsla[16]	

stretching of the ICA tissues will result in the narrowing of the gonioscopic and histologic appearance of the ICA over time.[40,41]

POAG is a much less common form of primary glaucoma in which goniodysgenesis is absent, and the ICA appears anatomically normal when gonioscopy is completed before IOP elevations.[30–38] This disorder is inherited in the Beagle and Norwegian elkhound as an ADAMTS10 mutation; in the basset hound, Basset Fauve de Bretagne, and Petite Basset Griffin Vendeen as a mutation of ADAMTS17; in the Shih-Tzu and Shiba Inu as a mutation of SRBD1; and in the Beagle and Shiba Inu as a myocilin mutation. [31–34,36–38] In POAG, the appearance of the ICA in the glaucomatous globe will narrow with disease progression. Similar to GDAG, this ICA narrowing/closure observed in POAG is likely related to alterations in the ICA morphology with repeated or progressive IOP elevation.[41] It is important to note that the terminology used here for open- versus closed-angle glaucoma is a clinically applied designation and this differs from the descriptive terminology used to describe the appearance of an open or closed ICA on histopathology.[39]

The pathogenesis of primary glaucoma is complex and poorly understood. In most forms there is an anatomic abnormality of the main outflow pathway (goniodysgenesis); however, this is not the cause of aqueous outflow obstruction, because glaucoma occurs in a subset of dogs with this anomaly and manifests later in life. It is likely that there are morphologic, physiologic, and biochemical changes that occur with age and tissue remodeling that affect the movement of aqueous humor into the aqueous collecting veins, which contributes to the onset of glaucoma in affected dogs.[1,6]

Table 2
Ocular tissue changes in acute and chronic glaucoma and assumed pathophysiology

Tissue	Acute Glaucoma[a]	Chronic Glaucoma
Globe	Normal size	Enlarged (buphthalmia) • Pressure-induced stretching
Conjunctiva and episclera	Red • Vascular congestion	Red • Vascular congestion
Cornea	Edema • Pressure-induced dysfunction of endothelial pump function	Edema • Pressure-induced dysfunction of endothelial pump function Striae • Globe stretching causing breaks in Descemet membrane Keratitis • Exposure due to buphthalmia
Iris and Pupil	Mydriasis • Pressure-induced paralysis	Mydriasis • Pressure-induced paralysis • Iris atrophy • Retinal and optic nerve degeneration
Lens	Normal	Subluxation and luxation • Zonular breakage due to globe stretching Cataract • Lens fiber degeneration due to reduced nutrition/waste removal by aqueous humor
Retina	Normal	Degeneration (tapetal hyperreflectivity, vascular attenuation) • Pressure-induced damage
Optic nerve	Normal	Degeneration (darkened, smaller), cupping (recessed) • Pressure-induced damage to nerve fiber layer and ganglion cells

[a] Changes described are most typical of primary glaucoma because secondary glaucoma will have additional clinical manifestations.

The clinical manifestations of primary glaucoma occur due to pressure exerted on all ocular tissues (**Table 2**). In the acute phase of glaucoma, elevated IOP interferes with the vascular circulation of the globe causing congested episcleral vessels. The function of the corneal endothelium is reduced, and diffuse corneal edema develops. The severity of edema is generally in proportion to the degree of pressure elevation. The pupillary constrictor muscle becomes paralyzed, and pupillary dilatation results (**Fig. 3**). Pressure on the retina will initially affect its function causing temporary vision loss; however, sustained elevations of IOP will induce necrosis and apoptosis of retinal ganglion cells.[42] There are many mechanisms that may contribute to retinal ganglion cell death including axonal transport failure, neurotrophic factor deprivation, toxic proneurotrophins, mitochondrial dysfunction, excitotoxic damage, oxidative stress, reactive glia, and loss of

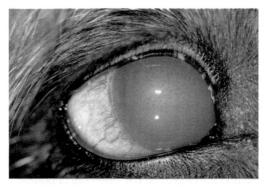

Fig. 3. Acute primary glaucoma in the right eye of a 5-year-old cocker spaniel. Note vascular congestion, diffuse corneal edema, and mydriasis.

synaptic connectivity.[43] In the acute phase, if the IOP can be normalized quickly, vision loss may be reversed to some degree, at least until the glaucoma progresses. In primary glaucoma, ocular examination does not reveal evidence of preexisting ocular disease, which is helpful to differentiate it from secondary glaucoma.

With sustained, elevated IOP, permanent changes develop. The globe begins to expand, and buphthalmos develops. Globe enlargement causes stretching of all tissues; breaks in Descemet membrane may develop, and these are called corneal striae or Haab striae. Stretching of the lens zonules can result in their breakage, and lens subluxation or luxation can develop (**Fig. 4**). Sustained, increased IOP will cause complete retinal and optic nerve degeneration. Initially, this involves the ganglion cells and nerve fiber layer; however, eventually all layers of the retina will die. The retina will develop vascular attenuation, and regions of tapetal hyperreflectivity will develop. The optic nerve will become atrophied and cupped and will appear smaller and recessed on the fundic examination. These pathologic changes are permanent, and vision will not be restored even when normal IOPs are sustained. The pupil will remain dilated due to the retinal and optic nerve degeneration as well as neurologic and muscle damage. With prolonged and continual elevated IOP the uvea atrophies, and the

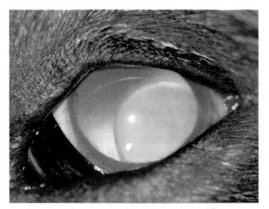

Fig. 4. Chronic primary glaucoma in the left eye of a 6-year-old Great Dane. The globe has buphthalmia and a posterior lens luxation due to zonular breakdown from globe stretching.

sclera thins to the point that the IOP may return to a normal range due to decreased aqueous humor production and filtering of aqueous humor through the sclera.

Secondary Glaucoma

Secondary glaucoma is acquired and develops because of an antecedent ocular condition that causes obstruction of aqueous humor drainage. Secondary glaucoma can present at any age, in any breed of dog, and may be unilateral or bilateral, depending on the underlying cause. In secondary glaucoma, the obstruction to aqueous humor circulation and outflow generally occurs at 1 of 2 anatomic locations: the ICA and/or the pupil. In certain forms of secondary glaucoma, an obvious cause of the elevation of IOP is present on ocular examination; in others it may not be obvious. Causes of secondary glaucoma and the presumed pathogenesis of outflow obstruction associated with these are described in the following discussion and in **Table 3**.

The clinical manifestations of secondary glaucoma include those discussed for primary glaucoma earlier; however, there are additional clinical findings depending on the underlying cause.

Many of the causes of secondary glaucoma discussed later involve the formation of preiridal fibrovascular membranes (PIFMs) that contribute to the pathogenesis of glaucoma. These membranes are challenging to detect clinically unless the iris and pupillary margins are examined carefully with a biomicroscope. Ectropion uveae, the outward curling of the pupillary margin, is an excellent indication of the presence of a PIFM; they are readily detected with light microscopic examination of sections of enucleated globes. Ectropion uveae develop with the budding of iris stromal blood vessels and deposition of supportive fibrous tissue by fibroblasts on the face of the iris.[44] PIFMs form in response to angiogenic cytokines released as a response to inflammation or ischemia of ocular tissues. Vascular endothelial growth factor (VEGF) is known to be a major mediator of PIFM development. Increased levels of VEGF in aqueous humor and positive immunohistochemical staining for VEGF in histologic samples have been reported for dogs with uveitis, retinal detachment, lens luxation, intraocular neoplasia, hyphema, and various forms of secondary glaucoma.[45,46] PIFMs contribute to development of glaucoma because they can grow over and occlude the pupil, and more commonly, span and contract the ICA. PIFMs contain fragile blood vessels, and therefore, hyphema is another common clinical sign of their presence.

Anterior Uveitis

Inflammation of the anterior uvea (iris and ciliary body) is the most common cause of secondary glaucoma. Anterior uveitis has many causes, but all are associated with breakdown of the blood-aqueous barrier and leakage of protein and cells into the aqueous humor. Anterior uveitis will commonly obstruct the pupil or the ICA with posterior and anterior synechiae. Proteins in the aqueous humor contribute to the formation of these adhesions of the iris to the lens (posterior synechia) or at the ICA (peripheral anterior synechia). Miosis (constriction of the pupil) occurs due to the action of prostaglandins on the iris constrictor muscle and brings the pupil in contact with the anterior surface. Blockage of aqueous humor circulation through the pupil if complete (360°) posterior synechiae develop results in buildup of aqueous humor in the posterior chamber and induces iris bombe, which narrows or closes the ICA. The ICA may also become obstructed by inflammatory or neoplastic cells or cellular debris, fibrin, and so on. Chronic uveitis also promotes the development of PIFMs on the iris surface, which also grow to cover and obstruct the ICA.

Table 3
Causes, mechanisms, and clinical manifestations of secondary glaucoma

Cause	Mechanism of IOP Obstruction	Clinical Manifestations Suggestive of cause	Breed or other Predispositions
Anterior uveitis	Pupil obstruction: • Complete posterior synechia ICA obstruction: • Inflammatory cells, and so on • Peripheral anterior synechia • PIFM formation	Aqueous flare, hypopyon, hyphema, iris hyperemia, iris hyperpigmentation, variable miosis, posterior synechia, iris bombe	None
Primary lens luxation	Pupil obstruction: • Block by lens and vitreous ICA obstruction: • Mechanical obstruction by prolapsed vitreous • Chronic uveitis due to physical irritation (see earlier for mechanisms)	Phacodenesis, iridodenesis, aphakic crescent (subluxation or posterior luxation), lens in anterior chamber (anterior luxation), vitreous strands in pupil or anterior chamber	Terrier breeds (mainly) Shar-Pei Border collie
Intumescent cataract	Pupil obstruction: • Enlarged lens fills pupil ICA obstruction: • Enlarged lens narrows and closes ICA	• Dense cataract with separation at the Y-sutures, anterior displacement of iris and anterior lens capsule, shallow anterior chamber	Diabetic dogs
Intraocular neoplasia	ICA obstruction: • Infiltration by tumor • PIFM formation	Mass within the iris or ciliary body, changes in iris shape and color, hyphema	None
Melanocytic Glaucoma	ICA obstruction: • Infiltration by pigment and pigment-containing cells	Hyperpigmentation of the iris, thickening of the iris base, pigment plaques in episclera and choroid	Cairn Terrier
Pigmentary/cystic glaucoma chronic retinal detachment	ICA obstruction: • Anterior displacement of iris by cysts • PIFM formation	• Aqueous flare, fibrin, hyphema, uveal cysts, radial pigment on anterior lens capsule, posterior synechia, iris hyperemia	Golden Retriever (main breed affected) American bulldog Great Dane

Although there are many causes of uveitis, the most common cause of secondary glaucoma in the dog is related to chronic cataracts[47]; this is termed phacolytic uveitis and is the result of leakage of soluble lens protein through the lens capsule. Phacolytic uveitis may not be clinically apparent, because the typical signs of uveitis such as episcleral injection, miosis, and aqueous flare may not be evident. However, lymphocytic-plasmocytic uveitis is present on light microscopic examination and exists to some degree in all eyes with cataract, regardless of the cataract stage.[1,47] The mean age at presentation of glaucoma secondary to phacolytic uveitis is 10.0 ± 2.0 years.[48] In addition to returning vision, cataract surgery can dramatically reduce the incidence of secondary glaucoma when successful. However, topical anti-inflammatory therapy is recommended in all eyes diagnosed with cataract, regardless of if the owner chooses to pursue cataract surgery because this measure alone can decrease the incidence of secondary glaucoma due to phacolytic uveitis.[47]

Clinical manifestations of uveitis-related secondary glaucoma may include corneal edema, corneal vascularization, aqueous flare, hypopyon, hyphema, and changes in iris shape and color. The pupil size and shape may be variable. Miosis is usually present with uveitis; however, with elevation of IOP, mydriasis may occur and formation of posterior synechia will also change the shape of the pupil. Glaucoma secondary to phacolytic uveitis will also have cataract present (**Fig. 5**).

PRIMARY LENS LUXATION

Primary lens luxation (PLL) is an inherited condition most commonly diagnosed in terrier and related breeds. Breeds known to have PLL include the Sealyham, Jack Russell, wirehaired fox, miniature bull terrier, Tibetan terrier, Shar-Pei, and Border collie; however, PLL is suspected to be inherited in more than 50 canine breeds.[1] The condition presents most commonly in young- to middle-aged dogs and is bilateral; however, lens luxation may not present concurrently.

Lens luxation occurs due to breakdown of the fibers (lens zonules) attaching the equatorial lens capsule to the ciliary body. Dogs with PLL are born with ultrastructural abnormalities of the lens zonules.[49,50] The mean age of dogs presenting with glaucoma secondary to PLL is 7.1 ± 2.7 years.[48] Progressive weakening of the zonules initially results in lens instability and eventually complete lens dislocation. Anterior lens luxation is the complete dislocation of the lens into the anterior chamber, whereas posterior luxation implies complete dislocation into the vitreous. Glaucoma occurs

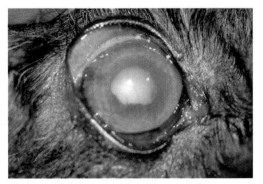

Fig. 5. Secondary glaucoma due to chronic phacolytic uveitis in an 11-year-old Labradoodle. Note mature cataract, and a midrange irregular pupil shape due to posterior synechia formation. There is mild cornea edema and peripheral corneal pigmentation.

more commonly and more acutely with anterior lens luxation than with posterior luxation or subluxation. Anterior displacement of the lens and vitreous face may occlude the flow of aqueous humor through the pupil causing pupillary block glaucoma.[1,5,39] Large amounts of prolapsed vitreous in the anterior chamber may also cause mechanical obstruction to aqueous outflow through the ICA.[1,51] Chronic uveitis due to physical irritation of the iris by an unstable lens may also contribute to development of glaucoma in subluxated or posteriorly luxated lenses.

wThe clinical manifestations of lens instability include tremors of the lens (phacodonesis) or iris (iridodonesis). The lens equator may become visible within the dilated pupil giving rise to a clinically detectable aphakic crescent. Degenerative vitreous strands are often visualized within the anterior chamber as fine, wispy white fibers. Changes in symmetry in the depth of the anterior chamber are also common. In anterior lens luxation there is an obvious change in the position of the lens as it may move completely through the pupil into the anterior chamber (**Fig. 6**), or it may cause forward displacement of the iris leaflets if it remains in the posterior chamber resulting in a narrowed anterior chamber depth. Corneal edema occurs due to irritation of the corneal endothelial cells from lens friction. In posterior lens luxation the lens often falls into the ventral vitreous, which has undergone syneresis or liquefaction, resulting in a deep anterior chamber.

Note that chronic glaucoma leads to buphthalmos, and this will also cause stretching and breakdown of the lens zonules and secondary lens luxations. Differentiating the inciting cause (other types of glaucoma vs PLL) in an eye with chronic glaucoma is difficult; however, consideration of breed in these cases may be most helpful. Many, but not all breeds with PLL have a genetic mutation of the ADAMTS17 gene.[52] Interestingly, mutations in ADAMTS17 are also associated with POAG in several breeds.[32,33,36] In the Chinese Shar-Pei both PLL and POAG have been associated with a mutation in this gene.[33] A DNA test for the mutation is available, which may also aid in diagnosis of the cause in these cases.

INTUMESCENT CATARACTS

Intumescent cataracts are swollen cataracts, which most often occur because of diabetes mellitus and the osmotic draw of fluid into the lens. In severe cases, extensive

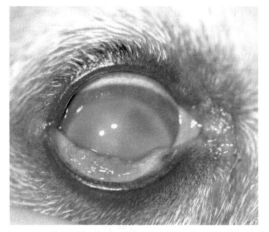

Fig. 6. Secondary glaucoma due to anterior lens luxation in a 6-year-old toy fox terrier. The lens is visualized in the anterior chamber in front of the iris, and there is marked corneal edema associated with the lens touching the corneal endothelium.

swelling can occur, which significantly displaces the iris forward; this can lead to secondary glaucoma via acute pupillary block as well as narrowing and closure of the ICA. In some cases, in which swelling occurs rapidly, the peripheral lens capsule may rupture contributing to severe uveitis, which also promotes the development of secondary glaucoma.[1]

Clinical manifestations of intumescent cataract include dense opacity of the lens with separation at the anterior suture lines. Swelling of the lens will displace the iris and anterior lens capsule forward leading to a shallow anterior chamber. In some cases, the lens may swell so much that there is virtually no detectable anterior chamber, and this can be mistaken as an anterior lens luxation.

Intraocular Neoplasia

Intraocular neoplasia may be primary, meaning developing from ocular tissues, or metastatic to the globe. The most frequently occurring primary intraocular neoplasia in the dog are melanocytic tumors of the uvea. In the dog these are typically benign in their behavior and therefore are called melanocytomas.[53] Canine uveal melanocytomas are usually nodular, and progressive growth and infiltration of the ICA results in glaucoma as they obstruct aqueous outflow. Clinical manifestations of uveal melanocytomas include darkly pigmented, nodular masses within the iris. These masses may bulge forward and typically induce abnormalities of the pupil (dyscoria). When glaucoma develops, episcleral congestion, corneal edema, and ocular discomfort are noted.

Iridociliary epithelial tumors (iris or ciliary body adenomas and adenocarcinomas) are the second most common primary intraocular tumor in the dog. Most behave in a benign nature regardless of the histopathologic designation of adenoma versus adenocarcinoma.[54] These are epithelial tumors, and as they grow, they will produce VEGFs. These chemical mediators are by the iris and promote formation of PIFMs. The growth of these membranes on the surface of the iris and ICA is the likely cause for obstruction of aqueous humor outflow and development of secondary glaucoma with these tumors.[44]

Iridociliary epithelial tumors usually grow as solitary nodules in the posterior chamber (behind the iris) or vitreous space. The nodules will eventually expand into the iris stroma and anterior chamber; they are often nonpigmented. Because these tumors incite PIFM formation, and these membranes are fragile and bleed easily, hyphema is a common presenting clinical manifestation with iridociliary epithelial tumors.

Although the most frequent type of intraocular neoplasia causing glaucoma in dogs are primary uveal melanocytic tumors and adenoma/carcinomas, any tumor that infiltrates or causes obstruction of the ICA will cause glaucoma. The most common ocular site for hematogenous spread of metastatic tumors is the uveal tract. Metastatic pulmonary and mammary carcinomas, as well as histiocytic sarcomas and lymphosarcoma are also known causes of secondary glaucoma[48]; this underscores the importance of submitting all enucleated globes for histopathology to evaluate the cause for the glaucoma because this may denote the need for further systemic workup.

Glaucoma Secondary to Melanocytosis

This condition is inherited in the cairn terrier breed but has also been reported in the boxer, Labrador retriever, and Dachshund.[55–57] The mean age of cairn terriers with ocular melanocytosis and secondary glaucoma is 10.9 ± 2.0 years.[46] This unique condition is also known as ocular melanosis because it is characterized by bilateral, progressive proliferation and aggregation of melanocytes and melanophages within the uvea.[56] Release of pigment-laden cells into the anterior chamber and deposition along the aqueous humor outflow pathways leads to the development of secondary glaucoma. Clinical manifestations include a darkened iris and thickening of the iris base with gradual development of pigment plaques in the episcleral as well as the choroid.

Pigmentary/Cystic Glaucoma

Pigmentary/cystic glaucoma occurs as an end stage of pigmentary uveitis (PU), which is an inherited condition of the golden retriever.[58] PU is also known as golden retriever uveitis due to the incidence in the breed; however, similar conditions have been reported to occur in other breeds including the American bulldog and Great Dane.[59,60]

PU normally occurs in middle-aged to older dogs and is usually bilateral but is not usually symmetric in its presentation. The pathogenesis of the condition is unknown. The term "uveitis" is applied due to the clinical manifestations typical of blood-aqueous barrier breakdown. However, there are surprisingly minimal inflammatory changes seen on light microscopic examination of enucleated globes.[61]

Uveal cysts are considered a risk factor or an early marker for PU.[58,62,63] The uveal cysts are typically thin walled, translucent, and attached to the ciliary body and posterior iris and contact the anterior lens capsule (**Fig. 7**). These cysts are most easily seen after pupil dilation because they extend into the pupil from the posterior chamber.[58] The diagnosis of PU is applied when there is radial deposition of pigment on the anterior lens capsule.[62] Additional clinical manifestations of PU include conjunctival hyperemia, aqueous flare, darkened irides, posterior synechiae formation, corneal edema, fibrinous debris in the anterior chamber, hyphema, and cataract formation.[62] Glaucoma occurs in up to 50% of dogs with PU.[64] The pathogenesis of glaucoma in these cases is not completely understood; however, it may to be due to posterior synechia formation, or by occlusion of the ICA, which may be due to the mechanical effect

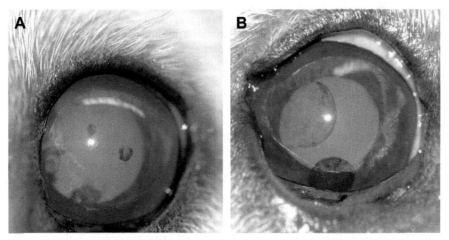

Fig. 7. Pigmentary uveitis and secondary glaucoma in an 11-year-old golden retriever. The right eye (*A*) has developed secondary glaucoma; note the diffuse corneal edema, dilated pupil, and pigment deposition on the anterior lens capsule and inner cornea. The left eye (*B*) has a normal IOP but shows signs of pigmentary uveitis with iris hyperpigmentation and cysts in the posterior and anterior chamber.

of forward pressure by cysts, presence of pigment or other debris in the ICA, or development of PIFMs and peripheral anterior synechia.[61,65]

Chronic Retinal Detachment

Rhegmatogenous retinal detachments are separations of the neurosensory retina from the retinal pigment epithelium (RPE) occurring due to a tear in the retina. Certain breeds such as Shih Tzus, Boston terriers, and Italian greyhounds are predisposed to spontaneous complete retinal tears secondary to vitreous degeneration. Liquefied vitreous enters a retinal hole and dissects between the neurosensory retina and RPE causing enlargement of the tear and the development of complete detachment.[66] Rhegmatogenous retinal detachments are also a complication of lens luxation, ocular trauma, and intraocular surgery.[67] Separation of the retina from the RPE results in outer retinal ischemia, which stimulates release of angiogenic growth factors in the globe; this promotes development of vascular membranes in the vitreous as well as PIFMs that will obstruct the ICA leading to secondary glaucoma.

The clinical manifestations of glaucoma secondary to retinal detachment may include signs of uveitis. Hyphema is likely the most common sign that develops secondary to hemorrhage from the PIFM. If the posterior segment is visible, the torn retina may be seen draped over the optic nerve head (ONH) and extending into the vitreous. As a result, the retinal vessels will not be visible over the tapetum and the tapetum will be very bright due to direct visualization without the overlying retina. Corneal edema and hyphema may obscure ability to examine intraocular structures. Ocular ultrasonography may be used to diagnose the retinal detachment in those cases in which hyphema or pupillary occlusion precludes posterior segment examination.

Diagnosis of Glaucoma

The initial diagnosis and classification of glaucoma requires a complete ocular examination including a neuro-ophthalmic examination, tonometry, and systematic assessment of all ocular structures. Gonioscopy or examination of the ICA is important; however, this requires specialized equipment (slit lamp biomicroscope and goniolens) and training to accurately perform and interpret, and given the importance of these diagnostics in determining the category of glaucoma, referral of all cases of glaucoma to a veterinary ophthalmologist is recommended.

The ophthalmic examination begins with a distant assessment of globe size and symmetry. Globe size is important, because enlarged globes (buphthalmos) confirm chronic glaucoma and these eyes are usually blind or severely visually impaired. The components of the neuro-ophthalmic examination that are particularly important in the assessment of visual potential include a menace response, dazzle reflex, assessment, and comparison of resting pupil size in both eyes, and direct and consensual pupillary light reflexes (cPLR). These assessments will help to define if the eye has potential for vision or is permanently blind. Elevated IOP will usually result in an absent menace response, and a dilated pupil, often unresponsive to light in both blind and potentially visual canine eyes. However, if there has been permanent retinal and optic nerve damage, the dazzle reflex and the cPLR to the contralateral eye will also be absent. The dazzle reflex is a subcortical reflex elicited by shining a bright light into the eye; if the visual pathway is intact, a blink or squint response occurs in that eye. The consensual pupillary light reflex is elicited by shining a bright light in the affected eye and observing the other eye for pupil constriction. The reflex occurs because of the decussation of afferent fibers at the optic chiasm and the pretectal region and will remain intact until the retina and optic nerve are damaged from glaucoma.

Tonometry is always an essential component of every ocular examination, and all veterinary practices should have access to at least one type of tonometer. The normal range for IOP for the dog is approximately 10 to 25 mm Hg.[1] Glaucoma is diagnosed when the IOP exceeds 30 mm Hg in the dog. There is diurnal variation in IOP, and various factors can affect this measurement. It is important to avoid pressure on the neck during restraint as well as the globe itself, for example, while opening the eyelids, to prevent erroneously high readings. There are 3 basic types of tonometry: indentation, applanation, and rebound. Indentation tonometry uses the Schiotz tonometer, which is a mechanical device that has 3 components (a threaded pin, a main handpiece with scale, and a 5.5–10 g weight) that must be assembled before use. Topical corneal anesthesia is required before measurements. Applanation tonometry works on the principal that a predetermined area of anesthetized cornea is flattened, and the instrument converts the pressure required to flatten the curvature to the IOP in mm Hg. An examples of an applanation tonometers is the Tono-Pen Avia Vet® (Reichert Technologies, NY). Rebound tonometry uses the processing of the rebound movement of a rod probe resulting from its interaction with the eye to estimate the IOP. This method has the advantage over indentation and applanation tonometry of not requiring use of topical corneal anesthesia before using the instrument and that they are inherently easier to master in the examination room. The Tonovet (Joregensen Laboratories, CO) and AccuPen Vet (Automated Ophthalmics, MD) are the 2 commercially available rebound tonometers used in veterinary medicine today.

Systematic examination of the globe is important to evaluate all ocular tissues for any abnormalities that might help confirm changes associated with chronicity as well as indications of antecedent ocular disease. The clinical manifestations of acute versus chronic glaucoma and those associated with the different causes of secondary glaucoma are summarized in **Tables 2** and **3**.

Gonioscopy is the clinical examination of the ICA; this requires use of a specially designed corneal contact lens (a goniolens) and a source of illumination and magnification such as a slit-lamp biomicroscope. Gonioscopy is usually performed in the non-glaucomatous globe because the presence of corneal edema associated with glaucoma will obstruct visualization. Because PLD is a bilateral condition, the presence of PLD in the normal globe is an indication of primary glaucoma.[15] A veterinary ophthalmologist at referral will confirm the cause of glaucoma and provide advice regarding ongoing management and therapy for the affected and contralateral globe.

OCT is a high-resolution optically based imaging system that uses low-coherence interferometry to provide high-resolution (4-5um) cross-sectional images of ocular tissues in vivo. OCT can be used to image the ONH and retina. Owing to the high-resolution capabilities, the layers of the retina can be differentiated and thickness of these layers can be measured (**Fig. 8**). In humans, OCT is used to evaluate the ONH and retinal nerve fiber layer (RNFL) as part of the monitoring and management of glaucoma.[68] Access to OCT technology is currently limited in veterinary ophthalmology and is more common in academic institutions. However, preliminary studies have shown that the predisposed, fellow eyes of dogs with unilateral primary glaucoma have statistically significant decreases in total retinal and RNFL thicknesses compared with normal eyes.[69] This observation suggests that damage to the inner retina may occur before the clinical diagnosis of glaucoma based on recognition of elevated IOP. OCT imaging may therefore be valuable in identifying early disease, and gauging response to therapy. Future studies are likely to validate the utilization of OCT as a diagnostic and management tool in canine glaucoma.

Ultrasound biomicroscopy (UBM) uses high-frequency (40–100 MHz) ultrasound energy to provide cross-sectional images of the anterior segment, including anatomic

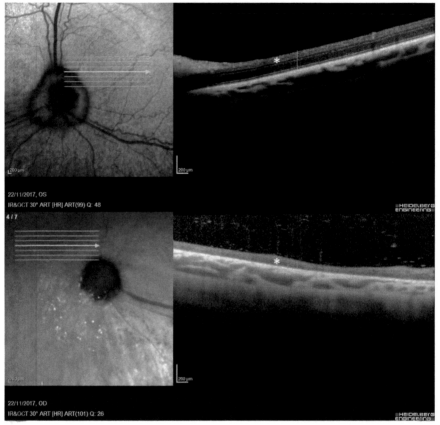

Fig. 8. OCT image of canine with primary glaucoma. The bottom image is of the glaucomatous retina, and the top image is the fellow eye. The retina is depicted with an asterisk in both images. Note the markedly decreased retinal thickness in the glaucomatous globe.

structures of the ICA. This modality can be used to estimate measurements of the angle opening, area, and width of the ciliary cleft area of the AAP. In a study comparing normal dogs with those with primary glaucoma, the fellow eye of dogs with unilateral primary glaucoma had significantly lower values for the width and angle of the ciliary cleft compared with normal dogs.[70] In addition, the opening of the ciliary cleft and the area of the AAP were significantly larger in dogs that responded to glaucoma therapy compared with those that did not. UBM is therefore another clinical tool that may be used in the management and monitoring of glaucoma in dogs.

Advanced imaging techniques such as UBM and OCT provide objective quantitative information about the ICA. As these technologies continue to be refined in the field of veterinary ophthalmology, they are likely to aid in further understanding of the pathogenesis of canine glaucoma, as well as establishing new diagnostic criteria and improved strategies for glaucoma management and monitoring.

Glaucoma Therapy

Glaucoma treatment can be separated into emergency and long-term therapy. Glaucoma therapy may involve both medical and surgical treatment. Decisions regarding the most appropriate treatment must take into account the cause (congenital, primary, or secondary), the stage of glaucoma (acute or chronic), and if the eye is permanently blind or has potential for vision. A simplified algorithm is presented in **Fig. 9** that may help guide the initial approach for assessment and therapy following a diagnosis of glaucoma.

Emergency Medical Management

The goal of emergency therapy is to reduce the IOP quickly to reduce damage to the retina and optic nerve. This approach is most appropriate in acute-onset glaucoma when there is evidence of visual potential (positive dazzle reflex, presence of a consensual pupillary light reflex in the contralateral eye).

There are many different topical antiglaucoma medications on the market, and the details of each are beyond the scope of this article. The most commonly used are summarized in **Table 4**. The medications used in emergency management may differ depending on the cause (primary vs secondary glaucoma). Emergency treatment has traditionally been hyperosmotic therapy with intravenous mannitol 1 to 2 g/kg administered over 20 minutes. This therapy will draw water from the vitreous and reduce the IOP quickly but temporarily. Longer-acting specifically targeted medical therapies (such as prostaglandin analogues and carbonic anhydrase inhibitors [CAI]) must be initiated in conjunction with mannitol. This approach is useful for most causes of glaucoma but is complicated by a requirement for hospitalization and placement of an intravenous catheter. Since the development of effective, rapidly acting topical antiglaucoma medications, the use of mannitol in the emergency management of glaucoma has markedly waned. Prostaglandin analogues are topical antiglaucoma mediations that are very potent and can reduce the IOP in dogs as quickly and effectively as mannitol in most cases. These analogues can be used as emergency therapy

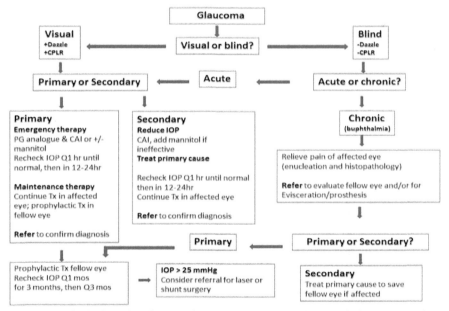

Fig. 9. Simplified algorithm for initial assessment and treatment of glaucoma in dogs. q, every; PG, prostaglandin; CAI, Carbonic anydrase inhibitor; Tx, treatment.

Table 4
Commonly used medications for treatment of canine glaucoma

Medication	Mechanism of Action	Onset of Action	Relative Potency	Frequency of Administration	Side Effects or Contraindications
Mannitol	Osmotically draws fluid from vitreous	1-2 h	High	1-2 g/kg over 20 min Can repeat 1-2 times	Emergency use only
Prostaglandin analogues, eg, latanoprost, travoprost, bimatoprost	Increased outflow	1-2 h	High	q 12-24 hours	Miosis in dogs. Avoid with anterior lens luxation
CAI, eg, dorzolamide, brinzolamide	Decreased aqueous humor production	2-4 h	Moderate	q 8 hours q 12 hours (prophylactic therapy)	Rarely, periocular sensitivity reactions
Beta-adrenergic antagonists, eg, 0.5% timolol maleate	Decreased aqueous humor production	6-8 h	Minimal	q 8-12 h	Cardiac and pulmonary effects. Avoid in asthma and heart failure
Combination CAI and beta-adrenergic antagonsits, eg, dorzolamide/timolol brinzolamide/timolol	Decreased aqueous humor production	2-4 h	Moderate	q 8 hours q 12 hours (prophylactic therapy)	See earlier

Abbreviations: PIFM, preiridal fibrovascular membranes; q, every.

in place of mannitol, especially in acute primary glaucoma. However, prostaglandin analogues cause marked miosis, which may exacerbate pupillary block in anterior lens luxation and can promote posterior synechia in uveitis and should therefore be avoided in these types of secondary glaucoma. During the emergency treatment period, the IOP should be reevaluated every 1 to 2 hours until it returns to normal range. Topical antiglaucoma mediations such as prostaglandins and CAI can be administered hourly during this time. Once the IOP has returned to normal, the frequency of topical medications can be returned to maintenance frequency (every 8–12 hours) and IOP should be re-evaluated in 12 to 24 hours.

Medical Management and Maintenance Therapy

If emergency therapy is successful in returning the IOP to normal range, the goal becomes maintaining normal IOP to preserve vision and comfort for as long as possible; this requires ongoing medical management and may include surgical interventions. Referral to an ophthalmologist is warranted at this stage to confirm suspected diagnosis and consider prognosis for the affected and fellow eye.

Maintenance treatment often requires using more than one of the topical agents described. For example, the authors commonly use a prostaglandin analogue every 12 hours, in addition to a CAI/beta-adrenergic agonist every 8 hours for initial maintenance of IOPs in dogs with primary glaucoma. Frequent measurement of the IOP is also required to monitor for disease progression. There is no set frequency for which reevaluation should occur. We typically recommend an IOP measurement within 5 to 7 days of the initial episode and then every 3 to 4 weeks for the first 3 months. If the IOP is maintaining within normal range, IOP measurements can be extended to every 3 months.

Congenital Glaucoma and Those Associated with Anterior Segment Dysgenesis

The treatment of congenital glaucoma will depend on if the globe is visual or blind. Therapy for visual globes can include a prostaglandin analogue every 12 hours, in addition to a CAI/beta-adrenergic agonist every 8 hours. Buphthalmic globes that retain vision may develop exposure keratitis, and topical lubricants may be beneficial to reduce corneal desiccation. Topical antibiotics are required if corneal ulceration develops. Blind globes should be treated surgically by enucleation or evisceration with placement of an intrascleral prosthesis as noted in later discussion, and the globe should be submitted for histopathology.

Primary Glaucoma

Primary glaucoma is a bilateral disease, even though it usually presents with one eye affected initially. The first eye often presents at the chronic and buphthalmic stage because the acute phase goes unnoticed or is disregarded by the owner. The other eye will usually develop glaucoma within several months. Studies have shown that prophylactic treatment of the fellow eye will delay the onset of glaucoma.[71,72] The most used medications for prophylaxis are a topical CAI or CAI/beta-adrenergic agonist combination every 12 to 24 hours. Concurrent treatment with topical corticosteroid or nonsteroidal anti-inflammatory agents may also help prolong the disease-free interval.[72] It is important to note that in primary glaucoma, the response to medical management is variable and usually short lived. The disease will progress beyond the ability for medications to control the IOP. Referral to a veterinary ophthalmologist is warranted in all cases to confirm the diagnosis and direct ongoing therapy, which may include surgery.

Secondary Glaucoma

The treatment of secondary glaucoma does depend on the underlying cause and can be complex to manage. Referral to an ophthalmologist is always recommended for these reasons. Most require specialized treatment of the underlying cause; however, topical CAI or CAI/beta-adrenergic agonist is useful and safe for most causes of secondary glaucoma while awaiting referral. Glaucoma secondary to uveitis (including PU) will also require topical corticosteroid and/or nonsteroidal anti-inflammatory therapy, possibly in addition to mydriatics. Glaucoma occurring secondary to anterior lens luxation is treated by surgical removal of the lens. Treatment of intumescent cataract requires phacoemulsification. Melanocytic and pigmentary/cystic glaucomas may respond to topical antiglaucoma therapy for a period. Intraocular neoplasia does not respond well to antiglaucoma therapy, and these usually require enucleation.

Surgical Options for Glaucoma

There are 3 basic categories of surgical therapy: those that improve the outflow of aqueous humor (anterior chamber implants), those that decrease the rate of formation of aqueous humor (laser photocoagulation, intraocular injections), and those considered to be end-stage procedures for blind eyes (enucleation and evisceration with placement of an intrascleral prosthesis). Aside from enucleation, surgical therapy requires referral to a veterinary ophthalmologist because these require specialized training and equipment to perform.

Surgical Therapy for Visual Eyes

Surgical treatments to improve aqueous humor outflow involve placement of implants that shunt aqueous humor from the anterior chamber out of the eye. Most of the commercially available devices divert aqueous humor to the subconjunctival tissue. Unfortunately, these develop fibrosis of the drainage end of the shunt due to cytokine-laden aqueous humor draining into mesenchymal tissues within weeks of surgery. Surgical use of antimetabolite drugs such as mitomycin C and 5-fluorouracil can reduce or slow fibrotic capsule formation.[73,74] However, these are toxic to the cornea and conjunctival epithelium and can cause additional severe complications. Shunts that divert to the frontal sinus avoid fibrosis, but the surgery to place them is more complex.[75,76] In the early postoperative period, the intraocular portion of a shunt may become obstructed by fibrin leading to IOP elevation; this can require intracameral injection of tissue plasminogen activator to dissolve the fibrin. Therefore, frequent postoperative monitoring is required, especially in the early stages. Long-term success rates for shunts vary from 65% to 90% at 1 year.[73,77,78,] Aside from eventual shunt failure, potential complications of anterior chamber shunts include hypotony, uveitis, cataract formation, infection, and migration of the shunt.[79,80]

Cyclophotocoagulation uses laser energy to destroy the ciliary epithelium to reduce production of aqueous humor. Transscleral cyclophotocoagulation (TSCP) is a noninvasive approach using a laser probe applied over several sites in sclera over the approximate region of the ciliary body. Complications can include postoperative uveitis, hyphema, phthisis bulbi, cataract formation, retinal detachments, and even acute elevations in IOP.[81–85] Using a high-power/short-duration protocol the efficacy in IOP control at 1 year is reported to be 53%.[84] Recently a low-power/long-duration protocol reported a more promising efficacy in IOP control of 92% at 1 year.[83] Endoscopic cyclophotocoagulation (ECP) is a newer technology that allows direct visualization and application of laser energy to the ciliary processes from within the eye; this has a reported efficacy in IOP control at 1 year of 80%.[86] ECP directly targets the tissue and therefore has fewer complications than TSCP. The most common complication of ECP is postoperative uveitis, and there is a high incidence of cataract formation. ECP is therefore most commonly performed in combination with cataract surgery.[86,87] It is common for eyes to develop acute elevation in the IOP after any of these laser procedures, and frequent postoperative monitoring is required. Topical antiglaucoma medications as well as anti-inflammatories are often continued for several weeks after surgery and modified according to clinical examination findings at follow-up. The effects of laser therapies are transient due to ciliary epithelium regeneration, and the procedures often need to be repeated weeks to months later to maintain the normal IOPs.

End-Stage Glaucoma Surgery

Unfortunately, medical and surgical interventions often eventually fail in all types of glaucoma. Uncontrolled IOP is a source of pain, and chronic IOP elevation will lead to buphthalmos and often exposure keratitis and corneal ulceration. End-stage procedures for glaucoma are aimed at removing the source of pain and the need for continued medical therapy. The most common end-stage surgeries are enucleation or evisceration and intrascleral prosthesis. The former is a relatively easy surgery to perform in general practice and has few complications. The latter requires referral to a veterinary ophthalmologist.

Some owners are resistant to the idea of eye removal surgery, mainly for cosmetic reasons.

An intrascleral prosthesis is a potentially more cosmetic alternative end-stage procedure for blind glaucomatous globes with the exception of those caused by intraocular neoplasia or intraocular infection.[88] This surgery involves removal of the intraocular contents and placement of a silicone ball into the fibrous corneoscleral shell. The fibrous tissue will conform to the size and shape of the ball. It is common for marked corneal vascularization to develop between 3 and 6 weeks during the healing process; however, this will resolve. In the long-term, the cornea usually develops diffuse gray opacity due to fibrosis. The potential complications of evisceration include infection, corneal ulceration, and reduced tear production due to decreased corneal sensation.[89]

Chemical ablation of the ciliary body via intravitreal injection of gentamicin or cidofovir has been described as an option for end-stage glaucomatous eyes. This procedure is most commonly used to avoid general anesthesia in high-risk patients. Because these drugs are toxic to the ciliary body epithelium, they will cause ciliary body degeneration and therefore reduced IOP. These drugs also lead to retinal degeneration and are reserved for blind eyes. Extreme care must be taken to avoid the lens capsule, because lens capsule punctures lead to a devastating phacoclastic uveitis. Although ciliary body ablation has a high success rate for reduction of IOP, complications of this procedure are common and include severe unresponsive uveitis, cataract formation, and phthisis bulbi.[90,91] Phthisis bulbi develops from chronic inflammation causing atrophy and shrinkage of the globe.[75] In humans phthisis bulbi is reported to cause chronic pain secondary to endophthalmitis,[92] and most dogs with phthisis also have chronic ocular pain. More importantly, other intraocular disease is commonly present in these shrinking globes. One study identified intraocular tumors in 40% of enucleated canine eyes that had been previously treated with intravitreal gentamicin injection.[93] It is not clear if there was a causal correlation between injection and development of neoplasia; however, this remains a significant concern. For these reasons, the authors do not recommend intravitreal injections as a treatment of glaucoma. Permanently blind glaucomatous eyes are best treated by enucleation or evisceration with silicone prosthesis implant.

It is important to submit all enucleated globes or eviscerated contents for histopathologic examination. Histopathology may not be able to confirm PLD in chronic/buphthalmic globes because globe stretching will change the morphology of the ICA.[41] However, it will usually establish an accurate categorization of ASD/congenital, secondary, or primary canine glaucoma, which is incredibly important for the clinician to establish the prognosis and guide therapy for the fellow eye.

Histopathologic Features of Glaucoma

The histopathologic features of glaucoma are vast and include those that are associated with the cause of glaucoma as well as those that are caused by the glaucoma.[12] The histologic features of the ICA are important to describe, because this is the location of aqueous humor outflow; however, these features alone cannot be used to determine cause. Rather, assessment of the pathologic changes to the globe as a whole, with consideration of signalment and evaluation of the fellow eye are important in establishing a cause for the glaucoma. Interpretation of ocular histopathology benefits from an experienced ocular pathologist, and there are several ocular several ocular pathology services available in North America.

Histopathologic Changes Caused by Glaucoma

Sustained elevation of IOP will result in damage to all ocular tissues. Prolonged elevations of IOP cause stretching of the globe (buphthalmos). The extent of globe stretching is age dependent because young animals have a greater tendency for stretching due to elasticity of the connective tissue. Buphthalmos is associated with scleral thinning and is most obvious anterior to the equator but can develop circumferentially. The cornea develops exposure keratitis with epithelial thinning, keratinization of the stratified squamous epithelium, rete peg formation, pigmentation, and often corneal ulceration.[39,94] Corneal stromal edema is characterized histologically by loss of the artifactual separation of the collagen lamellae that is normally present with fixation. The stroma may also develop vascularization in the periphery, which may extend centrally. Globe stretching may lead to ruptures in Descemet membrane (called striae or Haab striae). These appear as focal disruptions in the membrane and develop a fibrotic bridge with time. [39,94]

In the early acute stages of glaucoma there will be a neutrophilic infiltration within the anterior uvea and filtration angle; this is usually replaced quickly by a lymphocytic-plasmocytic inflammation in the uvea, filtration angle, and ciliary cleft.[29] Pressure atrophy of the entire uveal tract will occur with time. In the iris this manifests with stromal thinning, cystic degeneration, and atrophy of the posterior iris epithelium. The ciliary body appears reduced in size with fewer ciliary processes and thinning of the pars plana. The choroid becomes thinner and tapetal degeneration may occur.

Changes in the ICA that occur with chronic glaucoma include closure of the ciliary cleft, flattening of the pectinate ligament against the trabecular meshwork, stretching and recession of the ICA (**Fig. 10**), as well as alterations in the termination of Descemet membrane, also known as descemetization, a continuous or noncontinuous thickening of terminal Descemet membrane with fingerlike extensions in the ciliary cleft along the uveoscleral or uveal trabecular meshwork.[41,94]

Glaucoma-induced changes in the lens are less recognizable with light microscopy than they are clinically. Buphthalmos often leads to zonular breakdown and lens subluxation. Alterations in lens position are difficult to confirm on gross section and histologic section because lens displacement often occurs as an artifact of processing.[94] Cataracts may occur with chronic glaucoma associated with stagnation of aqueous

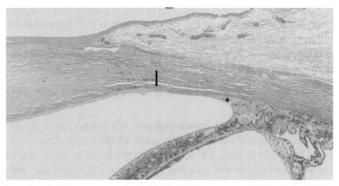

Fig. 10. Light microscopic appearance of ICA changes common in chronic glaucoma. The angle is open, and the ciliary cleft is collapsed. Note the termination of Descemet membrane (*arrow*) compared with the base of the iris (*asterisk*) indicating angle recession. (Hematoxylin and eosin stain, 4x magnification)

humor circulation or pressure necrosis of lens and cortical fibers.[94] Vitreous syneresis or liquefaction is also commonly noted in globes with chronic glaucoma. [94]

Pressure on the retina leads to initial thinning of the inner retina. There may be a mild neutrophilic infiltrate in the retina in the first few days of elevated IOP.[95] Necrosis of ganglion cells gives them hypereosinophilic appearance with loss of nuclear detail.[95] Ganglion cell loss and segmental degeneration of the nerve fiber layer occurs rapidly and progresses to scattered full-thickness retinal attenuation and disorganization often within days (**Fig. 11**).[42,95] End-stage full-thickness generalized retinal atrophy eventually occurs, and the retina becomes what is called a glial scar.[42,95] The ventral or nontapetal retina is consistently more degenerate than the dorsal or tapetal counterpart.[42,94,95] Hypertrophy of the RPE and displacement of RPE pigment into the neuroretina is common with prolonged glaucoma; this may be associated with focal separation of the neuroretina from the RPE but can also be present in areas of nondetachment. RPE changes are likely evidence that elevated IOP induces disruption of the RPE, permeability of the vascular endothelium, and inflammation within the retina.[96]

In the acute stages of elevated IOP, there may be mild optic nerve (ON) edema and neutrophilic papillitis; however, these progress within days to ON atrophy.[95] The

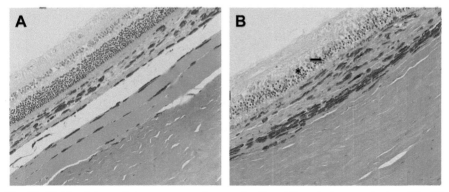

Fig. 11. Light microscopic appearance of normal retina (*A*) and glaucomatous retina (*B*). Note loss of ganglion cells and marked thinning of the inner nuclear layer (*asterisk*), as well as thinning of the outer nuclear layer and photoreceptors (*arrow*). (Hematoxylin and eosin stain, 10x magnification).

pressure atrophy leads to cupping or ectasia in which there is depression of the entire nerve head and posterior bowing of the lamina cribrosa.[94,95] Schnabel cavernous atrophy is another occasional phenomenon of severe glaucoma in which cavities containing alcian blue-positive proteinaceous material (vitreous in origin) are forced into the retrolaminar optic nerve.[39]

Histopathology of Congenital Glaucoma and Those Associated with Anterior Segment Dysgenesis

Histologic features of globes with congenital and ASD-associated glaucoma include those caused by elevated IOP discussed earlier in addition to anomalies of the anterior segment structures, which may be subtle. Buphthalmos is often marked in these globes due to the elasticity of the sclera in young animals. Thus, corneal edema and striae are common in addition to features of exposure keratitis such as vascularization, fibrosis, and ulceration. Features of ASD can include small lenses, elongated ciliary processes, ciliary body muscle hypoplasia, and hypoplastic or recessed filtration angles. Glaucomatous retinal and optic nerve atrophy are also present.[12,39]

Differentiating Primary and Secondary Glaucoma Histologically

Globes with primary glaucoma principally display the histologic lesions caused by elevated IOP on the ocular tissues as noted earlier without evidence of antecedent ocular disease. Globes with secondary glaucoma usually reveal additional lesions associated with the underlying cause.

One of the most common histopathologic findings in globes with secondary glaucoma is PIFM.[97–99] PIFMs are characterized by multiple layers of small blood vessels with supporting fibroblasts, arising from the anterior stroma of the iris, with subsequent deposition of collagen.[44] These membranes may cover both the anterior and posterior surfaces of the iris and often cause inward or outward curling of the pupillary region of the iris known as entropion and ectropion uveae, respectively. PIFMs contribute to the pathogenesis of glaucoma through obstruction of aqueous humor circulation and outflow; they can grow to cover the pupil and the ICA, and they contribute to development of peripheral anterior synechia, which is adhesion of the iris base to the inner cornea (**Fig. 12**). In addition, they may contribute to development of posterior synechia in which the iris is attached to the anterior lens capsule. Posterior

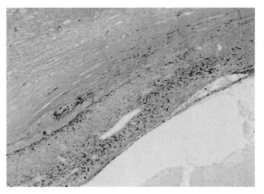

Fig. 12. Light microscopic appearance of a preiridal fibrovascular membrane (*asterisk*) resulting in a closed ICA. A peripheral anterior synechia has formed causing the base of the iris to adhere to the inner aspect of the cornea (*double-sided arrow*). (Hematoxylin and eosin stain, 10x magnification)

synechia may be focal or involve the entire pupillary margin causing iris bombe, a forward bowing of the iris leaflets that develops when the pupil is obstructed and aqueous humor builds up in the posterior chamber behind the iris.[94] PIFMs develop in response to angiogenic factors released within the globe secondary to conditions such as retinal detachment, intraocular neoplasia, and chronic uveitis.[44,45]

Histopathologic features of retinal detachment include separation of the neurosensory retina from the RPE, development of RPE hypertrophy, as well as photoreceptor degeneration and thinning of the outer nuclear layer.[39] Photoreceptor degeneration is a consequence of loss of metabolic support of the RPE and underlying choroid caused by the separation of the neurosensory retina from these structures. It is primarily the rhegmatogenous retinal detachments and intraocular neoplasia that lead to development of PIFMs. Rhegmatogenous detachments are related to a tear or a hole within the retina. Dissection of liquefied vitreous may then enter the space between the photoreceptors, and RPE may lead to development of a giant retinal tear and complete disinsertion of the dorsal retina.[90] It is postulated that the marked dislocation of the retina from the underlying RPE and choroid in this form of detachment results in ischemia and release of VEGFs that stimulate PIFM development, ultimately leading to the obstruction of aqueous outflow and glaucoma.[44]

Ocular neoplasia may cause secondary glaucoma through tumor infiltration and obliteration of the ICA, by stimulation of PIFM formation, or by causing marked secondary uveitis. The most common primary intraocular neoplasms in dogs are melanocytic uveal tumors. Melanocytic uveal tumors most often arise within the iris and cause glaucoma by local expansion, infiltration, and obliteration of the ICA. Histologic features of these tumors include sheets of spindle cells and clusters of deeply pigmented, large, polyhedral "plump" cells. Most are histologically benign with a mitotic index of 2 or less. [53] The second most common primary intraocular tumor in dogs is ciliary adenomas or adenocarcinomas; these typically induce PIFM formation, and secondary glaucoma develops secondarily to closure of the filtration angle and ciliary cleft. Histologic features include sheets, clusters, and cords of neoplastic epithelial cells with presence of basement membrane material.[54] Metastatic neoplasms are most often located within the anterior uvea, and these may infiltrate and obliterate the ICA as well as incite a severe inflammatory response.[48]

Common features of glaucoma associated with uveitis include evidence of the inflammatory response including protein (called plasmoid aqueous) and/or inflammatory cell infiltrate within the anterior chamber and uvea. In some cases, hemorrhage may also be present. There are multiple underlying causes of uveitis; however, phacolytic uveitis due to chronic cataract is one of the most common. Phacolytic uveitis is associated with cataract and is characterized by mild to moderate lymphocytic-plasmocytic infiltration of the anterior uvea. Histologic features of cataract include posterior migration of lens epithelium, cortical liquefaction, and wrinkling of the lens capsule associated with leakage of liquefied lens protein.[94] Phacoclastic uveitis a more severe form of lens-induced uveitis associated with traumatic lens rupture is characterized by disruption of the lens capsule and presence of a predominantly neutrophilic inflammatory response at the site of the rupture and extending between the lens fibers. This inflammation is usually severe and often extends throughout the globe.[39]

Another lens condition that is often associated with secondary glaucoma is primary lens instability. Mechanical irritation from an unstable lens may result in hypertrophy and/or hyperplasia of the posterior pigmented iris epithelium and subsequent cellular exfoliation and release of melanin pigment.[50] Mechanical irritation from an unstable lens may also cause uveal inflammation with variable degrees of mononuclear cell infiltration and PIFM development. Presence of melanophages within the ciliary cleft is also common in these globes.[50] Unfortunately, lens positional changes are difficult to confirm with histopathology because lens displacement is a common artifact of processing. Special stains may be used to evaluate the zonular fibers. Dysplastic zonular fibers have a protein morphology characterized by being tightly adherent to the non-pigmented ciliary body epithelium, having a distinct lamellar and cross-hatched pattern, and staining strongly with (periodic acid-schiff stain) PAS and Masson trichrome and negatively with elastin stain.[99] This pattern contrasts with zonular fiber collagenization in which zonular fibers are not tightly adherent to the ciliary body epithelium and stain positive with PAS, Masson trichrome, and elastin stain.[99] Zonular fiber dysplasia pattern is more likely to be associated with PLL than lens luxation caused by other ocular diseases.

Glaucoma secondary to melanocytosis of cairn terriers is characterized by pigment deposition in the perilimbal zone of the sclera, and extensive infiltration of melanin-containing cells with an eccentric nucleus located in the iris, ciliary body, retina, choroid, and sclera. These cells are effete melanocytes and melanophages.[57]

The common histologic features of glaucoma associated with PU include large thin-walled iridociliary cysts lined by attenuated cuboidal epithelium (corresponding to ciliary body epithelium) filling posterior chamber and PIFM formation. Additional findings can include thick-walled cysts containing hyaluronic acid, deposition of a hyaluronic acid and collagen-rich material on the equatorial and anterior lens capsule, free pigment within the trabecular meshwork, peripheral anterior synechia, posterior synechia, iris bombe, and anterior chamber hemorrhage.[61,64,65] Most intriguingly, despite having clinical characteristics of uveitis, few globes have discernible inflammatory cells in the uvea on light microscopic examination.[65]

Histopathology of the Iridocorneal Angle in Glaucoma

Histopathologic descriptions of globes with glaucoma usually include an assessment of the morphology of the aqueous outflow pathway. The ICA may be described as being open, closed, or obstructed. The angle is described as open unless there is apposition of the iris base to the endothelium or to Descemet membrane. The ICA is usually histologically open in primary glaucoma (see **Fig. 10**).[12,39,94] A closed angle implies adhesion of the iris base to the cornea and occurs with peripheral anterior synechia (see **Fig. 12**). Obstruction of the ICA structures may be seen with inflammatory cell infiltration, covering by a PIFM, or invasion and destruction by neoplasia. Therefore, histologically closed ICA is more common with secondary glaucoma. The ciliary cleft is usually collapsed in both primary and secondary glaucoma due to compression of the trabecular meshwork.[94]

Certain histologic features involving the termination of Descemet membrane and the iris root have conventionally been implied as diagnostic of goniodysgenesis-related primary glaucoma. [94] These features include an open ICA but closed ciliary cleft, absence of a clearly defined pectinate ligament, presence of solid uveal tissue spanning from iris root to the termination of Descemet membrane, thickening of the trabecular meshwork beams, alterations in the termination of Descemet membrane, extension of pigmented spindle cells into the deep corneal stroma adjacent to Descemet membrane, and extension of uveal tissue onto the posterior surface of the peripheral Descemet membrane. [94]

Despite attention paid to the histologic features described earlier, there is no set of histologic criteria for the ICA that can be relied upon for the diagnosis of chronic primary glaucoma associated with goniodysgenesis. Similar changes to the termination of Descemet membrane and iris root are seen in both primary and secondary glaucoma.[41,94] As the ciliary cleft collapses the pectinate ligament flattens against the trabecular meshwork giving the appearance of a thin band of tissue similar to a dysplastic pectinate ligament.[94] In addition, both primary and secondary glaucoma show descemetization, which is a continuous or noncontinuous thickening of terminal Descemet membrane with fingerlike extensions in the ciliary cleft along the uveoscleral or uveal trabecular meshwork.[94] A masked comparative evaluation of globes diagnosed with secondary glaucoma with globes with primary glaucoma corroborated with gonioscopically diagnosed PLD in the fellow eye confirmed that the ICA changes traditionally presumed to be characteristic for PLD/goniodysgenesis-associated primary glaucoma are indeed common in secondary glaucoma of various causes.[41] Therefore, just as for all other ocular tissues, chronically elevated IOP causes alterations to the ICA morphology such that ICA morphology alone cannot be used to establish the etiologic diagnosis for goniodysgenesis.[41] Experienced ocular pathologists will assess all histologic changes in the globe in conjunction with clinical information to postulate the most likely cause.

SUMMARY

Glaucoma is a common blinding and painful condition in the dog that occurs due to decreased exit of aqueous humor from the eye. There are 3 basic categories of glaucoma: ASD/congenital, primary, and secondary. ASD/congenital glaucoma occurs in young animals and may be unilateral or concurrently bilateral and the diagnosis is confirmed histologically by identification of ASD. Primary glaucoma is inherited in many breeds and most often is associated with goniodysgenesis/PLD, which is an abnormality of the ICA. Secondary glaucomas are those that occur when another ocular condition causes obstruction of aqueous humor exit and are the most common form of canine glaucoma. The most common cause of secondary glaucoma is uveitis. Other causes include anterior lens luxation, ocular melanocytosis, PU, intumescent cataract, intraocular neoplasia, and rhegmatogenous retinal detachments. When a diagnosis of glaucoma is made, a systematic ocular examination is required to evaluate if the eye has potential for vision and for signs of antecedent ocular disease. This examination is important for clinical decision making regarding the most appropriate therapy and prognosis. Eyes with acute glaucoma may continue to have the potential for vision, whereas those with chronic glaucoma are most often blind. Emergency medical therapy is indicated in acute glaucoma where there is potential for vision. Glaucoma can be a challenging disease to manage in veterinary medicine, and most cases benefit from referral to a veterinary ophthalmologist. Ophthalmic specialists will perform gonioscopy, as well as other advanced diagnostic techniques to establish a cause and can offer advanced surgical therapy when indicated that may prolong IOP control and vision. The prognosis for glaucoma is always guarded to poor regardless of the cause; the condition will most often progress beyond the ability of medications to control the IOP and therapies are rarely successful long term. Therefore, the goal is to maintain vision and comfort as long as possible. Blind eyes with chronic glaucoma are best treated by enucleation or referral for evisceration and intrascleral prosthesis placement, and all enucleation and evisceration samples should be fixed and evaluated histologically.

CLINICS CARE POINTS

- Glaucoma can be congenital, primary, or secondary, and evaluation of age, breed, and clinical manifestations will help to differentiate these categories.

- Therapeutic decisions can be guided by deciding what category the glaucoma is, if it is acute or chronic, and if there is potential for vision.
- Lack of a dazzle reflex or consensual pupillary light reflex is indication that the eye is blind.
- Buphthalmos is an indication that the glaucoma is chronic and most likely permanently blind.
- Emergency therapy is used for eyes that have potential for vision.
- Topical carbonic anhydrase inhibitors are safe to use in all forms of glaucoma as a part of emergency and maintenance therapy.
- Prostaglandin analogues are safe and effective for primary glaucoma but should not be used when anterior lens luxation or anterior uveitis is present.
- Glaucoma is a referral disease once IOP is stable.
- The long-term prognosis for all glaucoma is poor and end-stage, blind, glaucomatous eyes should be removed, and histopathology performed.

REFERENCES

1. Plummer CE, Komaromy AM, Gelatt KN. The Canine Glaucomas. In: Gelatt KN, editor. Vet Ophthalmol1, 6th edition. Hoboken: John Wiley & Sons; 2021. p. 1173–255.
2. Pizzirani S, Gong H. Functional anatomy of the outflow facilities. Vet Clin Small Anim 2015;45:1101–26.
3. Tripathi RC. Ultrastructure of the exit pathway of the aqueous in lower animals. Exp Eye Res 1971;12:311–4.
4. Samuelson DA, Gelatt KN. Aqueous outflow in the Beagle. II. Postnatal morphologic development of the iridocorneal angle: corneoscleral trabecular mesh work and angular aqueous plexus. Curr Eye Res 1984;3:795–807.
5. Barrie KP, Gum GG, Samuelson DA, et al. Quantitation of uveoscleral outflow in normotensive and glaucomatous Beagles by 3H-labeled dextran. Am J Vet Res 1985;46:84–8.
6. Gum GG, Do Samuelson, Gelatt KN. Effect of hyaluronidase on aqueous humor outflow resistance in normotensive and glaucomatous eyes of dogs. Am J Vet Res 1992;53:109–14.
7. Peiffer RL Jr, Fischer CA. Microphthalmia, retinal dysplasia, and anterior segment dysgenesis in a litter of Doberman Pinschers. J Am Vet Med Assoc 1983;183:875–8.
8. Shaw GC, Tse MPY, Miller AD. Microphthalmia with multiple anterior segment defects in Portuguese water dogs. Vet Path 2018;56:269–73.
9. Halenda RM, Grahn BH, Sorden SD, et al. Congenital equine glaucoma: clinical and light microscopic findings in two cases. Vet Comp Ophthalmol 1997;7:105–9.
10. Cullen CL, Grahn BH. Congenital glaucoma in a Llama (Lama glama). Vet Comp Ophthalmol 1997;7:253–7.
11. Beckwith-Cohen B, Hoffman A, McLellan GJ, et al. Feline neovascular vitreoretinopathy and anterior segment dysgenesis with concurrent glaucoma in domestic cats. Vet Path 2018;56:259–68.
12. Grahn BH, Peiffer RL, Wilcock BP. Histologic basis of glaucoma. In: Histologic Basis of ocular disease in animals. Hoboken, NJ: Wiley-Blackwell; 2019. p. 255–87.
13. Komáromy AM, Petersen-Jones SM. Genetics of canine primary glaucomas. Vet Clin Small Anim 2015;45:1159–82.

14. Gelatt KN, MacKay EO. Prevalence of the breed-related glaucomas in pure-bred dogs in North America. Vet Ophthalmol 2004;7:97–111.
15. Bedford PG. A gonioscopic study of the iridocorneal angle in the English and American breeds of Cocker Spaniel and the Basset Hound. J Small Anim Pract 1977;18:631–42.
16. Oliver JA, Ekiri AB, Mellersh CS. Pectinate ligament dyslplasia in the Border Collie, Hungarian Vizsla, and Golden Retriever. Vet Rec 2017;180:279.
17. Dublin AJ, Bentley E, Buhr KA, et al. Evaluation of potential risk factors for development of primary-closure glaucoma in the Bouviers des Flandres. J Am Vet Med Assoc 2017;250:60–7.
18. Corcoran KA, Koch SA, Peiffer RL. Primary glaucoma in the Chow Chow. Vet Comp Ophthal 1994;4:193–7.
19. Oliver JA, Ekiri A, Mellersh CS. Prevalence of pectinate ligament dysplasia and associations with age, sex and intraocular pressure in the Basset hound, Flat-coated retriever, and Dandie Dinmont terrier. Canine Genet Epidemiol 2016;3:1.
20. Bjerkas E, Eksesten B, Farstad W. Pectinate ligament dysplasia and narrowing of the iridocorneal angle associated with glaucoma in the English Springer Spaniel. Vet Ophthalmol 2002;5:49–54.
21. Wood JL, Lakhani KH, Read RA. Pectinate ligament dysplasia and glaucoma in Flat Coated Retrievers. II. Assessment of prevalence and heritability. Vet Ophthalmol 1998;1:91–9.
22. Cottrell BD, Barnett KC. Primary Glaucoma in the Welsh Springer Spaniel. J Small Anim Pract 1988;29:185–99.
23. Wood JL, Lakhani KH, Mason IK, et al. Relationship of the degree of goniodysgenesis and other ocular measurements to glaucoma in Great Danes. Am J Vet Res 2001;62:1493–9.
24. Bedford PGC. The aetiology of primary glaucoma in the dog. J Small Anim Pract 1975;16:217–39.
25. Fricker GV, Smith K, Gould DJ. Survey of the incidence of pectinate ligament dysplasia and glaucoma in the UK Leonberger population. Vet Ophthalmol 2016;19:379–85.
26. Eksesten B, Bjerkas E, Kongengen K, et al. Primary glaucoma in the Norwegian elkhound. Vet Comp Ophthalmol 1997;7:14–8.
27. Eksesten B, Narfström K. Correlation of morphologic features of the iridocorneal angle to intraocular pressure in samoyed dogs. Am J Vet Res 1991;52:1875–8.
28. Kanemaki N, Tchedre KT, Imayasu M, et al. Dogs and humans share a common susceptibility gene SRBD1 for glaucoma risk. PLoS One 2013;8(9):e74372.
29. Reilly CM, Morris R, Dubielizig RR. Canine goniodysgenesis-related glaucoma: a morphologic review of 100 cases looking at inflammation and pigment dispersion. Vet Ophthalmol 2005;8:2553–8.
30. Gelatt KN, Gum GG, Gwin RM, et al. Primary open angle glaucoma: inherited primary open angle glaucoma in the Beagle. Am J Pathol 1981;102:292–5.
31. Kuchtey J, Olson LM, Rinkoski T, et al. Mapping of the disease locus and identification of ADAMTS10 as a candidate gene in a canine model of primary open angle glaucoma. Plos Genet 2011;7(2):e1001306.
32. Oliver JA, Forman OP, Pettitt L, et al. Two independent mutations in ADAMTS17 are associated with primary open angle glaucoma in the Basset hound and Basset Fauve de Bretagne breeds of dog. PLoS One 2015;10:e0140436.
33. Oliver JA, Rustidge S, Pettit L, et al. Evaluation of ADAMTS17 in Chinese Shar-Pei with primary open-angle glaucoma, primary lens luxation, or both. Am J Vet Res 2018;79:98–106.

34. Ahonen SJ, Kaukonen M, Nussdorfer FD, et al. A novel missense mutation in ADAMTS10 in Norwegian elkhound primary glaucoma. PLoS One 2014;9(11): e111941.

35. Bedford PG. Open-angle glaucoma in the Petit Basset Griffon Vendeen. Vet Ophthalmol 2017;20:98–102.

36. Forman OP, Pettitt L, Komaromy AM, et al. A novel genome-wide association study approach using genotyping by exome sequencing leads to the identification of a primary open angle glaucoma associated inversion disrupting ADAMTS17. PLoS One 2015;10(12):e0143546.

37. Hart H, Samuelson DA, MacKay E, et al. Immunolocalization of MYOC protein within the anterior eye of normal and primary open-angle glaucomatous dogs. Invest Ophthalmol Vis Sci 2005;46(13):3697.

38. Kato K, Sasaki N, Matsunaga S, et al. Cloning of canine myocilin cDNA and molecular analysis of the myocilin gene in Shiba Inu dogs. Vet Ophthalmol 2007; 10(suppl 1):53–62.

39. Grahn BH, Peiffer RL. Veterinary ophthalmic pathology. In: Gelatt KN, editor. Vet Ophthalmol1, 6th edition. Hoboken: John Wiley & Sons; 2021. p. 479–563.

40. Ekesten B, Torrang I. Age-related changes in ocular distances of normal eyes of Samoyeds. Am J Vet Res 1995;56:127–33.

41. Bauer BS, Sandmeyer LS, Philbert H, et al. Chronic glaucoma in dogs: relationship between histologic lesions and the gonioscopic diagnosis of pectinate ligament dysplasia. Vet Path 2016;53:1197–203.

42. Whiteman AL, Klauss G, Miller PE, et al. Morphologic features of degeneration and cell death in the neurosensory retina in dogs with primary angle-closure glaucoma. Am J Vet Res 2002;63:257–61.

43. Almasieh M, Wilson AM, Morquette B, et al. Prog Ret Eye Res 2012;31:152–81.

44. Peiffer RL, Wilcock BP, Yin H. The pathogenesis and significance of preiridal fibrovascular membrane in domestic animals. Vet Pathol 1990;27:41–5.

45. Zarfoss MK, Breaux CB, Whiteley HE, et al. Canine pre-iridal fibrovascular membranes: morphologic and immunohistochemical investigations. Vet Ophthalmol 2010;13:4–13.

46. Sandberg CA, Herring IP, Huckle WR, et al. Aqueous humor vascular endothelial growth factor in dogs: association with intraocular disease and the development of pre-iridal fibrovascular membrane. Vet Ophthalmol 2012;15:21–30.

47. Lim CC, Bakker Sc, Waldner CL, et al. Cataracts in 44 dogs (77 eyes): a comparison of outcomes for no treatment, topical medical management, or phacoemulsification with intraocular lens implantation. Can Vet J 2011;52:283–8.

48. Refstrup Strom A, Hassig M, Iburg T, et al. Epidemiology of canine glaucoma presenting to the University of Zurich from 1995 to 2000. Part 2: secondary glaucoma (217 cases). Vet Ophthalmol 2011;14:127–32.

49. Curtis R, Barnett KC, Lewis SJ. Clinical and pathological observations concerning the etiology of primary lens luxation in the dog. Vet Rec 1983;12:238–46.

50. Alario AF, Pizzirani S, Pirie CG. Histopathologic evaluation of the anterior segment of eyes enucleated due to glaucoma secondary to primary lens displacement in 13 canine globes. Vet Ophthalmol 2013;16:34–41.

51. Pumphrey S. Canine secondary glaucomas. Vet Clin Small Anim 2015;45: 1335–64.

52. Gould D, Pettitt L, McLaughlin B, et al. ADAMTS17 mutation associated with primary lens luxation is widespread among breeds. Vet Ophthalmol 2011;14: 378–84.

53. Wilcock B, Peiffer RL. Morphology and behavior of primary ocular melanomas in 91 dogs. Vet Pathol 1986;23:418–24.
54. Dubielzig RR, Steinberg H, Garvin H, et al. Iridociliary epithelial tumors in 100 dogs and 17 cats: a morphological study. Vet Ophthalmol 1998;1:223–31.
55. Peterson-Jones SM, Forcier J, Mentzer AL. Ocular melanosis in the Cairn Terrier: clinical description and investigation of mode of inheritance. Vet Ophthalmol 2007;10:63–9, supp 1.
56. Peterson-Jones SM, Mentzer AL, Dubielzig RR, et al. Ocular melanosis in the Cairn Terrier: histopathological description of the condition, and immunohistological and ultrastructural characterization of the characteristic pigment-laden cells. Vet Ophthalmol 2008;11:260–8.
57. Van de Sandt RR, Boeve MH, Stades FC, et al. Abnormal ocular pigment deposition and glaucoma in the dog. Vet Ophthalmol 2003;6:273–8.
58. Holly VL, Sandmeyer LS, Bauer BS, et al. Golden retriever cystic uveal disease: a longitudinal study of iridociliary cysts, pigmentary uveitis, and pigmentary/cystic glaucoma over a decade in western Canada. Vet Ophthalmol 2016;19:237–44.
59. Spiess BM, Bolliger JO, Guscetti F, et al. Multiple ciliary body cysts and secondary glaucoma in the Great Dane: a report of nine cases. Vet Ophthalmol 1998;1:41–5.
60. Pumphrey SA, Pizzirani S, Pirie CG, et al. Glaucoma associated with uveal cysts in American Bulldogs: a case series. Vet Ophthalmol 2013;16:377–85.
61. Esson D, Armour M, Mundy P, et al. The histopathological and immunohistochemical characteristics of pigmentary and cystic glaucoma in the Golden Retriever. Vet Ophthalmol 2009;12:361–8.
62. Townsend WM, Huey JA, McCool E, et al. Golden retriever pigmentary uveitis: Challenges of diagnosis and treatment. Vet Ophthalmol 2020;3:774–84.
63. Townsend W, Gornik K. Prevalence of uveal cysts and pigmentary uveitis in Golden Retrievers in three midwestern states. J Am Vet Med Assoc 2013;243:1298–301.
64. Sapienza JS, Simo FJ, Prades-Sapienza A. Golden Retriever uveitis: 75 cases (1994–1999). Vet Ophthalmol 2000;3:241–6.
65. Deehr AJ, Dubielzig RR. A histopathological study of iridociliary cysts and glaucoma in Golden Retrievers. Vet Ophthalmol 1998;1:153–8.
66. Plummer CE, Regnier A, Gelatt KN. The canine glaucomas. In: Gelatt KN, Gilger BC, Kern TJ, editors. Veterinary ophthalmology. 5th edition. Ames (IA): Wiley-Blackwell; 2014. p. 1050–145.
67. Vainisi SJ, Wolfer JC, Hoffman AR. Surgery of the canine posterior segment. In: Gelatt KN, Gilger BC, Kern TJ, editors. Veterinary ophthalmology. 5th edition. Ames (IA): Wiley-Blackwell; 2014. p. 1393–431.
68. Quigley HA, Katz J, Derick RJ, et al. An evaluation of optic disc and nerve fiber layer examinations in monitoring progression of early glaucoma damage. Ophthalmology 1992;99:19–28.
69. Graham KL, McCowan CL, Caruso K, et al. Optical coherence tomography of the retina, nerve fiber layer, and optic nerve head in dogs with glaucoma. Vet Ophthalmol 2020;23:97–112.
70. Hasegawa T, Kawata M, Ota M. Ultrasound biomicroscopic findings of the iridocorneal angle in live healthy and glaucomatous dogs. J Vet Med Sci 2015;77:1625–31.
71. Miller PE, Schmidt GM, Vainisi SJ, et al. The efficacy of topical prophylactic anti-glaucoma therapy in primary closed angle glaucoma in dogs: a multicenter clinical trial. J Am Anim Hosp Assoc 2000;36:431–8.

72. Dees DD, Fritz KJ, Maclaren NE, et al. Efficacy of prophylactic antiglaucoma and anti-inflammatory medications in canine primary angle-closure glaucoma: a multi-center retrospective study (2004-2012). Vet Ophthalmol 2014;17:195–200.

73. Westermeyer HD, Hendrix DV, Ward DA. Long-term evaluation of the use of Ahmed gonioimplants in dogs with primary glaucoma: nine cases (2000-2008). J Am Vet Med Assoc 2011;238:610–7.

74. Palmberg P. The failing filtering bleb. Ophthalmol Clin North Am 2000;13(3):517–29.

75. Cullen CL. Cullen frontal sinus valved glaucoma shunt: preliminary findings in dogs with primary glaucoma. Vet Ophthalmol 2004;7:311–8.

76. Cullen CL, Allen AL, Grahn BH. Anterior chamber to frontal sinus shunt for the diversion of aqueous humor: a pilot study in four normal dogs. Vet Ophthalmol 1998;1:31–9.

77. Graham KL, Donaldson D, Billson FA, et al. Use of a 350-mm^2 Baerveldt glaucoma drainage device to maintain vision and control intraocular pressure in dogs with glaucoma: a retrospective study (2013-2016). Vet Ophthalmol 2017;20:427–34.

78. Graham KL, Hall E, Caraguel C, et al. Comparison of diode laser transscleral cyclophotocoagulation versus implantation of a 350-mm2 Baerveldt glaucoma drainage device for the treatment of glaucoma in dogs (a retrospective study: 2010-2016). Vet Ophthalmol 2018;21:487–97.

79. Bentley E, Nasisse MP, Glover T, et al. Implantation of filtering devices in dogs with glaucoma: preliminary results in 13 eyes. Vet Comp Ophthalmol 1996;6:43–6.

80. Tinsley DM, Betts DM. Clinical experience with a glaucoma drainage device in dogs. Vet Comp Ophthalmol 1994;4:77–84.

81. Nassise M, Davidson M, McLachian N, et al. Neodymium:yttrium, aluminum, and garnet laser energy delivered transsclerally to the ciliary body of dogs. Am J Vet Res 1988;49. 1972–8.

82. Sapienza J, Miller T, Gum G, et al. Contact transscleral cyclophotocoagulation using a neodymium:yttrium aluminum garnet laser in normal dogs. Prog Vet Comp Ophthalmol 1992;2:147–53.

83. Nassise M, Davidson M, English R, et al. Treatment of glaucoma by use of transscleral neodymium:yttrium aluminum garnet laser cyclocoagulation in dogs. J Am Vet Med Assoc 1990;197:350–3.

84. Cook C, Davidson M, Brinkmann M, et al. Diode laser transscleral cyclophotocoagulation for the treatment of glaucoma in dogs: results of six and twelve months follow-up. Vet Comp Ophthalmol 1997;7:148–54.

85. Hardman C, Stanley R. Diode laser transscleral cyclophotocoagulation for the treatment of primary glaucoma in 18 dogs: a retrospective study. Vet Ophthalmol 2001;4:209–15.

86. Lutz EA, Sapeinza J. Diode endoscopic cyclophotocoagulation in pseudophakic and aphakic dogs with secondary glaucoma. Vet Ophthalmol 2008;11:423.

87. Bras D, Maggio F. Surgical treatment of canine glaucoma: cyclodestructive techniques. Vet Clin Small Anim 2015;45:1283–305.

88. Naranjo C, Dubielzig RR. Histopathological study of the causes for failure of intrascleral prostheses in dogs and cats. Vet Ophthalmol 2014;17:343–50.

89. Blocker T, Hoffman A, Schaeffer DJ, et al. Corneal sensitivity and aqueous tear production in dogs undergoing evisceration with intrascleral prosthesis placement. Vet Ophthalmol 2007;10:147–54.

90. Bingaman DP, Lindley DM, Glickman NW, et al. Intraocular gentamicin and glaucoma: a retrospective study of 60 dog and cat eyes (1985-1993). Vet Comp Ophthalmol 1994;4:113–9.

91. Low MC, Landis ML, Peiffer RL. Intravitreal cidofovir injection for the management of chronic glaucoma in dogs. Vet Ophthalmol 2014;17:201–6.

92. Tripathy K, Chwala R, Temkar S, et al. Phthisis Bulbi – a clinicopathological perspective. Semin Ophthalmol 2018;33:788–803.

93. Duke FD, Strong TD, Bentley E, et al. Canine ocular tumors following ciliary body ablation with intravitreal gentamicin. Vet Ophthalmol 2013;16:159–62.

94. Smith RIE, Peiffer RL, Wilcock BP. Some aspects of the pathology of canine glaucoma. Prog Vet Comp Ophthalmol 1993;3:16–28.

95. Scott EM, Boursiquot N, Beltran WA, et al. Early histopathologic changes in the retina and optic nerve in canine primary angle-closure glaucoma. Vet Ophthalmol 2013;16(suppl 1):79–86.

96. Mangan BG, Al-Yahya K, Chen CT, et al. Retinal pigment epithelial damage, breakdown of the blood-retinal barrier, and retinal inflammation in dogs with primary glaucoma. Vet Ophthalmol 2007;10(suppl 1):117–24.

97. Bedos L, Grahn BH, Philibert H, et al. Histologic, immunohistochemical, and scanning electron microscopic comparison of pre-iridal monocellular and fibrovascular membranes in normal and glaucomatous canine globes. Vet Ophthalmol 2021;24:361–73.

98. Grahn BH, Barnes LD, Breaux CB, et al. Chronic retinal detachment and giant retinal tears in 34 dogs: outcome comparison of no treatment, topical medical therapy, and retinal reattachment after vitrectomy. Can Vet J 2007 Oct;48:1031–9.

99. Morris RA, Dubielzig RR. Light-microscopy evaluation of zonular fiber morphology in dogs with glaucoma: secondary to lens displacement. Vet Ophthalmol 2005;8:81–4.

Glaucoma Associated with Anterior Segment Dysgenesis in Dogs and Cats

Marina L. Leis*, Bruce Grahn

KEYWORDS

- Anterior segment dysgenesis • Congenital glaucoma • Canine • Feline

KEY POINTS

- Glaucoma associated with anterior segment dysgenesis (ASD) presents similarly in both dogs and cats within the first few years of life.
- Characterization of the clinical and histopathologic manifestations of glaucoma associated with ASD is challenging due to the paucity of reports in the veterinary literature.
- Ophthalmologists and pathologists should be familiar with the clinical and histopathologic framework needed to make a diagnosis of ASD-associated glaucoma.
- An established breeding colony has facilitated the study of congenital glaucoma in cats caused by a specific mutation in the LTBP2 gene.

DEFINITIONS

Anterior segment dysgenesis: a sporadic, congenital syndrome presenting at birth with a constellation of anomalies including but not limited to filtration angle and anterior uveal hypoplasia, iris to lens and iris to cornea persistent pupillary membranes, elongated ciliary processes, microphakia, lenticonus, and cataract.

Glaucoma: elevation of intraocular pressure secondary to reduced aqueous outflow via the trabecular meshwork and uveoscleral pathways.

Congenital glaucoma: glaucoma present at birth or within the first year of life occurring because of ASD.

Anterior segment dysgenesis associated glaucoma: later onset (>1 year), juvenile glaucoma occurring because of ASD.

Introduction

Glaucoma in dogs and cats is a group of conditions characterized by elevations of intraocular pressure due to limited aqueous humor outflow through the trabecular

These authors have no commercial or financial conflicts of interest to disclose.
Western College of Veterinary Medicine, 52 Campus Drive, Saskatoon, Saskatchewan S7N 5B4, Canada
* Corresponding author.
E-mail address: marina.leis@usask.ca

meshwork and uveoscleral pathway. The resulting changes in the retinal ganglion cells and optic nerve caused by sustained increases in intraocular pressure ultimately lead to irreversible vision loss and pain. Globe enlargement (buphthalmos), filtration angle recession, corneal opacification secondary to exposure keratitis, and optic nerve and retinal and vitreous degeneration are the product of chronic, end-stage glaucoma, and are not specific to the underlying etiologic diagnosis.

Glaucoma has been categorized according to etiologic diagnosis (primary glaucoma, secondary glaucoma, congenital glaucoma), by gonioscopic appearance of the filtration angle (open, closed, narrow iridocorneal angle, and/or ciliary cleft), and finally by stage of disease (acute, chronic). Although primary and secondary glaucoma have been well characterized in companion animal species due to their relative higher frequency, reports of congenital glaucoma in veterinary medicine are sparse.[1–6]

Congenital glaucoma in veterinary species has conventionally been thought to present within the first year of life and be associated with multiple anomalies of the anterior segment (anterior segment dysgenesis [ASD]).[1,4–6] Causes of ASD are often idiopathic, related to genetic mutations, or result from in utero exposure to nutritional deficiencies, toxins, or infectious agents.[7] Microscopic manifestations include varying degrees of ASD including ciliary and filtration angle hypoplasia, elongated ciliary processes, incomplete separation of the lens from the cornea, and dysplastic uveal tissue that attaches to the corneal stroma where endothelium and Descemet's membrane are lacking (Peter's anomaly).[7,8] Congenital glaucoma results in either unilateral or bilateral disease, and the affected eye may be blind or sighted. Intraocular pressure is usually elevated (>30 mm Hg); however, it may be normal or even low related to buphthalmos and scleral thinning. Vitreous degeneration, retinal degeneration, and optic nerve degeneration may be present as the result of sustained elevations of intraocular pressure occurring in utero or within the perinatal period.[8]

Given the variety of presentations for ASD, clinical classification and description of ASD in veterinary ophthalmology remains challenging. Combine this with a paucity of reports in the literature, and it becomes clear that there are large knowledge gaps not only regarding the differing clinical presentations of ASD but also regarding what forms of ASD lead to the development of glaucoma.

Embryology of the Anterior Segment and Dysgenesis

Anterior segment dysgenesis disorders manifest with abnormalities of the cornea, iris, ciliary body, anterior chamber, and/or lens. Changes are caused by a lack of induction and differentiation of neural crest and surface ectoderm tissues or an obstruction to migration by delayed separation of the lens from surface ectoderm.[7] Normally, following the formation of the embryonic optic cup and separation of the lens vesicle from surface ectoderm at day 25 in the dog, cells from the posterior portion of the lens vesicle give rise to the primary lens fibers, and the cells from the anterior portion of the lens vesicle give rise to secondary lens fibers.[9] The mesenchyme anterior to the developing lens divides into 2 layers where the outer mesenchymal layer eventually forms the corneal stroma.[9] The corneal epithelium develops from surface ectoderm, the corneal endothelium develops from neural crest cells, and mesenchyme forms the iridopupillary membrane, which must regress in order to form the pupil.[9] The epithelium of the iris and the ciliary body originates from the optic cup (neuroectoderm), the stroma of the iris and the ciliary body originates from neural crest cells, the iris dilator and sphincter muscles develop from neuroectoderm, and the ciliary muscle develops from mesenchyme.[9]

Embryologic errors at these critical steps results in differing presentations of ASD including microphakia (small lens), spherophakia (round lens), lenticonus (abnormal anterior or posterior lens shape) cataract, a failure of the iris and cornea to separate, microcornea, and corneal opacification.[7,9] When present, uveal and filtration angle hypoplasia may contribute to the development of congenital glaucoma.[7] Both clinical and histological interpretations of the filtration angle are challenging or impossible due to marked angle recession secondary to tissue stretching and buphthalmos.[7,10]

Congenital and Developmental Glaucoma in Humans

Primary congenital glaucoma in humans is relatively uncommon and has been divided into different subtypes depending on the age of onset.[11–13] In true congenital or newborn glaucoma, individuals are born with an enlarged globe or globe enlargement within the first month of life. Infantile glaucoma and juvenile glaucoma manifest within 1 to 36 months and after 3 years of age, respectively. Although the majority of cases seem to be sporadic, several autosomal recessive mutations are reported to be responsible for disease development and the disease is more commonly apparent in consanguineous populations.[11,13]

A second approach to the classification of congenital glaucoma in pediatric patients is based on the type of anterior segment anomalies.[12] In its least severe form, trabeculodysgenesis refers to dysgenesis of the trabecular meshwork only.[12] Iridotrabeculodysgenesis refers to uveal hypoplasia, anomalous iridal vessels, or uveal defects (colobomas or aniridia).[12] The more severe forms of ASD are under the umbrella of corneotrabeculodysgenesis, which includes syndromes such as Axenfeld-Rieger anomaly and Peter's anomaly. Within the syndromes Axenfeld-Rieger anomaly and Peter's anomaly, several subcategories have been described. In short, Axenfeld-Rieger anomaly is most commonly bilateral and presents with varying degrees of iridal abnormalities including hypoplasia, polycoria (more than one pupil), colobomas, filtration angle abnormalities, and congenital systemic anomalies including heart and dental defects.[11,14] Peter's anomaly can be unilateral or bilateral, and is characterized by adhesions of the iris and cornea and a central corneal opacity associated with a defect in the corneal endothelium and Descemet membrane, and can be present with concomitant congenital ocular and systemic lesions.[15] Regardless of the type and subtype of ASD, all affected individuals are considered high risk for the development of glaucoma.

Anterior Segment Dysgenesis Associated Glaucoma in the Dog

ASD in dogs is underreported and manifests sporadically as a spectrum of disease. Peter's anomaly has been reported in a Springer Spaniel having iris-to-cornea persistent pupillary membranes and a corneal leukoma where Descemet's membrane and corneal endothelium were lacking.[16] Persistent pupillary membranes, congenital cataract, and a range of other anterior segment anomalies have been reported in a Basenji, Saint Bernard, and Cocker Spaniel.[2,17,18] These initial investigations do not thoroughly describe the appearance of the filtration angles nor the presence of glaucoma, either clinically or histopathologically.

In a more recent histologic study of Portuguese Water Dogs with multiple anterior segment defects, 15/32 eyes demonstrated a lack of both ciliary cleft and trabecular meshwork with or without an identifiable scleral venous plexus.[19] In this study, only one dog is described to have retinal changes consistent with glaucoma; however, the authors acknowledge that a detailed examination of the retina was not always possible and that they likely underdiagnosed glaucoma.[19] An additional limitation of the study was the lack of correlation with the clinical findings at the time of ophthalmic examination. Conversely, another recent, purely clinical study that lacked histopathologic data reported 4 cases of congenital glaucoma in dogs aged less than 1 year.[1] Of these 4 cases, only 2 were reported to have features consistent with ASD, again underscoring the paucity of well-described literature in this area.

Anterior Segment Dysgenesis Associated Glaucoma in the Cat

Similar to dogs, reports of domestic cats with spontaneously occurring ASD and congenital glaucoma are rare. Bilateral ASD including Peter's anomaly in a 7-month-old cat was associated with congenital glaucoma in one eye but not the other.[20] A young Siamese cat with bilateral congenital glaucoma was described to have an open iridocorneal angle and ciliary cleft in both eyes and an apparently normal appearance of the uveal trabecular meshwork.[3] The authors concluded that the cause of the glaucoma was due to the corneoscleral trabecular meshwork that was markedly compressed.[3] Anterior segment dysgenesis associated glaucoma has also been reported to present concurrently with an avascular peripheral retina, gliosis, and epiretinal neovascularization of the central retina, which the authors termed "feline neovascular retinopathy."[21] In this report, the authors acknowledge that the cause underlying glaucoma in these cases could also be secondary to peripheral anterior synechiae and intraocular inflammation.[21]

The most thoroughly investigated type of feline congenital glaucoma stems from a breeding colony of Siamese cats.[22–24] This colony originated from a cat with spontaneously occurring congenital glaucoma, has an autosomal recessive and fully penetrant mode of inheritance, and is associated with a point mutation in the LTBP2 gene.[22] In this subtype of feline congenital glaucoma, elevated intraocular pressure, buphthalmos and elongated ciliary processes occur by 8 weeks of age.[22,25] Gonioscopy typically reveals an open or slightly narrowed iridocorneal angle, with subtle dysplasia of the pectinate ligament. Ultrasound biomicroscopy of the anterior segment reveals severe narrowing of the ciliary cleft.[26] Other clinical features observed in affected animals include prominent, elongated ciliary processes, spherophakia, iris hypoplasia, and iridodonesis (trembling of the iris).[22] Light microscopy reveals the presence of few intrascleral blood vessels, hypoplasia of the iris stroma and ciliary body, elongated ciliary processes, and trabecular meshwork and angular aqueous plexus hypoplasia.[22] As expected with chronic glaucoma, inner retinal degeneration and optic nerve atrophy are observed.[22]

UPDATE ON ANTERIOR SEGMENT DYSGENESIS–ASSOCIATED GLAUCOMA IN DOGS AND CATS: CASE SERIES REVIEW

Given the scarcity of reports regarding glaucoma associated with ASD in veterinary ophthalmology, we sought to review the clinical, gross, and histopathological findings among dog and cat submissions to the Prairie Ocular Pathology Service at the Western College of Veterinary Medicine. Cases included canines and felines aged less than 3 years with histopathological changes consistent with glaucoma defined by the presence of loss of retinal ganglion cells, inner retinal degeneration, and optic nerve atrophy. Cases included also had histopathology consistent with ASD defined by the presence of one or more of the following congenital anomalies: uveal and filtration angle hypoplasia, elongated ciliary processes, ciliary hypoplasia, microphakia, spherophakia, and uveal adhesion to the corneal stroma where endothelium and Descemet membrane were lacking. Five age-matched dogs diagnosed with secondary glaucoma served as a control group. Age matching was not possible for cats and therefore 6 adult cats with secondary glaucoma served as controls.

All globes were sectioned and stained with hematoxylin-eosin and periodic acid–Schiff. It remains challenging to differentiate between uveal hypoplasia and atrophy

Table 1
Histopathologic findings for 17 dogs with congenital glaucoma

Case	Signalment	Uveal Hypoplasia	Thin and Elongated Ciliary Processes	Filtration Angle Hypoplasia	Filtration Angle Recession	Corneal Opacification or Striae	Microphakia	Cataract	Comments	Lens Surface Area (mm²)
1	Boxer X (3 m; MI)	X	X		X	X				No lens visible in block
2	Chinese Pug (5 m; MI)	X	X		X	X			Fused iris and corneal tissue	No lens visible in block
3	Great Dane (12 m; FI)	X	X		X	X	X			54.5
4	Golden retriever (18 m; MN)	X	X	X		X	X	X		54.2
5	Bouvier des Flandres X (12 m; FI)	X	X		X	X	X			37.9
6	Samoyed (4 m; MI)	X	X		X	X	X			29.3
7	Newfoundland (8 m; MI)	X	X		X	X				Lens improperly sectioned
8	Unknown breed (12 m; FS)	X	X		X	X	X	X		32.2
9	Husky (5 m; MN)	X	X		X	X				No lens visible in block
10	Bull terrier (24 m; FI)	X	X		X	X	X		PPM to cornea	51.0
11–1OD	English springer spaniel (12 m; MI)	X	X		X	X			Dysplastic retina	38.2

(continued on next page)

Table 1
(continued)

Case	Signalment	Uveal Hypoplasia	Thin and Elongated Ciliary Processes	Filtration Angle Hypoplasia	Filtration Angle Recession	Corneal Opacification or Striae	Microphakia	Cataract	Comments	Lens Surface Area (mm²)
11–2OS	English springer spaniel (12 m; MI)	X	X		X	X			Dysplastic retina	Lens improperly sectioned
12	Afghan hound (36 m; FS)	X	X	X	X	X				42.6
13	Welsh springer spaniel X (12 m; MN)	X	X		X	X	X	X	Iris-iris PPM	51.4
14	Poodle (9 m; MN)	X	X		X	X	X	X		24.9
15	Husky (35 m; MN)	X	X		X	X	X			53.0
16–1 OD	Australian shepherd X (36 m; FS)	X	X	X		X	X			50
16–2 OS	Australian shepherd X (36 m; FS)	X	X	X		X	X			39.8
17	Shih tzu (3 m; FI)	X	X		X	X	X		Inflammation in filtration angle	39.3

Abbreviations: FI, female intact; FS, female spayed; MI, male intact; MN, male neutered; OD, right eye; OS, left eye; PPM, persistent pupillary membranes.

in globes with chronic intraocular pressure elevation; therefore, we labeled sections with smooth muscle actin to help distinguish between the two. In addition, although microphakia is often reported clinically, it is a subjective assessment, therefore when quality sections of the lens were available, we measured lens surface area of fixed globes within the wax block using Image-Pro Premier Image Analysis software (Meyer Instruments Inc, Houston TX). Sections were evaluated under light microscopy by a board-certified pathologist and board-certified ophthalmologist. Data were determined to be parametric and using SPSS Statistics (IBM SPSS Statistics Version 24), a standardized unpaired t-test was used to determine the statistical significance of lens size variation between ASD associated and secondary glaucomatous globes, with P less than .05 being considered significant.

Canines

Clinical findings in dogs with anterior segment dysgenesis–associated glaucoma

A total of 17 canine cases met the inclusion criteria corresponding to ASD and glaucoma where it was unilateral in 15 and bilateral in 2 dogs. The average age at enucleation in dogs with glaucoma associated with ASD was 16 months (range = 3–36 months). There were 10 males (5/10 neutered) and 7 females (3/7spayed). Breeds affected included a boxer cross (n = 1), Chinese pug (n = 1), great Dane (n = 1), golden retriever (n = 1), Bouvier des Flandres cross (n = 1), Samoyed (n = 1), Newfoundland (n = 1), Siberian husky (n = 2), bull terrier (n = 1), English springer spaniel (n = 1), Afghan hound (n = 1), Welsh springer spaniel cross, standard poodle (n = 1), Australian shepherd cross, shih tzu (n = 1), and one dog of unknown breed (**Table 1**). Clinical examination findings in dogs with glaucoma associated with ASD varied. Elevated intraocular pressures that could not be controlled with medical therapy were noted in all cases (17/17) and other clinical findings recorded included buphthalmos (4/17), corneal edema (4/17), uveitis (3/17), cataract (3/17), and lens luxation/instability (2/16) (**Fig. 1A**).

Five dogs diagnosed with secondary glaucoma affected unilaterally were enucleated at an average age of 28 months (range = 7 months to 36 months). There were 4 females (2/4 spayed) and 1 male. Breeds affected included a Rottweiler (n = 1), French bulldog cross (n = 1), American bulldog (n = 1), Labrador retriever (n = 1), and Labrador retriever cross (n = 1; **Table 2**). Dogs with secondary glaucoma presented following a suspected traumatic event to the globe (2/5), uveitis (2/5), or an ocular tumor noted before enucleation (1/5).

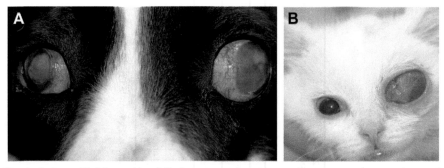

Fig. 1. A dog with bilateral buphthalmos secondary to anterior segment dysgenesis associated glaucoma (*A*) and a kitten with unilateral buphthalmos secondary to congenital glaucoma (*B*). Exposure keratitis is a common feature of globe enlargement.

Table 2
Histopathologic findings for 5 dogs with secondary glaucoma

Case	Signalment	Corneal Edema	Corneal Ulceration	Inflammatory Infiltrate into Filtration Angle	Lens Rupture	Comments	Lens Surface Area (mm²)
18	Rottweiler (23 m; FI)	X	X		X		No lens visible in block
19	French bulldog (7 m; FI)	X		X	X		No lens visible in block
20	Labrador retriever (36 m; FS)					Iridociliary adenocarcinoma	No lens visible in block
21	American bulldog (36 m; FS)	X		X		Ciliary body atrophy	54.4
22	Labrador retriever (36 m; MN)	X		X			53.8

Abbreviations: FI, female intact; FS, female spayed; MI, male intact; MN, male neutered.

Histopathologic findings in dogs with anterior segment dysgenesis–associated glaucoma

Consistent changes noted on histological evaluation of canine globes with glaucoma associated with ASD included corneal edema, vascularization, scarring, or striae (19/19), incomplete separation of the lens and cornea (1/19; **Fig. 2A**), elongated ciliary processes (19/19), ciliary hypoplasia (19/19), hypoplastic (15/19) or recessed (4/19) filtration angles, and retinal/choroidal atrophy (19/19; **Fig. 3**). Minimal smooth muscle actin immunoreactivity was noted in ciliary bodies associated with elongated ciliary processes in all globes, consistent with ciliary muscle hypoplasia (see **Fig. 3D**).

In contrast, control globes with secondary glaucoma presented clinically with a corneal laceration or ulcer (1/5), an iridociliary adenocarcinoma (1/5), and uveitis (3/5). Histologic manifestations included lens rupture (2/5), endophthalmitis (3/5; **Fig. 4A**), and glaucomatous retinal and uveal atrophy (5/5). Smooth muscle actin highlighted the presence of multiple layers of smooth muscle in all ciliary bodies under the ciliary processes despite mild glaucomatous atrophy (**Fig. 4B**). The average lens surface area in globes with ASD-associated glaucoma was 42.7 mm^2 (range = 24.9–54.5 mm^2), whereas the average lens surface area in globes with secondary glaucoma was 54.1 mm^2 (range = 53.8–54.4 mm^2; P = .13; see **Tables 1** and **2**).

Felines

Clinical findings in cats with anterior segment dysgenesis–associated glaucoma

A total of 9 feline cases affected unilaterally met the inclusion criteria for glaucoma associated with ASD. The average age at enucleation was 18 months (range = 2–36 months), and there were 6 neutered males and 3 females (2/3 spayed). Breeds affected included domestic shorthairs (n = 6), the domestic medium hair (n = 1), and 2 did not have a recorded breed (**Table 3**). Cats most commonly presented clinically with signs of buphthalmos (7/9) and corneal ulceration/perforation (5/9; **Fig. 1B**).

For cats with secondary glaucoma, the average age at enucleation was 11.7 years (range = 9–15 years). The majority of cases were male [n = 5; (5/5 neutered)] as compared with female [n = 1; (1/1 spayed)]. Breeds affected included domestic shorthairs (n = 4), a Siamese cross (n = 1), and a domestic longhair (n = 1; **Table 4**). Secondary glaucoma was unilateral in 5 and bilateral in 1 of these cats. Cats with secondary glaucoma presented clinically with uveitis, vitritis, or endophthalmitis (4/6), and lens luxation (4/6).

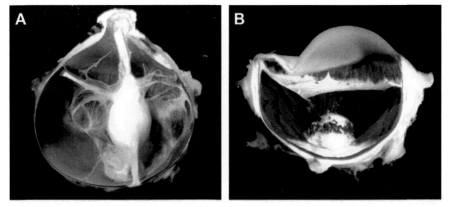

Fig. 2. Gross images demonstrating incomplete separation of the lens from the cornea in a dog (*A*) and elongated ciliary processes in a cat (*B*) affected by ASD-associated glaucoma.

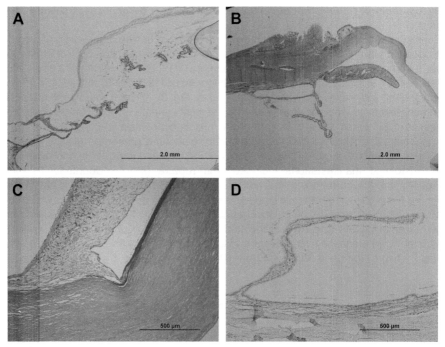

Fig. 3. H&E section illustrating elongated ciliary processes (*A*) and hypoplastic filtration angles (*B, C*) in dogs with glaucoma associated with ASD. Smooth muscle actin-labeled section demonstrating ciliary hypoplasia in a dog with ASD-associated glaucoma (*D*).

Histopathologic findings in cats with anterior segment dysgenesis–associated glaucoma

Consistent findings on gross sections included buphthalmos with filtration angle recession, microphakia, and elongated ciliary processes (**Fig. 2**B). Histological evaluation of feline globes with ASD-associated glaucoma revealed corneal opacification (9/9), elongated hypoplastic ciliary processes (9/9), hypoplastic uvea (9/9), mild-to-moderate glaucomatous retinal atrophy (9/9), hypoplastic filtration angles (3/9), and

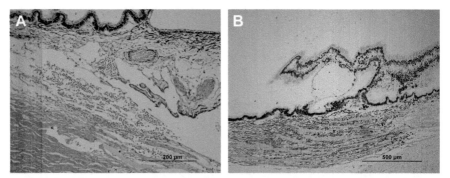

Fig. 4. H&E section revealing neutrophilic infiltration of the iris, ciliary body, and filtration angle in a dog with secondary glaucoma (*A*) and section of normal, robust musculature of the ciliary body in a dog with secondary glaucoma as labeled by smooth muscle actin (*B*).

Table 3
Histopathologic findings for 9 cats with congenital glaucoma

Case	Signalment	Uveal Hypoplasia	Thin and Elongated Ciliary Processes	Filtration Angle Hypoplasia	Filtration Angle Recession	Corneal Opacification or Striae	Microphakia	Cataract	Comments	Lens Surface Area (mm²)
23	DSH (2 m; MN)	X	X		X	X	X		Mild stromal melting	50.3
24	DMH (12 m; FS)	X	X	X		X			Dysplastic uvea attached to cornea	No lens visible in block
25	Feline (24 m; MN)	X	X		X	X		X	Spherophakia	79.4
26	DSH (18 m; MN)	X	X		X	X				No lens visible in block
27	Feline (36 m; MN)	X	X		X	X				62.3
28	DSH (24 m; MN)	X	X		X	X				76.8
29	DSH (19 m; FS)	X	X	X		X			Lens improperly sectioned	
30	DSH (19 m; MN)	X	X	X		X	X			10.0
31	DSH (5 m; FI)	X	X			X	X		Filtration angle open with mild inflammatory infiltrate	55.5

Abbreviations: DMH, domestic medium hair; DSH, domestic shorthair; FI, female intact; FS, female spayed; MI, male intact; MN, male neutered.

Table 4
Histopathologic findings for 6 cats with secondary glaucoma

Case	Signalment	Corneal Edema	Inflammatory Infiltrate into Filtration Angle	Cataract	Endophthalmitis	Lens Surface Area (mm²)
32	DSH (108 m; MN)	X	X		X	76.9
33	Siamese X (132 m; FS)	X	X	X	X	82.2
34	DSH (132 m; MN)	X	X		X	100.7
35	DSH (120 m; MN)	X	X	X	X	120.6
36	DLH (168 m; MN)	X	X		X	74.7
37	DSH (180 m; MN)	X	X	X	X	77.7

Abbreviations: DLH, domestic longhair; DMH, domestic medium hair; DSH, domestic shorthair; FI, female intact; FS, female spayed; MI, male intact; MN, male neutered.

marked angle recession (5/9; **Fig. 5**). Minimal smooth muscle actin immunoreactivity was noted in ciliary bodies and ciliary processes in all globes (see **Fig. 5**D).

Feline globes with secondary glaucoma commonly had corneal edema (6/6), open filtration angles with inflammatory cells that extended into the ciliary cleft (6/6), endophthalmitis or panophthalmitis (6/6), and glaucomatous retinal and optic nerve atrophy (6/6; **Fig. 6**). Smooth muscle actin highlighted the robust presence of smooth

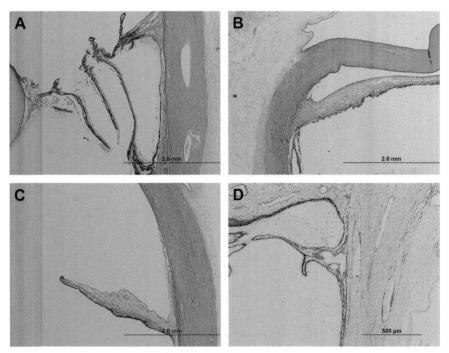

Fig. 5. H&E sections depicting elongated ciliary processes (*A*), hypoplastic filtration angle (*B*), and angle recession (*C*) in cats with anterior segment dysgenesis associated glaucoma. Uveal hypoplasia is also a consistent feature as illustrated in this section labeled with smooth muscle actin (*D*).

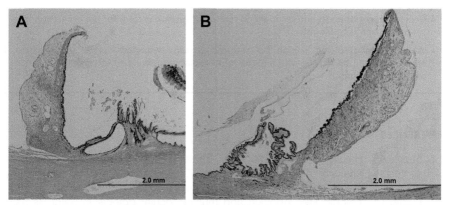

Fig. 6. H&E section of a feline globe with secondary glaucoma showing an open filtration angle infiltrated with lymphocytic, plasmacytic inflammation that extends into the ciliary cleft (*A*). Smooth muscle actin-labeled section highlighting normal and robust smooth ciliary musculature in a cat with secondary glaucoma, despite glaucomatous atrophy (*B*).

muscle in all ciliary bodies and processes, even in the presence of glaucomatous atrophy (see **Fig. 6**B). The average lens surface area in globes with glaucoma associated with ASD was 55.7 mm^2 (range = 10–79.4 mm^2) and was significantly smaller than the average lens surface area in globes with secondary glaucoma [88.8 mm^2 (range = 74.7–100.7 mm^2)] (*P* = .01; see **Tables 3** and **4**).

SUMMARY

The varying clinical and histopathologic presentations of sporadic ASD presented herein add to the body of evidence that ASD in dogs and cats represents a disease spectrum rather than a single disease entity and puts affected animals at risk of glaucoma development within the first years of life. Because overt signs of glaucoma such as elevated intraocular pressure and globe enlargement do not necessarily occur at birth or even within the first year, the term congenital glaucoma can be misleading. For this reason, it is preferred to designate the term "glaucoma associated ASD" for cases with a later (>1 year), juvenile onset of glaucoma presenting with compatible clinical and histopathologic signs of ASD.

Specifically, the anterior segment anomalies that put the neonatal or juvenile dog or cat at significant risk for the development of glaucoma are filtration angle and anterior uveal hypoplasia, elongated ciliary processes, and microphakia. Globe enlargement, exposure keratopathy, filtration angle recession, and retinal and optic nerve atrophy are present in glaucoma associated with ASD as a direct result of sustained elevated intraocular pressure, similar to other underlying causes of glaucoma.

CLINICS CARE POINTS

- Congenital and anterior segment dysgenesis–associated glaucoma may present unilaterally or bilaterally, and the affected eye(s) may be blind
- A constellation of concomitant anterior segment anomalies will be present such as filtration angle and anterior uveal hypoplasia, elongated ciliary processes, and microphakia
- Intraocular pressure is usually elevated (>30 mm Hg), or may be normal to low owing to buphthalmos and scleral thinning

- General practitioners should recommend referral of suspicious cases for the evaluation by a veterinary ophthalmologist
- When clinical suspicion is high for anterior segment dysgenesis–associated glaucoma, enucleation and submission of the globe for histopathology will be both therapeutic and confirm the diagnosis

REFERENCES

1. Strom AR, Hassig M, Iburg TM, et al. Epidemiology of canine glaucoma presented to University of Zurich from 1995 to 2009. Part 1: Congenital and primary glaucoma (4 and 123 cases). Vet Ophthalmol 2011;14(2):121–6.
2. Martin CL, Leipold HW. Aphakia and multiple ocular defects in Saint Bernard puppies. Vet Med Small Anim Clin 1974;69(4):448–53.
3. Brown A, Munger R, Peiffer RL. Congenital glaucoma and iridoschisis in a Siamese cat. Vet Comp Ophthalmol 1994;4(3):121–4.
4. Gelatt KN, Brooks DE, Kallberg ME. The canine glaucomas. Essentials Vet Ophthalmol 2008;2:155–87.
5. Cullen CL, Grahn BH. Congenital glaucoma in a llama (Lama glama). Vet Comp Ophthalmol 1997;7(4):253–7.
6. Halenda RM, Grahn BH, Sorden SD, et al. Congenital equine glaucoma: clinical and light microscopic findings in two cases. Vet Comp Ophthalmol 1997;7(2):105–9.
7. Grahn BH, Peiffer RL. Fundamentals of veterinary ophthalmic pathology. In: Gelatt KN, editor. Veterinary ophthalmology. 6th edition. NJ: Blackwell Publishing; 2007.
8. Grahn B, Peiffer R, Wilcock B. Histologic basis of ocular disease in animals. NJ: John Wiley & Sons; 2018.
9. Cook CS. Ocular Embryology and Congenital Malformations. In: Gelatt KN, editor. Veterinary ophthalmology. 4th ed. Blackwell Publishing; 2007. p. 3–36, chap 1.
10. Bauer BS, Sandmeyer LS, Philibert H, et al. Chronic Glaucoma in Dogs: Relationships Between Histologic Lesions and the Gonioscopic Diagnosis of Pectinate Ligament Dysplasia. Vet Pathol 2016;53(6):1197–203.
11. Lewis CJ, Hedberg-Buenz A, DeLuca AP, et al. Primary congenital and developmental glaucomas. Hum Mol Genet 2017;26(R1):R28–36.
12. Kaur K, Gurnani B. Primary congenital glaucoma. St Petersburg, FL: StatPearls; 2022.
13. Mocan MC, Mehta AA, Aref AA. Update in Genetics and Surgical Management of Primary Congenital Glaucoma. Turk J Ophthalmol 2019;49(6):347–55.
14. Zamora EA, Salini B. Axenfeld-rieger syndrome. St Petersburg FL: StatPearls; 2022.
15. Bhandari R, Ferri S, Whittaker B, et al. Peters anomaly: review of the literature. Cornea 2011;30(8):939–44.
16. Swanson HL, Dubielzig RR, Bentley E, et al. A case of Peters' anomaly in a springer spaniel. J Comp Pathol 2001;125(4):326–30.
17. Strande A, Nicolaissen B, Bjerkas I. Persistent pupillary membrane and congenital cataract in a litter of English cocker spaniels. J Small Anim Pract 1988;29(4):257–60.
18. Barnett KC, Knight GC. Persistent pupillary membrane and associated defects in the Basenji. Vet Rec 1969;85(9):242–8.

19. Shaw GC, Tse MPY, Miller AD. Microphthalmia with multiple anterior segment defects in portuguese water dogs. Vet Pathol 2019;56(2):269–73.
20. Park S, Kim K, Kim Y, et al. Bilateral ASD with the presumed Peters' anomaly in a cat. J Vet Med Sci 2018;80(2):297–301.
21. Beckwith-Cohen B, Hoffman A, McLellan GJ, et al. Feline Neovascular Vitreoretinopathy and ASD With Concurrent Glaucoma in Domestic Cats. Vet Pathol 2019; 56(2):259–68.
22. Kuehn MH, Lipsett KA, Menotti-Raymond M, et al. A Mutation in LTBP2 Causes Congenital Glaucoma in Domestic Cats (Felis catus). PLoS One 2016;11(5): e0154412.
23. Snyder KC, Oikawa K, Williams J, et al. Imaging Distal Aqueous Outflow Pathways in a Spontaneous Model of Congenital Glaucoma. Transl Vis Sci Technol 2019;8(5):22.
24. Telle MR, Chen N, Shinsako D, et al. Relationship between corneal sensitivity, corneal thickness, corneal diameter, and intraocular pressure in normal cats and cats with congenital glaucoma. Vet Ophthalmol 2019;22(1):4–12.
25. McLellan GJ, Miller PE. Feline glaucoma–a comprehensive review. Vet Ophthalmol 2011;14(Suppl 1):15–29.
26. Gomes FE, Bentley E, Lin TL, et al. Effects of unilateral topical administration of 0.5% tropicamide on anterior segment morphology and intraocular pressure in normal cats and cats with primary congenital glaucoma. Vet Ophthalmol 2011; 14(Suppl 1):75–83.

A Review of Canine Episclerokeratitis and Scleritis

Bruce Grahn, DVM

KEYWORDS

- Canine • Episclerokeratitis • Nodular episclerokeratitis • Diffuse episclerokeratitis
- Granulomatous scleritis • Posterior scleritis • Anterior scleritis • Necrotic scleritis

KEY POINTS

- Episclerokeratitis is unique to dogs and manifests as a hyperemic and edematous limbal swelling, which may be nodular and involve the cornea and third eyelid in collie breeds, or be discrete and involve just a few clock hours of the limbal tissues, or be diffuse and cause a generalized swelling of most of the limbus, episclera, and adjacent cornea.
- Episclerokeratitis responds to topical anti-inflammatory therapies.
- Scleritis is a rare canine disorder. and the most appropriate collective term is granulomatous scleritis.
- Granulomatous scleritis is a challenging disorder to treat and requires early diagnosis and therapeutic management with long-term systemic immune suppression.

Embryology and anatomy of the sclera and episclera: A brief review of the embryology and anatomy of the episclera and sclera will aid all clinicians in their understanding of these 2 apparently confusing inflammatory disorders of dogs. It will also facilitate the clinical and histologic differentiation of these apparently nonrelated conditions. Neurocrest tissue is induced to form the sclera and the episcleral tissues relatively late in ocular development by cellular messengers from the retinal pigment epithelium. Only the nerves (neuroectoderm origin) and blood vessels (mesodermal origin) that traverse the sclera have different derivations within the sclera and episclera. The sclera composes most of the fibrous tunic of the eye and it joins the cornea at the limbus (**Fig. 1**A, B). It varies significantly in pigment content from none at all, to patches of lightly pigmented melanocytes, which are usually on the inner (suprachoroidal region), and the outer region where it is covered by the well-vascularized episcleral

The author has nothing to disclose.
Department of Small Animal Clinical Sciences, Prairie Ocular Pathology Service, Prairie Diagnostic Laboratory, Western College of Veterinary Medicine, University of Saskatchewan, 52 Campus Drive, Saskatoon, Saskatchewan S7N 5B4, Canada
E-mail address: bruce.grahn@usask.ca

Vet Clin Small Anim 53 (2023) 439–454
https://doi.org/10.1016/j.cvsm.2022.10.007

and conjunctival tissues. Most of the sclera is made of collagen that is continuous with the corneal stroma at the limbus. The precise organization of the collagen bundles of the corneal stroma is lost in sclera where multiple randomly interlacing collagen bundles, some elastin fibers, melanocytes, and occasional fibrocytes are present (**Fig. 2**). The sclera is variable in color from white to yellow to pale blue. In young animals, the sclera will be thin and bluish and as they mature, it will become thicker and develops a white to yellow color noted in the canine species. Blood supply is minimal, and long and short ciliary vessels traverse the sclera around the equator and beside the optic nerve, respectively. The sclera is thinnest at the equator (see **Fig. 1A, B**). The sclera anchors the extraocular muscles and is posteriorly enveloped externally by Tenon capsule and the episcleral tissues anteriorly, and inside by the choroid and the anterior uvea. The episclera is composed of fibrocytes, multiple blood vessels, and nerves, and it is continuous with Tenon capsule. Bulbar conjunctiva overlies the episcleral tissue to the fornix where it reflects back to line the eyelids as palpebral conjunctiva. Lymphatic drainage vessels from the episclera, and conjunctiva and eyelids drain lymph to the parotid and retropharyngeal lymph nodes via the lateral canthus. The sclera, orbit, and intraocular tissues are all devoid of lymphatics. The inexperienced veterinarian clinician and pathologist often less appreciate the episclera. It lies under the translucent bulbar conjunctiva (**Figs. 3** and **4**) and fuses with Tenon capsule that surrounds the posterior pole. This tissue is rich in collagen strands, which are loosely apposed and traversed by multiple capillaries, blood vessels, and nerves. Primary inflammatory conditions predominate uniquely in the dog, and only occasional parasitic (Onchocerca) and neoplastic conditions (limbal melanocytoma, lymphosarcoma, hemangioma) that invade it or originate in the pigmented or vascular or nerve supply within it. This review will focus on immune-mediated inflammatory episcleritis and scleritis.

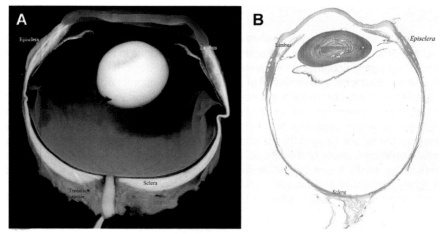

Fig. 1. (A) The gross section of a pinniped eye that clearly defines the anatomy of the sclera and episclera. Note that the sclera forms the majority of the fibrous tunic of the eye. It merges with the cornea at the limbus. The sclera is covered by episclera from just behind the limbus. The episclera is enveloped externally by bulbar conjunctiva to the fornix where it transitions to palpebral conjunctiva. The sclera is also wrapped posteriorly by Tenon capsule, which is continuous with the episclera anteriorly. The inner surface of the sclera is adherent to the uvea (choroid, ciliary body, iris). (B) This is a subgross histologic section of a canine eye stained with hematoxylin and eosin. Note that the sclera is thinnest at the equator and the sclera transitions to cornea at the limbus.

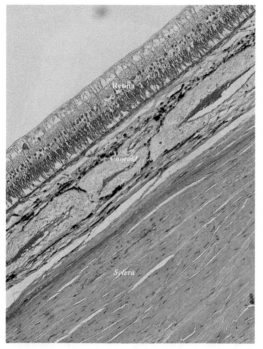

Fig. 2. Masson trichrome–stained photomicrograph reveals the histologic features of the sclera and its junction with the choroid.

AN INTRODUCTION TO EPISCLEROKERATITIS AND ITS MANY SYNONYMS

Immune-mediated inflammatory episcleral disorders are unique to dogs and much of the confusion surrounding this disorder has stemmed from a variety of names listed in previous publications during the last 5 decades. These include nodular fasciitis,[1,2] fibrous histiocytoma,[3] nodular granulomatous episcleritis,[4–6] episclerokeratitis,[7] variant nodular episclerokeratitis,[8–10] and proliferative episcleritis.[11] This variable nomenclature is the result of variable clinical manifestations (episclerokeratitis can be unilateral or bilateral at initial presentation or become bilateral later); they affect the limbal region as a focal, diffuse, or nodular lesions and they may affect other ocular tissues (eyelids etc). We prefer based on its most common manifestation at the limbus where both the episcleral and cornea tissues are affected that these conditions all be classified as episclerokeratitis. This is supported by the consistent histologic manifestation of mixed inflammation for all the forms as either episcleritis (**Fig. 5**) or episclerokeratitis (**Fig. 6**). Lesions that involve only the episclera are more appropriately term episcleritis (Barnes and colleagues, 2010). Additional clarification is useful for the clinician only, by adding the adjectives denoting 3 distinctive manifestations focal, diffuse, or nodular as these vary slightly in their cell types and responses to therapy.[7,12]

DISTINCTIVE CLINICAL CATEGORIES OF EPISCLEROKERATITIS AND DIFFERENTIATING THESE FROM PANNUS AND SCLERITIS

We classify episclerokeratitis and episcleritis based on its clinical manifestations as focal, nodular, and diffuse lesions (**Figs. 7–9**). These conditions are assumed

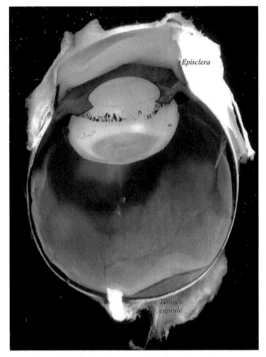

Fig. 3. A gross section of a canine eye photographed under water to reveal the thick loose texture of the episclera and fragments of Tenon capsule.

immune-mediated based on the histologic features, response to topical immune suppression, and the lack of infective agents or foreign material detectable in any of these on microscopic examination of biopsies.[12] Episcleritis and scleritis are distinct, and although the scleritis cases will have inflammatory infiltrates in episclera, these are bystander lesions. Moreover, episclerokeratitis has not been reported to progress to scleritis. In contrast to episclerokeratitis, scleritis is a rare fulminant immune-mediated granulomatous disorder of dogs that will always induce bystander extraocular episcleral and conjunctival hyperemia and congestion, and significant panuveitis. Scleritis manifests most commonly as panophthalmitis. Episclerokeratitis induces conjunctival hyperemia and inflammatory infiltrates in the episclera and limbal cornea but little to no scleritis and a complete absence of endophthalmitis.

Primary immune-mediated episclerokeratitis has only been reported in dogs. The clinical manifestations are limited and considered diagnostic by many veterinary ophthalmologists. These include discrete subtle perilimbal swelling with hyperemia and edema of the conjunctiva, episclera and cornea, characteristically at the limbus (see **Figs. 5–9**). Focal canine episclerokeratitis may be unilateral or bilateral and typically only affects a discrete region of the limbus. In contrast, nodular episclerokeratitis is 2 to 4 mm tumor on the cornea just inside the limbus that is most often bilateral and usually manifests with similar inflammatory masses on the palpebral surface of the nictitans (see **Fig. 8**). In contrast, diffuse limbal episclerokeratitis cases involve much of the limbal tissues circumferentially, and they may be unilateral or bilateral (see **Fig. 9**). Diffuse episclerokeratitis shares some similarities to anterior scleritis but it is a much milder disease without uveitis or panophthalmitis, which are consistently seen with scleritis. Pannus (canine superficial keratitis) at least in acute stages shares

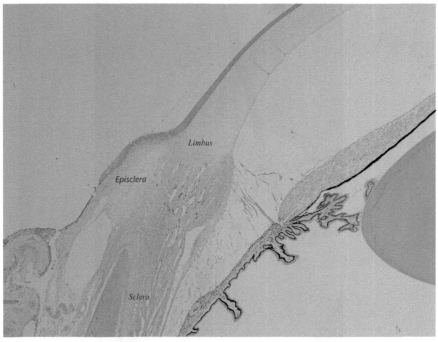

Fig. 4. A high-power hematoxylin-eosin–stained photomicrograph reveals the microscopic anatomy of the junction of the sclera with the cornea (limbus), and the overlying episclera and bulbar conjunctiva, and the apposition of the anterior uvea inside the eye to the sclera of a bird.

some resemblance to episclerokeratitis, and it is differential diagnosis. It is, however, breed-specific (German shepherd and other large breeds of dogs) bilateral condition that usually begins only at the temporal limbus and extends across the cornea to the medial side (**Fig. 10**). Pannus requires a lifelong topical therapy, and it will recrudesce when topical immune suppressive medications are reduced too far. Most cases of episclerokeratitis cases will not recrudesce after complete therapeutic remission.

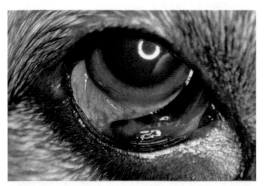

Fig. 5. A dog has a focal episcleritis. Note the small-inflamed area of bulbar conjunctiva and underlying episclera. The cornea is essentially normal with a small rim of limbal edema. Contrast this with the episclerokeratitis in **Fig. 6**.

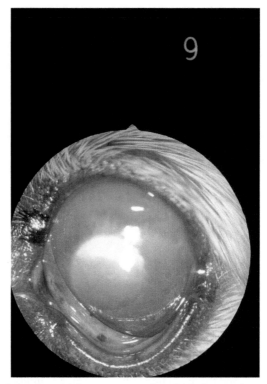

Fig. 6. The term episclerokeratitis is most appropriate for lesions such as noted in this canine globe, where the cornea and limbus an episclera are all involved in this inflammatory limbal-based disorder.

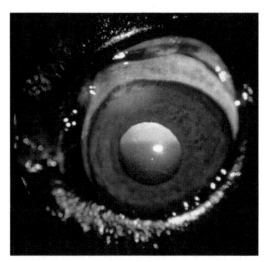

Fig. 7. The subtle focal limbal episclerokeratitis in an American cocker spaniel.

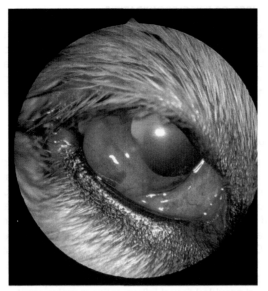

Fig. 8. The unique clinical manifestations of nodular episclerokeratitis in the Collie dog. Note the limbal corneal tumor and swelling of the third eyelid of this often-bilateral condition.

Similarly, anterior manifestations of scleritis although a rare condition can be challenging to differentiate from episclerokeratitis and episcleritis. The important clinical clue to differentiate anterior forms of granulomatous scleritis is the fulminant nature and associated uveitis and histologic confirmation of granulomatous scleritis, contrasted with the mixed inflammatory infiltrate note in episclerokeratitis.

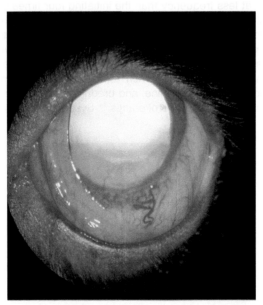

Fig. 9. The clinical manifestations of diffuse episclerokeratitis mimic that of focal lesions (see **Fig. 8**); however, they involve much larger areas of the limbus, cornea, and episcleral tissues.

HISTOLOGIC FEATURES OF EPISCLEROKERATITIS

Despite the unique clinical manifestations of episclerokeratitis, the histologic manifestations are not unique, rather the inflammatory infiltrate found in biopsies of episclera of all 3 forms of episclerokeratitis are identical. The inflammation that is seen histologically is mixed. There are lymphocytes, plasma cells, macrophages, neutrophils, and fibroblasts (**Figs. 11** and **12**). When the biopsies are harvested properly, the underlying sclera if attached will be devoid of any significant inflammation.

Therapeutic Options and Prognosis for Canine Episclerokeratitis

All forms of episclerokeratitis usually respond to topical immune suppression. Usually topical corticosteroids are recommended at 3 to 4 times per day on the affected eye(s). A significant response should be apparent in 3 weeks, provided that the owner is compliant and completes the treatment as instructed. The topical medications can be tapered based on response during several months, and then, they may be discontinued. The most effective therapies include topical applications of either 1% prednisolone acetate or 0.1% dexamethasone applied 4 times per day on the affected eye until all inflammation subsides.[13] The frequency is then reduced gradually on a monthly basis until alternative day therapy is achieved, and then, all medications can be discontinued provided limbal inflammation remains resolved.[12] Topical T cell suppressors (calcineuron inhibitors) are also commonly used successfully although they induce remission less quickly and are more costly to use. The prognosis for episclerokeratitis is excellent with most cases responding within a few weeks and most dogs are off therapy in 2 to 6 months. Focal often unilateral episclerokeratitis responds the quickest and usually does not recrudesce after all limbal inflammation is suppressed.[12] Most nodular episclerokeratitis cases benefit from surgical debulking with submission of these tissues for histologic examination. This facilitates a prompt resolution to topical corticosteroids; however, longer term topical therapy is usually required, although at less frequency than the initiating four times per day (QID) therapy. Similarly, diffuse episclerokeratitis is often bilateral and generally slower to respond and often will recrudesce if topical corticosteroids are withdrawn too soon. Systemic calcineuron inhibitors may also be used in combination with topical corticosteroids to suppress the T-cell rich inflammation in the more resistant bilateral diffuse and nodular forms that recrudesce when topical immune suppressive therapy is reduced. Oral niacinamide, tetracycline, and prednisone have also been used occasionally to systemically treat episclerokeratitis.[14] Systemic therapy with azathioprine

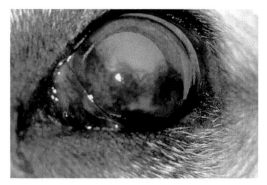

Fig. 10. The typical corneal manifestation of the pigmented form of canine pannus.

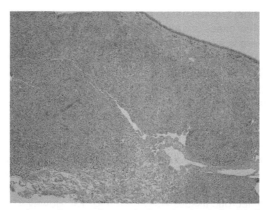

Fig. 11. A low-power photomicrograph reveals the mixed episcleral inflammation that typifies focal, diffuse, and nodular forms of canine episclerokeratitis and episcleritis.

administered orally at 2 mg/kg body weight, until clinical improvement is detected and then reduced to 1 mg/kg body weight and then reduced to alternate day therapy and discontinued when remission is achieved has also been reported.[15] When treating dogs with systemic azathioprine weekly hemograms need to be reviewed. Debulking followed by adjunctive cryotherapy was reported as a successful therapy.[16]

The cause and pathogenesis of episclerokeratitis remains unknown. However, collie breeds are overrepresented with the nodular forms and cocker spaniels with bilateral diffuse episclerokeratitis, perhaps indicating some genetic predisposition. Based anecdotal discussions about episclerokeratitis by veterinarian ophthalmologists there seems to be significant geographic variations in the regional case numbers of the 3 clinical forms episclerokeratitis.

CATEGORIZATION OF SCLERITIS

Sclera diseases are limited to a scant number of congenital (colobomata), parasitic infestation of the superficial sclera with Onchocerca, and primary granulomatous

Fig. 12. A high-power photomicrograph allows the identification of the mixture of lymphocytes, macrophages, plasma cells, neutrophils, and fibroblasts found in biopsies of episclerokeratitis.

scleritis[17,18] The former two will not be reviewed here as our focus will be on the latter where only a scant few cases of canine scleritis are reported.[5,7,9,19–22] It is important to appreciate that sclera is a tough relatively resistant barrier to neoplasia or inflammation within the globe or orbit. Primary neoplasia has not been reported in this tissue, if you exclude limbal melanocytoma. These limbal tumors are categorized as corneal neoplasms as they originate from pigmented cells in deep limbus next to Descemet membrane. Granulomatous forms of scleritis have only been reported in dogs. Similar to episcleritis, there remains much confusion regarding the classification and differentiation of scleritis among ophthalmologists and pathologists in the past and today. Peer-reviewed literature includes the terms necrotic scleritis,[7,20,22–24] granulomatous scleritis,[18,21] nonnecrotizing scleritis,[25] orbital nodular granulomatous scleritis,[26] scleritis,[5] posterior scleritis, and anterior scleritis.[9] The term necrotic scleritis is in reference to the characteristic patches of eosin staining scleral collagen. These have similarities to necrotic tissues elsewhere (**Fig. 13**). However, collagen is an inert protein, and it does not become necrotic.[18] The cause of this unusual staining pattern noted histologically in some cases is unknown. In addition, there is a lack of consistent identification of this histologic finding in scleritis cases and allows one to speculate that it may develop or resolve over time. So negating that term leaves one to consider anterior, posterior, and orbital granulomatous scleritis. Based on our collaborative article on this scleral pathologic condition,[18] we continue to suggest that all the forms of scleritis are best characterized simply as granulomatous scleritis. This is based on our observations that all the reported cases manifest histologically with predominantly histiocytic inflammation, which induces most commonly a severe progressive proliferative disorder[18] and the much less commonly a lytic form where extraocular muscles dehisce from the sclera.[27] These lesions usually present to the pathologist with general scleral involvement in enucleated globe, likely indicating a progressive disease from either anterior or posterior lesions.

In conclusion, scleritis is easiest to understand as a primary immune-mediated granulomatous scleral inflammation that is mediated by histiocytes, it may develop focally or generally and be unilateral or bilateral, and although rare, it is a very challenging disease to treat successfully. Secondary scleritis related to ocular perforation or penetration does occur[28] but is readily controlled by the anti-inflammatories and

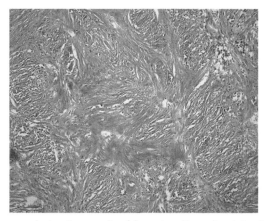

Fig. 13. A high-power photomicrograph of hematoxylin-eosin–stained section of canine sclera that reveals the bright eosin staining of collagen that has been coined necrotic collagen.

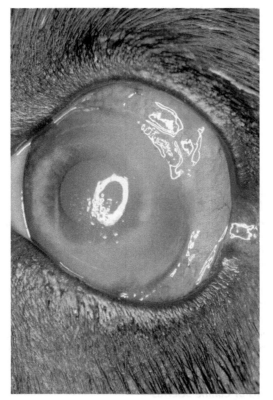

Fig. 14. A dog with granulomatous scleritis that involves most of the anterior sclera, and although reminiscent of episclerokeratitis, note the significant inflammation and the miosis, swollen iris, and although not evident in this photograph, there was a significant aqueous flare consistent with endophthalmitis secondary to scleritis.

antibiotics commonly used in the therapy for endophthalmitis or orbital cellulitis associated with these perforating or penetrating ocular and orbital conditions and therefore warrants no further comments or review.

Clinical Manifestations and Diagnosis of Granulomatous Scleritis

Granulomatous scleritis has only been reported in dogs, and the springer spaniel may be overrepresented as a breed, although there is very limited number of cases reported to date.[22,27] The transcleral inflammation may develop in any part or all of the sclera.[7] When the anterior sclera is involved, the cornea is also often involved (**Fig. 14**).[18] When the lesions of scleritis are small, focal, and just developing over the anterior visible sclera, the disorder will mimic episclerokeratitis and episcleritis as either a focal or a diffuse disease.[27] To differentiate these clinically, it is important to remember that scleritis is a fulminant disorder and without exception is associated with an endophthalmitis and aqueous flare, and episcleral and conjunctival inflammation.[18] Multiple white granulomas will develop within the choroid (**Figs. 15**). The ophthalmologist will consider multiple differential infectious causes for uveitis. The best diagnostic approach is ultrasonographic or sectional imaging and based on those a deep scleral biopsy should be submitted for histologic examination early in the disease.[19] When the affected globe is blind due to complications of panuveitis, exudative

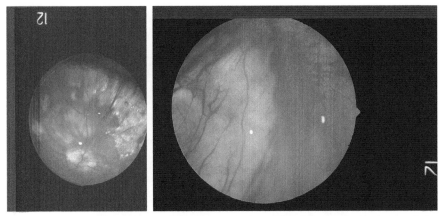

Fig. 15. Another important clinical manifestation that differentiates scleritis from episclerokeratitis is the presence of subchoroidal scleral granulomas noted in both fundi of this dog with granulomatous scleritis. They manifest as these pale yellow—white swellings in the inner sclera and suprachoroidal.

retinal detachment, glaucoma, and keratitis, enucleation should be completed promptly. The confirmed diagnosis always warrants a thorough ocular examination on the contralateral globe after mydriasis. Histologic examination of excisional biopsies is challenging when superficial predominantly episcleral tissues are harvested. It is advisable to refer all suspect cases of scleritis to an ophthalmologist to facilitate the sectional imaging analysis if required and the necessary deep scleral biopsy.

Histologic Diagnosis of Canine Scleritis

Gross (**Fig. 16**) and subgross (**Fig. 17**) and histologic findings (**Figs. 18** and **19**) confirm the diagnosis of scleritis. Histologic examination of biopsies and globes with scleritis reveal diffuse or focal lesions with marked granulomatous with some mixed inflammatory infiltration through the sclera (see **Figs. 18** and **19**). When examining affected globes this granulomatous to mixed inflammation will involve the uvea as well and choroidal effusions and exudative retinal detachments are common. Similarly, the optic nerve and its meninges are also commonly inflamed as bystander lesions.

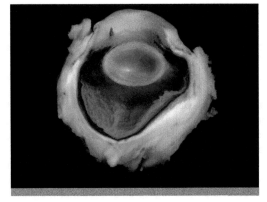

Fig. 16. A gross section of an enucleated dog's eye with granulomatous scleritis. Noted the generalized scleral thickening, the retinal detachment, and thickened uvea.

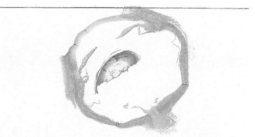

Fig. 17. A hematoxylin-eosin–stained subgross photomicrograph of the eye in **Fig. 17.** Note the thickened sclera and limbus and pan uveal thickness and the detached retina.

Infectious agents have not been detected despite the use of special stains.[18,22] The scleral inflammation is typically histiocytic (see **Fig. 19**). Previous reports of necrotic scleritis were based on histologic identification of hypereosinophilic patches of collagen and the presence or absence of this eosin staining collagen has limited significance to the confirmation of the diagnosis of granulomatous scleritis.[18] The lytic scleral lesions where the extraocular muscles have dehisced from their scleral attachments have similar granulomatous infiltration and lytic collagen and their histologic importance is of limited importance. Once the diagnosis of granulomatous scleritis is confirmed, prompt systemic immunosuppression should be initiated. Other systemic disorders have not been associated with scleritis in dogs to date.

Medical and Surgical Therapies for Granulomatous Scleritis

Oral prednisone given at immune suppressive doses (2 mg/kg) per day will usually suppress the inflammation, and cautious lowering of these dosages may be considered when all signs of uveitis subside. Additional medications such a systemic T cell suppressors (calcineuron inhibitors) may be considered and used in conjunction with oral steroids, as well as treatment with azathioprine and other immunesuppressive agents.[29] The prognosis for control and maintenance of a visual globe is guarded. Blind eyes that remain inflamed should be enucleated. The cause and

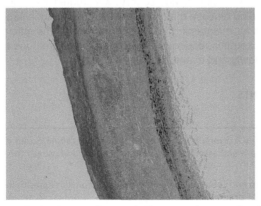

Fig. 18. A low-power photomicrograph reveals the pan sclera predominantly granulomatous scleritis. Note the full thickness scleral inflammation and secondary choroiditis and the exudative retinal detachment.

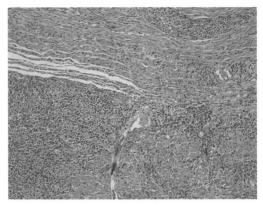

Fig. 19. A high-power Masson trichrome–stained photomicrograph that reveals the diffuse granulomatous scleritis that targets the scleral collagen fibers.

the pathogenesis of this disease remain unknown. To date despite diagnosing and treating multiple cases personally, only 1 dog has maintained bilateral vision with the retention of multiple bilateral chorioretinal scars during 3 years and is currently on a lifelong 0.5 mg/kg oral dose of prednisone, and the lesions are limited to bilateral multiple large chorioretinal scars.

SUMMARY

Episclerokeratitis and scleritis are primary disorders of the episclera and sclera, respectively, and they have only been reported in the canine. Other systemic disorders have not been associated with either episclerokeratitis or scleritis. Unfortunately, many terms describing both of these conditions has led to much clinician and pathologist confusion regarding both disorders and even mixing up or even integrating these distinct syndromes. For clarity we propose recognizing 3 clinical forms of episclerokeratitis but only 1 histologic diagnosis of episclerokeratitis (when the cornea is involved) and episcleritis when only the episclera is involved. Similarly, one term "granulomatous scleritis" to encompass the terms necrotic scleritis, anterior and posterior scleritis, nodular orbital scleritis, and so forth will create less confusion. This is a rare often-bilateral blinding disease that requires systemic immune suppression to control and the prognosis for maintaining vision and controlling the inflammation is poor. In contrast, episclerokeratitis responds promptly to topical immune suppression, which can be reduced slowly and eventually discontinued.

CLINICS CARE POINTS

- Episclerokeratitis is a common idiopathic inflammatory canine ocular disorder that always affects the episclera and associated bulbar conjunctiva, and usually the superficial limbal cornea.
- The most effective and common topical therapies for episclerokeratitis include topical ocular dexamethasone or prednisone.
- Once the lesions have recrudesced these may be slowly tapered and then discontinued.
- Granulomatous scleritis is a rare fulminant panophthalmitis of dogs.

- Granulomatous scleritis requires an early diagnostic biopsy and histologic examination that confirms granulomatous inflammation.
- Prompt and continued systemic immune suppression is required to attempt control of this immune mediated granulomatous panophthalmitis.

REFERENCES

1. Bellhorn RW, Henkind P. Ocular nodular fasciitis in a dog. J Am Vet Med Assoc 1967;170:611–4.
2. Lavignette AM, Carlton WW. A case of ocular nodular fasciitis in a dog. J Am Anim Hosp Assoc 1974;10:503–6.
3. Smith JS, Bistner S, Riis R. Infiltrative corneal lesions resembling fibrous histiocytoma: clinical and pathologic findings in six dogs. J Am Vet Med Assoc 1976;169: 722–6.
4. Paulsen ME, Lavach JD, Snyder SP, et al. Nodular granulomatous episcleritis in dogs: 19 cases (1973- 1985). J Am Vet Med Assoc 1987;19:1581–7.
5. Fischer CA, Lindley DM, Carlton WC, et al. Tumors of the cornea and sclera. In: Ocular tumors in animals and Humans. 2002. p. 149–202.
6. Hamzianpour N, Heinrich C, Jones R, et al. Clinical and pathological findings in three dogs with a corneocentric presentation of nodular granulomatous episcleritis. Vet Ophthalmol 2019;22:529–37.
7. Grahn BH, Sandmeyer LS. Canine eiscleritis, nodular episclerokeratitis, scleritis and necrotic scleritis. Vet Clin North Am SAP 2008;38:291–308.
8. Dugan SJ, Ketring KL, Severn GA, et al. Variant nodular granulomatous episclerokeratitis in four dogs. J Am Anim Hosp Assoc 1993;29:403–9.
9. Deykin AR, Guandalini A, Ratto A. A retrospective histopathologic study of primary episcleral and scleral inflammatory disease in dogs. Prog Vet Comp Ophthalmo 1997;7:245–8.
10. Gionfiddo JR, Krohne SG, Powell CC, et al. Idiopathic ocular and nasal granulomatous inflammatory disease in a dog. Vet Ophthalmol 2003;6:163–7.
11. Gwin RM, Gelatt KN Peiffer RL. Ophthalmic nodular fasciitis in the dog. J Am Vet Med Assoc 1977;170:611–4.
12. Breaux CB, Sandmeyer LS, Grahn BH. Immunohistochemical investigation of canine episcleritis. Vet Ophthalmol 2007;10:168–72.
13. Whitley RD, Hamor RE. Diseases and surgery of the canine cornea and sclera. In: Gelatt KN, editor. Veterinary Ophthalmology. 6th edition. Toronto: John Wiley and Sons; 2021. p. 1082–172.
14. Hurn S, McCowan C, Turner A. Oral doxycycline, niacinamide and prednisolone used to treat bilateral nodular granulomatous conjunctivitis of the third eyelid in an Australian Kelpie dog. Vet Ophthalmol 2005;8:349–52.
15. Latimer C, Wyman M, Szymanski C. Azothioprine in the management of fibrous histiocytoma in two dogs. J Am Anim Hosp Assoc 1983;19:155–8.
16. Wheller C, Blanchard G, Davidson H. Cryosurgery for treatment of recurrent proliferative Keratoconjunctivitis in five dogs. J Am Vet Med Assoc 1989;195:354–7.
17. Peiffer RL, Gelatt KN, Gwin RM. Proliferative episcleritis in the dog. Vet Med Sm Anim Clin 1976;1273–8.
18. Grahn BH, Peiffer RL, Wilcock BP. Histologic basis of ocular disease in animals. Wiley; 2019. p. 181–96.
19. Braga Sa MBP, Perlmann E, de Goes ACA, et al. Ultrasound diagnosis and monitoring of canine scleritis. Braz J Vet Res Anim Sci 2015;51:309–15.

20. Cazalot G, Lavergne SN. Investigation of anti-myeloperoxidase antibodies in a dog with bilateral necrotizing scleritis. Vet Sci 2015;2:259–69.
21. Day MJ, Mould JRB, Carter WJ. An immunohistochemical investigation of canine idiopathic granulomatous scleritis. Vet Ophthalmol 2008;11:11–7.
22. Denk N, Sandmeyer LS, Lim CC, et al. A retrospective study of the clinical, histological and immunohistochemical manifestations of 5 dogs originally diagnosed histologically as necrotizing scleritis. Vet Ophthalmol 2012;15:102–9.
23. Martin CL. Cornea and sclera. In: Ophthalmic disease in veterinary medicine. Manson Publishing; 2005. p. 241–97.
24. Otranto D, Giannelli S, Latrofa MS, et al. Canine infections with Onchocerca lupi nematodes, United states 2011-2014. Emerg Infect Dis 2015;5:868–71.
25. Best L, Newman SJ, Ward DA, et al. Scleral rupture secondary to idiopathic non-necrotizing scleritis in a dog. Case Reports Vet Med 2013;2013:1–5.
26. Barnes LD, Pearce JW, Berent LM, et al. Surgical management of orbital nodular granulomatous episcleritis in a dog. Vet Ophthalmol 2010;13:251–8.
27. Grahn BH, Cullen CL, Wolfer J. Diagnostic Ophthalmology; Necrotic scleritis in a Springer spaniel. Can Vet J 1999;40:679–80.
28. Welihozkiy A, Pirie CG, Pizzirani S. Scleral and suprachoroidal foreign body in a dog – a case report. Vet Ophthalmol 2011;14:345–51.
29. Li Puma MC, Diehl KA. The use of systemic mycophenalate in canine immune mediated ophthalmic disease. Vet Rec Case Rep 2021;9.

Blepharitis and Neoplasms of the Canine Eyelid Margin and Skin

Bruce Grahn, DVM

KEYWORDS

• Canine • Blepharitis • Eyelid neoplasia

KEY POINTS

- The most common blepharitis of young dogs is juvenile cellulitis (puppy strangles), which is effectively treated with systemic immune suppression (often oral corticosteroids).
- The most common blepharitis of middle aged to older dogs is pyogranulomatous blepharitis, which is also most effectively treated with systemically administered immune suppressive medications.
- The most common eyelid neoplasm of younger dogs is histiocytoma, which is often treated by excisional biopsy; however, it will recrudesce spontaneously without medical or surgical management.
- The most common eyelid neoplasms of older dogs are tarsal gland epitheliomas and adenomas, which are both benign and are treated by surgical resection.

INTRODUCTION: BLEPHARITIS AND NEOPLASMS OF THE CANINE EYELID SKIN

The clinical manifestations of canine blepharitis are quite diverse, and usually they are diagnosed in 2 age groups (younger dogs neonatal to 1 year of age) and older dogs (6-teenage years).[1] The clinical manifestations include tumor (**Fig. 1**), erythema and swelling, exudate, lacrimation, ulceration, and blepharospasm. Canine blepharitis has multiple causes, and similar to all aspects of dermatology, scrapings and cytological examination, and biopsies and histologic examination remain the gold standards for diagnosis. Treatment varies with the cause and usually involves systemic therapy as opposed to topical therapy, to maintain adequate medication concentrations within the eyelid tissues. This article reviews the most common forms of blepharitis organized from youngest to oldest age at onset. These include puppy strangles, allergic angiodermatic blepharitis, bacterial blepharitis, parasitic blepharitis, fungal

The author has nothing to disclose.
Western College of Veterinary Medicine, Prairie Ocular Pathology Service, Prairie Diagnostic Laboratory, University of Saskatchewan, 52 Campus Drive, Saskatoon, Saskatchewan S7N 5B4, Canada
E-mail address: bruce.grahn@usask.ca

Vet Clin Small Anim 53 (2023) 455–471
https://doi.org/10.1016/j.cvsm.2022.11.002
0195-5616/23/© 2022 Elsevier Inc. All rights reserved.

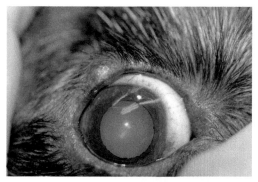

Fig. 1. Note the small upper eyelid tumor on this middle-aged mixed breed dog. Is this inflammatory or neoplastic and how would diagnose and treat this?

blepharitis, immune-mediated medial canthal ulceration, and pyogranulomatous blepharitis. Systemic dermatologic disorders such as atopy, pemphigoid, parasitic blepharitis, and Vogt-Koyangi-Harada-like syndrome will receive brief mention only because they affect many areas of the skin and are not usually unique to the eyelids only.

Eyelid neoplasms tend to develop later in life with the noted exception of histiocytomas, which manifest in young dogs. The clinical manifestations of palpebral neoplasia also include tumor or generalized eyelid swelling (**Fig. 2**), ulceration and ocular discharge, which make blepharitis and eyelid neoplasia important differential clinical diagnoses. Again the critical diagnostic step is excisional or a diagnostic incisional biopsy with histologic examination. Most eyelid neoplasms in the dog are benign and treated by surgical resection with or without adjunctive therapy. However, local recurrence occasionally happens with incomplete resection, or with adenomas, more commonly recurrence is simply the development of new primary neoplasm in an adjacent tarsal gland. We will review the most common and some uncommon palpebral neoplasms in order of most common to more rare. These include tarsal gland adenoma and epithelioma, melanocytoma and melanoma, histiocytoma, mast cell neoplasia, granular cell tumors, spindle cell neoplasms, peripheral nerve sheath tumors, squamous cell carcinoma, lymphosarcoma, and finally trichoblastoma. In

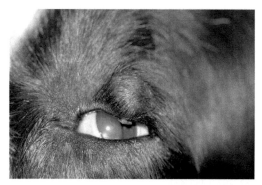

Fig. 2. Note the large swelling on the upper eyelid of this dogs left eye, and the subtle eyelid margin tumor. Are these related? How would you diagnosis and treat these?

conclusion, a brief review of eyelid dermoids and hamartomas will complete this section. We will not include reviews of the conjunctivitis and conjunctival neoplasms.

Blepharitis

Puppy strangles (juvenile cellulitis/pyoderma)

This disease commonly affects the facial skin and draining lymph nodes of puppies.[2] However, it occasionally involves predominantly the eyelids in puppies to young adult dogs. Occasionally, older dogs (aged 1–3 years) will manifest with this disease.[3–5] A key clinical manifestation is the marked enlargement of all of the draining facial lymph nodes, furunculosis, pustular draining tracts, and crusts.[6,7] The clinical diagnosis is usually based solely on these clinical manifestations. When biopsies are completed, they reveal a pyogranulomatous folliculitis, dermatitis, and lymphadenitis but usually there is no evidence of infectious organisms.[8–10] Bacterial cultures are typically negative and special stains for bacteria in lymph node and skin biopsies are reported to be negative.[8] The cause and pathogenesis remain unknown although some authors speculate a bacterial hypersensitivity.[11,12] The response to systemic immune-suppression is rapid and recrudescence is uncommon after complete remission. Response to systemic antibiotic therapy alone is generally poor[6]; hence most dogs receive the initial dose of systemic prednisone (2 mg/kg/d) with or without concurrent systemic antibiotics, which are often cephalosporin.

Allergic angioneurotic edema

This disorder is acute (minutes to hours), and the clinical manifestations include severe conjunctival and eyelid and facial edema (**Fig. 3**). General practitioners and emergency veterinarians often see this disorder, and it has received scant literature citations by ophthalmologists.[13] Usually, by the time referral to an ophthalmologist is completed, all clinical manifestations have subsided. Most of the affected dogs are seen sporadically, although in my experience many manifest in the fall and they are often young hunting dogs that are affected while they are active in the field. Angioneurotic edema is a clinical diagnosis and often biopsies and histologic findings are not completed. This hypersensitivity reaction of the facial skin and eyelids develops secondary to a large variety of toxins and insect stings. The facial edema is intense and when the eyelids are involved the affected dog is often visually impaired related to an inability to open the eyelids due to the concurrent edema. There is often self-trauma including

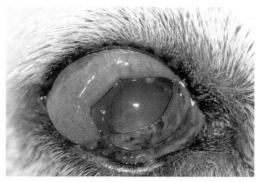

Fig. 3. Note the severe conjunctival edema in this dog. Twenty-four hours earlier, this dog was diagnosed with angioneurotic edema and neither eye could be examined due to the intense conjunctival and eyelid edema. The dog was treated with systemic and topical corticosteroids and responded completely 24 hours later.

hyperemia and ulceration due to rubbing and scratching, presumably secondary to pruritus. The most appropriate therapy includes systemic corticosteroids (1–2 mg/kg) and antihistamines until the swelling is gone, which is often within 24 to 48 hours. Warm or cold compresses and topical mast cell stabilizers maybe useful adjunctive therapies and E-collars will be needed in the acute phase to reduce self-trauma.

Allergic blepharitis

Atopic and food allergic diseases may affect the eyelids; however, most will involve significant other areas of the skin including face, feet, ears, axillary and ventral and dorsal trunk regions. Rarely is there just primary blepharitis or conjunctivitis. This is in contrast to what is often written in textbook articles and many web-based discussions. Primary allergic blepharitis secondary to inhalant, contact or food allergies that affects only the eyelids is likely uncommon in dogs and has not received significant peer review reports. When primary blepharitis due to inhalant or contact (related to topical ocular medications) or food allergies are diagnosed, they will respond to a topical mast cell stabilizers (chromolyn) given bid-qid and if necessary topical or if needed oral corticosteroids (prednisone) given at anti-inflammatory doses (1 mg/kg). These therapies will provide prompt relief until the offending allergen is identified and either removed from the diet or therapeutic regime or the dog is desensitized or treated long term with a systemic calcineuron inhibitor and so forth.

Bacterial blepharitis

Bacterial blepharitis dogs may also be over diagnosed in veterinary and ophthalmologists practices when juvenile cellulitis, parasitic and pyogranulomatous blepharitis are accurately diagnosed and excluded as differential diagnoses. Bacterial blepharitis does develop occasionally in older dogs, and most cases are secondary other ocular (**Fig. 4**) and periocular diseases and occasionally traumatic injuries.[14–16] Chronic bacterial blepharitis can develop secondary to chronic dry eye (Keratoconjunctivitis Sicca), chalazion, seborrhea, and hypothyroidism.[17] Staphylococcal and streptococcus infections of the tarsal glands have been reported.[17,18] These infections maybe the harbinger for pyogranulomatous blepharitis, described later, although negative cultures and lack of histologic evidence for a bacterial presence in that disorder has been reported.[19] The diagnosis of bacterial blepharitis is confirmed on histologic examination of eyelid skin biopsies coupled with culture and sensitivity. Systemic bactericidal antibiotic therapy is based on the culture and sensitivity and

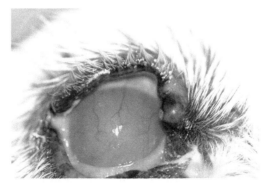

Fig. 4. This adult cocker spaniel has had Keratoconjunctivitis Sicca for many years now has a blepharitis associated with Staphylococcus infected tarsal glands. Multiple chalazion were present under the palpebral conjunctiva of both eyelids.

usually long-term (6–8 weeks) therapy is required when the blepharitis is chronic. Staphylococcal bacterin has been recommended for the treatment of chronic staphylococcal blepharitis in one dog.[20–22]

Parasitic blepharitis

The most common parasite that affects the canine eyelids is *Demodex canis*. This parasite is considered a normal inhabitant of the eyelid hair follicles, sebaceous, and apocrine glands of dogs. However, *Demodex* can induce blepharitis and may affect other facial skin (**Fig. 5**). Demodectic blepharitis is characterized as scaly, often nonpruritic blepharitis typically of young dogs. The diagnosis is confirmed most often by skin scraping and microscopic confirmation of the mite.

Sarcoptic mange may also affect the eyelids and facial skin and it is characterized by intense pruritus, moist secondary dermatitis and many areas of skin on the body will be infested. Similar to Demodex the diagnosis is confirmed by skin scrapings and mite identification.

The therapy for parasitic blepharitis is a systemic antiparasitic medication, which may include the effective

An uncommon eyelid parasite is Cuterebra that embeds itself and develops within eyelid tissues,[23] and this parasite is treated by surgical removal. Spot-on therapy with imidacloprid/modiectin.

Protozoa

For dogs with a travel history to the Mediterranean, India, and South and Central America, Leishmaniasis should remain on the differential diagnosis list because up to 25% of all cases involve periocular signs that include eyelid swelling, dermatitis, alopecia, draining tracts, and so forth. The diagnosis is confirmed by biopsy and histologic examination. Oral therapy with antimonials, amphotericin B, allopurinol, and paromomycin including other medications in highly variable treatment regimes.[24]

The current recommended therapy includes subcutaneous N-methylglucamine antimoniate (80 mg/kg) and allopurinol orally (10 mg/kg) antimonial for 10 to 12 months to be effective.[25]

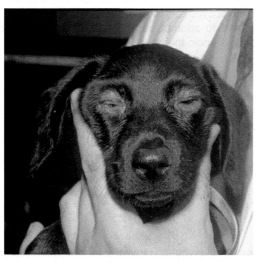

Fig. 5. This Dachshund puppy has Demodex associated blepharitis.

Fungal blepharitis
Dermatophyte infestation of only the eyelids is also a rare canine condition. However, when it does occur, it is accompanied by a generalized skin condition with scaly alopecic lesions with prominent facial involvement. *Microsporum* and *Trichophyton* species have been reported and the clinical signs are similar to parasitic blepharitis and include alopecia, scaling, and hyperemia and skin scrapings with cytological examination and culture confirm the diagnosis. Effective therapies include topical clotrimazole creams, iodine solutions, and miconazole ointments.[26,27]

Immune-mediated dermatologic disorders that affect the eyelids and skin of dogs
These conditions affect the skin near to mucocutaneous junctions but are not usually limited to just the eyelid skin (**Fig. 6**). These include pemphigus complex, and discoid and systemic lupus.

Pemphigus complex disorders include pemphigus vulgaris, pemphigus vegetans, and bullous pemphigoid. They are all characterized by the involvement of mucocutaneous junctions over the body, and their diagnosis is based on histologic examination and unique immunohistochemical antibody staining. They respond to systemic immune suppression.

Discoid lupus will induce local facial dermatitis with eyelid involvement characterized by poliosis and vitiligo. Systemic lupus can also induce similar eyelid disease but is systemic disorder that affects many organs including the kidney, joints, red blood cells, platelets, and so forth. Both of these disorders are immune mediated related to antinuclear antibodies, and the diagnosis is based on light microscopic examination of skin biopsies for discoid lupus and multisystem disease and biopsy systemic alterations in blood, serum, and urine for systemic lupus erythematosus (SLE). Both are treated by immune-suppression.

Canine Vogt-Koyangi-Harada-like syndrome manifests without exception with pan-uveitis (endophthalmitis) with depigmentation of the uvea (usually the choroid) initially. The skin lesions will usually appear weeks to months later and are typically characterized by depigmentation and dermatitis (vitiligo and poliosis) of the periocular skin and lips (**Fig. 7**). The diagnosis is based on typical signalment and clinical signs and the disease is confirmed by histologic findings, usually after an enucleation of a blind glaucomatous globe. The histologic findings that support the diagnosis include confirmation panuveitis with histiocytic targeting of the uveal melanocyte. Systemic immune suppression is required to attempt control of the panuveitis and often the eyelid lesions develop during chronic therapy.

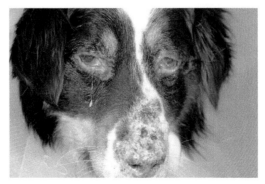

Fig. 6. This dog is manifesting with ulcerative disease that is affecting the mucocutaneous junctions, typical of several pemphigoid diseases.

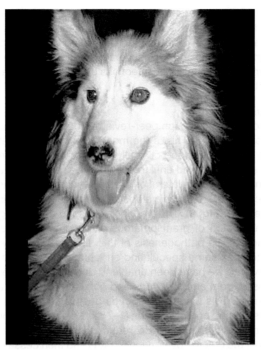

Fig. 7. Note the depigmentation, poliosis and vitiligo in this dog with chronic medically managed VKH-like syndrome.

Immune-mediated canthal ulceration

This disorder has received little peer-reviewed attention, yet it is frequently diagnosed by veterinary ophthalmologists. It is referenced predominantly based on textbook descriptions.[18,19,28,29] The disease manifests with medial canthal ulceration that is often bilateral. This condition has likely 2 distinct pathogeneses, and there are no other dermatologic abnormalities (**Fig. 8**). The secondary form is perhaps most common and develops secondary to poor medial canthal hygiene where there is a buildup of crusts and debris that predispose to secondary bacterial infections and ulceration. This is common in small breeds of dogs, usually brachycephalic breeds. Appropriate daily ocular hygiene and topical antibiotics easily treat this disorder. The less common form may be immune-mediated and is often noted in a variety of breeds of dogs. The ulceration is often quite severe and bilateral, and some affected dogs also have

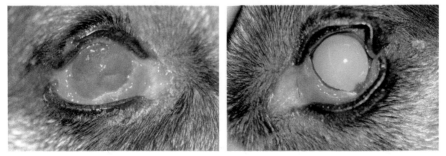

Fig. 8. Deep ulcerative medial canthal ulceration in a mature dog with chronic superficial keratitis (Pannus).

pannus (superficial chronic keratitis) but not all affected dogs have an associated immune-mediated keratitis. The cause and pathogenesis is unknown but most speculate that this is an immune-mediated disorder based on the response to systemic (prednisone 1–2 mg/kg orally) and topical corticosteroids to induce remission. Bacterial cultures are typically negative, and infectious organisms detected in biopsies have not been reported.

Pyogranulomatous blepharitis

This condition also lacks a thorough peer-reviewed description, and most references are found in textbooks.[18,19,28] This is the most common inflammatory blepharitis of older dogs. It can be misdiagnosed clinically as a benign neoplasm, or bacterial blepharitis. It is occasionally ignored until the condition is generalized and involves most of the eyelids. It manifests as unilateral or bilateral eyelid tumor (mass) with inflammation, and when the lesions are chronic alopecia and draining tracts in multiple areas of the eyelids can develop (**Fig. 9**). The diagnosis is based on histologic examination of biopsies with confirmation of granulomatous or pyogranulomatous blepharitis with loss of tarsal glands.[19] The pathogenesis of this disease is unknown but the curious loss of tarsal glands has some speculating on tarsal gland inflammation or infection as the cause. However, we have been unable to document infectious organisms histologically in biopsies from affected dogs and generally, systemic antibiotics are not effective as treatment. This disorder responds best to anti-inflammatory or immune suppression with systemic corticosteroids (1–2 mg/kg orally), and once the inflammation is responding, the dosage can be reduced to anti-inflammatory followed by gradual reduction of the dosage over many months and then cessation. The prognosis is excellent once the inflammation is completely resolved.

A Review of Canine Eyelid Neoplasia

Tarsal gland adenomas and epitheliomas

These are by far the most common eyelid neoplasms in the dog. Both of these tumors originate from the tarsal (Meibomian) glands, which line the upper and lower eyelids, and these glands are responsible for the sebaceous component of the tear film. The distinction of adenomas versus epithelioma is histologic and based on the predominance of basal cells versus the more differentiated sebocyte. Although the epithelioma variants tend to grow deeper within the eyelid, generally, there are no prognostic or therapeutic differences between these 2 variants. Many question the need for pathologists and ophthalmologists to differentiate these, and rather simply term them all tarsal gland adenomas, which based on the clinical disorder is appropriate. They

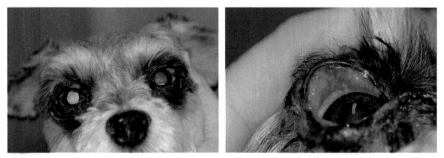

Fig. 9. Pyogranulomatous blepharitis may develop in one or all four eyelids. Note the hyperemic thickened eyelids, mucopurulent ocular discharge, and the swollen inflamed tarsal glands in this middle-aged dog.

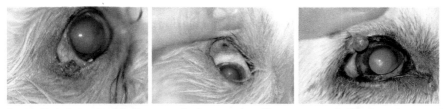

Fig. 10. Tarsal gland epitheliomas and adenomas manifest as an exophytic often pigmented tumors at the eyelid margin most commonly, occasionally through the palpebral conjunctiva, and less commonly through the palpebral skin.

manifest clinically in middle-aged to older dogs as sole or multiple tumors that most commonly grow outward (exophytic) from the eyelid margin. A smaller number grow inward through the conjunctival or even less commonly through the eyelid skin (**Fig. 10**). Typically the surface of these tumors are papillated, crusty, and reactive and when there is contact with the cornea, they will often induce keratitis that may be ulcerated or nonulcerated. Although tarsal gland adenocarcinomas are referenced,[30] they are rare and diagnosed based on invasive growth and anaplastic cellular features. The histologic features of the epithelioma and tarsal gland adenoma are quite varied. However, these are benign with limited to no mitotic figures, no invasive growth, just an expansile growth usually outward from the eyelid margin. Light microscopic examination will reveal that all tarsal gland tumors manifests with some reactive inflammation within and often at the exposed edges of these neoplasms. The clinical diagnosis is based on the typical appearance and origin from within the tarsal glands and a marginal eyelid tumor. Chalazion and focal pyogranulomatous blepharitis are common accompaniments to these neoplasms, presumably related to secretion of sebaceous material within the eyelid stroma. The treatment of choice for tarsal gland adenomas and epitheliomas is surgical resection, although adjunctive cryotherapy and laser photocoagulation and so forth are common adjunctive therapies. Provided the surgical margins are clean, excision is curative. Although recurrence is uncommon, new tarsal gland neoplasms will commonly develop within the eyelids.

Eyelid melanocytoma and melanoma
Eyelid melanocytoma is the second most common palpebral skin neoplasm of the dog. These manifest clinically in 2 forms: individual pedunculated heavily pigmented tumors (**Fig. 11**) and the less common chain of multiple pigmented tumors that extend

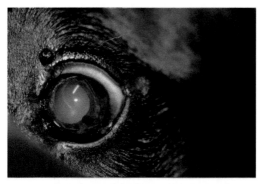

Fig. 11. The most common clinical manifestations of palpebral melanocytoma include a heavily pigmented exophytic often-pedunculated tumor.

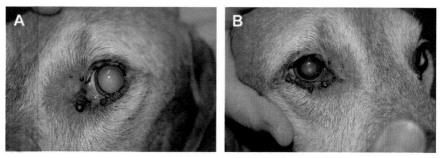

Fig. 12. The less common manifestation of eyelid dermal melanocytoma is the contiguous neoplasm that may present on multiple eyelids.(See above *A* and *B*)

along the eyelid margin (**Fig. 12** A and B). Malignant skin melanoma rarely if ever develops along the eyelid margin. The diagnosis of eyelid melanoma would be based on histologic documentation of anaplastic melanoma features with the invasion of eyelid tissues. In contrast, the melanocytoma has distinctive benign features histologically, which include large round heavily pigmented cells that vary from spindle to polygonal shapes, and they are arranged in clusters within the epidermis and below in the subcutaneous tissues. The lack of mitotic figures, infiltration of eyelid tissues, and benign histologic features (limited mitotic figures, mild anisocytosis, and anisokaryosis) confirm the benign nature of this marginal eyelid tumor. These tumors are usually slow growing and can be photographed and monitored. Surgical resection is curative for the individual pedunculated lesions, whereas more extensive surgical blepharoplasty is required to remove contiguous melanocytomas. The only significant clinical differential diagnosis is the pigmented tarsal gland adenoma that originates from the tarsal gland and has extended through the lid margin (see **Fig. 10**), whereas eyelid melanocytoma are pedunculated and extend off the skin only. Adjunctive therapy including laser or cryotherapy although commonly recommended is not required provided surgical margins are clean. The prognosis postexcision is excellent.

Eyelid histiocytoma. This is also a relatively common benign cutaneous neoplasm of young dogs, and there is a subtle preference for these to develop on the eyelids. The clinical manifestations are a solitary umbilicated usually hairless or alopecic pink tumor (**Fig. 13**). The diagnosis is confirmed by excisional biopsy, which reveals a

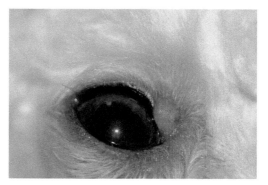

Fig. 13. This young dog has a typical eyelid histiocytoma. Note the alopecia, umbilicated shape and the mild hyperemia.

nonencapsulated dermal tumor that is composed of sheets of histiocytes with a variable population of lymphocytes and occasional neutrophils. This tumor originates from dermal Langerhans cells. These are occasionally misdiagnosed as cutaneous lymphosarcoma, or granulomatous inflammation, and immunohistochemistry can be used to confirm the diagnosis and rule out other cutaneous round cell tumors.[31–36] Although many histiocytomas are commonly treated by excisional biopsy, these will spontaneously regress, and the prognosis is excellent. Recently, lymph node metastasis has been reported in several dogs although long-term follow-up failed to reveal any evidence of systemic complications.[37]

Eyelid mast cell neoplasia

Although mast cell tumors are among the most frequent canine skin neoplasms, they are less commonly diagnosed on the palpebrae than adenomas, melanocytomas, and histiocytomas. The clinical manifestations in the dog include hyperemia, and diffuse edematous swelling of the affected eyelid (**Fig. 14**). These findings are very similar to the even less common infiltrative palpebral lymphosarcoma and the more common pyogranulomatous blepharitis, and these manifestations always warrant eyelid dermal biopsies with submission for light microscopic examination. Eosinophils commonly accompany mast cell neoplasms, and the neoplastic mast cells are round with cytoplasmic metachromatic granules that stain readily with toluidine blue. Eyelid mast cell neoplasms are graded similar to other dermal mast cell neoplasms. The grades include grade 1 (a bland oval to round cell neoplasm with prominent granules and few to no mitoses), grade 2 (similar oval to round cells with anisokaryosis and anisocytosis and occasional mitotic figures), and grade 3 (cells have marked anisocytosis and anisokaryosis with many mitotic figures and usually invasion of subcutaneous tissues). Surgical resection remains the treatment of choice, and benign forms are more common in the dog eyelid than malignant types.

Eyelid lymphosarcoma

Systemic lymphosarcoma will masquerade as primary blepharitis or other primary palpebral neoplasia occasionally in dogs (**Fig. 15**). This is usually a systemic neoplasm, and the diagnosis is through dermal biopsy and histologic examination. The diagnosis of palpebral lymphosarcoma warrants a thorough physical examination, complete blood count, serum biochemical analysis, urinalysis, and advanced imaging of the chest and abdominal cavities and staging. Once the lymphosarcoma is staged, referral for medical oncologist assessment and chemotherapy should be considered and the long-term prognosis is guarded.

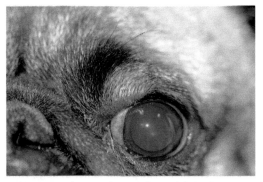

Fig. 14. Mast cell neoplasia manifests with a subtle eyelid thickening and mild to moderate hyperemia.

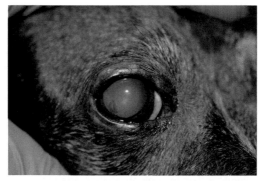

Fig. 15. Lymphosarcoma is the great mimicker of blepharitis and many eyelid neoplasms. Note the subtle thickened upper eyelid on this dog with palpebral lymphosarcoma.

Eyelid fibrosarcoma and peripheral nerve sheath tumors

The clinical manifestation of these 2 neoplasms is similar, usually a firm slowing enlarging eyelid tumor within the eyelid of older dogs. The diagnosis is based on histologic examination of excisional or incisional biopsies. Surgical removal remains the therapy of choice, and similar to all spindle cell neoplasms, local recurrence related to inadequate removal is the most common complication.

Squamous cell carcinoma

This is actually an uncommon neoplasm of the canine eyelids. It is reported here simply to be thorough and alert naïve veterinarians that dogs rarely get this eyelid neoplasm that is so common in horses and cattle, and is seen more occasionally in cats. Typically, as in other species, this neoplasm develops in poorly pigmented palpebral skin and manifests as a scaly erosive to ulcerative pale pink tumor. The diagnosis is confirmed by histologic examination of excisional or incisional biopsies. Surgical excision with clean surgical margins is curative, and adjunctive therapies including cryotherapy are commonly completed.

Trichoblastoma

This exophytic tumor is also uncommon and manifests as a slowly growing nodular to papillomatous mass, often with mild ulceration and discharge (**Fig. 16**). This is a

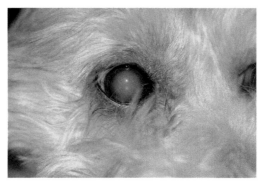

Fig. 16. Trichoblastoma is an uncommon palpebral tumor of dogs, which often manifests as an exophytic dermal tumor that is very similar in appearance to tarsal gland adenomas but it develops independent of the tarsal glands.

benign tumor of the hair follicle tissues. The diagnosis is confirmed usually by histologic examination of excisional biopsies. This benign dermal neoplasm is cured by complete surgical excision.

Granular cell neoplasia

This neoplasm develops usually as a hairless or mildly alopecia mass with a predilection to the medial canthus (**Fig. 17**). Most granular cell neoplasms develop within the oral cavity, lips, and some are reported in the calavarium and less commonly in the skin, lymph nodes, and vascular system.[38] The diagnosis is confirmed by histologic examination, which reveals acidophilic granules packed within the cytoplasm.[38] Complete surgical removal is curative and the lack of invasion, slow growth, and lack of mitotic figures strongly support that this is a benign neoplasm. The cell of origin for granular cell tumors has received considerable debate, and previous reports of a myoblastic origin have been refuted. Most pathologists today think these benign neoplasms originate from Schwann cells based on immunohistochemistry and electron microscopy.[38] However, negative immunohistochemical labeling with S100 and cytokeratin on palpebral canine granular cell tumors make Schwann cell or epithelial origins unlikely, and vimentin staining of these cells have suggested a possible mesenchymal origin.[39,40] The prognosis postsurgical resection remains excellent.

Eyelid hamartomas/dermoids (the conundrum of classification of hamartomas and choristomas revisited)

These palpebral tumors are nonneoplastic, and they may be classified as hamartomas of perhaps 2 types rather than a hamartoma and choristoma. The hamartoma of the eyelid is a collagen-rich mass that develops on the eyelid of middle-aged to older dogs, and the pathogenesis is unknown (**Fig. 18**). Palpebral hamartomas are rare, and one retrospective histopathologic report describes canine eyelid hamartomas in 10 dogs.[41] The age range at diagnosis of these dogs were aged 6 to 10 years, which is substantially older than the palpebral dermoids reported by others, which begs the question whether eyelid hamartomas and eyelid dermoids are different in their pathogenesis. However, the report by an earlier study[41] suggests that these lesions may have been present at a younger age and then enlarged. Hamartomas likely represent an intermediate disorder of tissue proliferation, where one tissue is overproduced and is between malformation and benign neoplasm.[41–47]

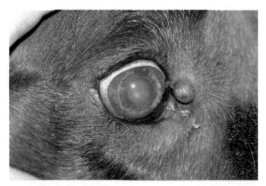

Fig. 17. Granular cell neoplasms are also uncommon palpebral tumors. They arise most frequently in the oral cavity and elsewhere in dogs. When they do develop on the eyelid, they are alopecic, slow growing tumor with a predisposition to the medial canthus.

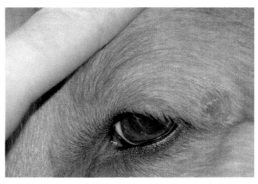

Fig. 18. Hamartoma of the canine eyelid is a rare palpebral tumor. Note the alopecia of this slow growing eyelid mass.

In contrast, the ocular choristoma (ocular dermoid), that are congenital and present on the limbus, cornea, and conjunctiva are misplaced normal tissues which develop during embryogenesis. This is the correct designation for all ocular surface dermoids but not for eyelid dermoids because most of these masses are composed of epithelial and mesodermal elements.[41,48] Therefore, the most commonly diagnosed dermoids, those that manifest on the limbal cornea and bulbar conjunctiva and limbus are choristomas because they are misplaced normal tissues.[49] However, when they are diagnosed on the palpebrae (**Fig. 19**), they may be better classified in this location as a congenital hamartoma, because they contain enlarged dermal elements and yet are located on the skin surface of the eyelid, refuting the classification that defines choristoma. Bandanes and Ledbetter reported more than 20% of their dermoids were palpebral, and it is quite likely that eyelid dermoids are missed by simply being hidden in eyelid hair or ignored as a tuft of longer hair. Similarly, many limbal, corneal, and conjunctival dermoids are overlooked in the first few months of life,[49] until the hair growth on the dermoid induces epiphora, keratitis, ulceration, and pigmentation.

The treatment of choice for ocular dermoids that are inducing irritation is surgical excision.[48,50–52] Ocular dermoids that are inducing no or minimal irritation can be ignored or treated with ocular lubrication.[49] Similarly, palpebral dermoids that are not inducing ocular irritation secondary to large hairs (trichiasis) may also be ignored

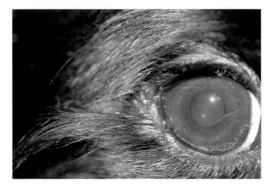

Fig. 19. Eyelid dermoids can go undetected in longhaired dogs. Note the tuft of long hair growing from the small eyelid mass, which is typical of an eyelid dermoid.

and considered a congenital blemish. Dermoids have been reported to have a genetic predisposition in dogs, cattle, and cats.[49] Systemic cardiac disease and hepatic portosystemic shunts have been reported in 20% of dogs with ocular dermoids.[49]

Having diagnosed both palpebral dermoids and palpebral hamartomas in the dog clinically and confirmed these with light microscopy, the clinical and histologic findings also differ significantly. Palpebral hamartomas are often hairless or alopecic and located often at the lateral canthus. Histologic examination reveals that they are composed of disorganized bundles of collagen, with some interlacing adipose and skeletal muscle bundles. These are rare incidental submissions of excisional or diagnostic biopsies from middle age to older dogs. In contrast, the palpebral dermoids are more appropriately classified a congenital hamartoma and they are more common, and manifest in young dogs. Veterinarians and ophthalmologists ignore many as palpebral masses with hypertrichosis. Histologic examination of these reveals small bundles of collagen, many large hair follicles, sebaceous and apocrine glands, and fat. The prognosis after surgical resection of palpebral hamartomas and dermoids is excellent.

CLINICS CARE POINTS

- Canine blepharitis and eyelid neoplasms both manifest as eyelid tumors (ie, masses), and therefore, they are clinical differential diagnoses.
- Differentiating blepharitis from eyelid neoplasia requires excisional or incisional biopsies and histologic examination.
- Canine eyelid neoplasms are usually benign, and their surgical excision with or without adjunctive therapy is usually curative.
- Most types of canine blepharitis respond to systemic medications with or without topical therapeutics.

REFERENCES

1. Aquino SM. Management of eyelid neoplasms in the dog and cat. Clin Tech Small Anim Pract 2007;22:46–54.
2. Bezerra JAB, Santos JPdS, Filgueira KD. Canine juvenile cellulitis: a retrospective study (2009-2016). Braz J Vet Res Anim Sci 2017;54:407–11.
3. Jeffers JG, Duclos DD, Goldschmidt MH. A dermatosis resembling juvenile cellulitis in an adult dog. J Am Anim Hosp Assoc 1995;31:204–8.
4. Neuber AE, van den Broek AH, Brownstein D, et al. Dermatitis and lymphadenitis resembling juvenile cellulitis in a four-year-old dog. J Small Anim Pract 2004;45: 254–8.
5. Newbold GM, Outerbridge CA, Kass PH, et al. Malassezia spp on the periocular skin of dogs and their association with blepharitis, ocular discharge, and the application of ophthalmic medications. J Am Vet Med Assoc 2014;244:1304–8.
6. White SD, Rosychuk RA, Stewart LJ, et al. Juvenile Cellulitis in dogs: 15 cases (1979-1988). J Am Vet Med Assoc 1989;195:1609–11.
7. Zibura AE, Henriksen MdL, Rendahl A, et al. Retrospective evaluation of canine palpebral masses treated with debulking and cryotherapy. Vet Ophthalmol 2019; 22:256–64.
8. Reimann KA, Evans MG, Chalifoux LV, et al. Clinic pathologic characterization of canine juvenile cellulitis. Vet Path 1989;26:499–504.

9. Romkes G, Klopfleisch R, Eule JC. Evaluation of one vs two-layered closure after wedge excision of 43 eyelid tumors in dogs. Vet Ophthalmol 2014;17:32–40.

10. Sansom J, Heinrich C, Featherstone H. Pyogranulomatous blepharitis in two dogs. J Small Anim Pract 2000;41:80–3.

11. Hutchings SM. Juvenile cellulitis in a puppy. Can Vet J 2003;44:418–9.

12. Helga K, Natalija MM, Tatjana L, et al. Traumatic blepharitis including cutaneous changes with a clinical appearance of immune-mediated disease. Acta Vet 2021; 71:120–30.

13. Bistner S. Allergic and immunologic mediated diseases of the eye and adnexa. Vet Clin North America 1994;24:711–34.

14. Wiggans KT, Hoover CE, Erhart EJ, et al. Malignant transformation of a putative eyelid papilloma to a squamous cell carcinoma in a dog. Vet Ophthalmol 2013; 16:105–12.

15. Weingart C, Kohn B, Siekierski M, et al. Blepharitis in dogs; a clinical evaluation in 102 dogs. Vet Dermatol 2019;30:222.

16. Whitley D 2000.

17. Whitley RD. Canine and feline primary ocular bacterial infections. Vet Clin North America 2000;30:1151–67.

18. Stades FC, van der Woerdt A. Diseases and Surgery of the canine eyelid. In: Gelatt KN, editor. Veterinary ophthalmology. 6th ed. Wiley Blackwell Hoboken NJ; 2021. p. 923–87.

19. Grahn B, Peiffer R, Wilcock B. Diseases of the eyelid, conjunctiva, lacrimal, and nasolacrimal systems. In: Histologic basis of ocular disease in animals, 2019. p. 105–42.

20. Chambers ED, Severin GA. Staphylococcal bacterin for treatment of chronic staphylococcal blepharitis in the dog. J Am Vet Med Assoc 1984;185:422–4.

21. Csaba J, Velovics J, Agnes Szabara A. Incidence of canine eyelid tumors. Retrospective pathological study. Magyar allatorvosok Lapja 2012;134:330–8.

22. Donaldson D, Day MJ. Epitheliotropic lymphoma (mycosis fungoides) presenting as blepharoconjunctivitis in an Irish setter. J Small Anim Pract 2000;41:317–20.

23. Rosenthal. 1975.

24. Olias-Molerno AI, Fontan-Matilla E, Cuquerella M, et al. Scientometric analysis of chemotherapy of canine leishmaniasis (2000-2020). Parasites & Vectors 2021; 14:1–8.

25. Stades F, van der Woerdt. 2019.

26. Moriello KA, Coyner K, Paterson S, et al. Diagnosis and treatment of dermatophytosis in dogs and cats: Clinical consensus. Vet Dermatol 2017;28:266–8.

27. Munoz-Duque JD, Ramirez-Rojas MC, Duque-Arias S, et al. Eye-related neoplasms in dogs a retrospective study. Revista Colombiana de Ciencias Pecuarias 2019;32:298–311.

28. Pena MR, Leiva M. Canine conjunctivitis and blepharitis. Vet Clin North America, SAP 2008;3:233–49.

29. Pena MT, Roura X, Davidson MG. Ocular and periocular manifestations of leishmaniasis in dogs: 105 cases (1993-1998. Vet Ophthalmol 2000;3:35–41.

30. Dubielzig R et al 2010.

31. Fernandez NJ, west KH, Jackson ML, et al. Immunohistochemical and histochemical stains for differentiating canine cutaneous round cell tumors. Vet Path 2005;42:437–45.

32. Furiani N, Scarampella F, Piera AM, et al. Evaluation of the bacterial microflora of the conjunctival sac of healthy dogs and dogs with atopic dermatitis. Vet Dermatol 2011;22:490–6.

33. Stilwell JM, Rissi DR. Immunohistochemical labelling of multiple myeloma onco-gene1/interferon regulatory factor 4 (MUM1/IRF-4) in canine cutaneous histiocy-toma. Vet Path 2018;55:517–20.
34. Vercelli A, Cornegliani L, Portigliotti L. Eyelid eosinophilic granuloma in a Siberian husky. J Small Anim Pract 2005;46:31–3.
35. Wang AL, Kern T. Melanocytic ophthalmic neoplasms of the domestic veterinary species: A review. Topic Comp Anim Pract 2015;43:111–2.
36. Wang SL, Dawson C, Wei LN, et al. The investigation of histopathology and loca-tion of excised eyelid masses in dogs. Vet Rec 2019;6:12–8.
37. Faller M, Lamm C, Affolter VK, et al. Retrospective characterization of solitary cutaneous histiocytoma with lymph node metastasis in eight dogs. J Small Anim Pract 2016;57:548–52.
38. Meuten DM 2002.
39. Lu JE, Dubielzig R. Canine eyelid granular cell tumor: a report of eight cases. Vet Ophthalmol 2012;15:406–10.
40. Mikkelsen LH, Holm F, Clasen-Linde E, et al. T cell lymphoma in the eyelid of a 9-year old English setter. Acta Vet Scandinavia 2018;60:79.
41. Kafarnik C, Calvarese S, Dubielzig RR. Canine mesenchymal hamartoma of the eyelid. Vet Ophthalmol 2010;13:94–8.
42. Kim Y, Kim H-J, Kim JH, et al. A case of blepharoconjunctivitis associated with atopic dermatitis. J Biomed Translational Res 2021;22:100–4.
43. Komnenou A, Thomas A, Kyriazis AP, et al. Ocular manifestations of canine trans-missible venereal tumor: a retrospective study of 25 cases in Greece. Vet Rec 2015;176:523.
44. Krehbiel JD, Langham RF. Eyelid neoplasms of dogs. Am J Vet Res 1975;36:115–9.
45. Ledbetter EC. Canine herpesvirus-1 ocular diseases of mature dogs. N Z Vet J 2013;61:193–201.
46. Lourenco-Martins AM, Delgado E, Neto I, et al. Allergic conjunctivitis and conjunctival provocation tests in atopic dogs. Vet Ophthalmol 2011;14:248–56.
47. Schorfield D Cotran RS 1999.
48. Balland O, Raymond I, Mathieson I, et al. Canine bilateral conjunctivo-palpebral dermoid; Description of two clinical cases and discussion of the relevance of the terminology. Case Rep Vet Med 2015;2015:1–6.
49. Bandanes Z, Ledbetter EC. Ocular dermoids in dogs: a retrospective study. Vet Ophthalmol 2019;22:760–6.
50. Erdikmen Do, Aydin D, Saroglu M, et al. Surgical correction of ocular dermoids in dogs: 22 cases. Kafkas Uni Vet Fak Derg 2013;19(Suppl-A A41-A47).
51. Esson DW. Autoimmune blepharitis. In: Esson D, Calvarose S, editors. Clinical atlas of canine and feline ophthalmic disease. Google Books; 2015. p. 44–5.
52. Esson DW. Demodex-associated blepharitis. In: Clinical atlas of canine and feline ophthalmic disease. Google Books; 2015. p. 52–3.

Topical Ocular Therapeutics in Small Animals

Elizabeth M. James-Jenks, BVSc (Hons)*, Chantale L. Pinard, DVM, MSc

KEYWORDS

- Topical ocular therapeutics • Antimicrobials • Anti-inflammatories
- Antiglaucoma medications • Lacrostimulants

KEY POINTS

- Topical ocular medications penetrate the eye via corneal and noncorneal routes.
- Bioavailability is affected by composition of the preparation as well as interactions with the tear film.
- Systemic absorption of topical medications does occur, with potential adverse effects.

BACKGROUND

Topical ophthalmic medications are widely used to treat a variety of ocular diseases. The topical route of administration is often chosen over systemic, due to its relative ease of administration and potential for reduced systemic side effects. Considerations of topical administration should include the desired target ocular structure within the anterior segment of the eye, potential barriers to absorption, the ability to achieve therapeutic concentrations at the target site, potential adverse effects, and patient compliance. This article aims to discuss the administration of topical ophthalmic mediations as well as the indications, pharmacology, and adverse effects of commercially available topical ocular therapeutic agents used in the therapy for anterior segment diseases.

CONSIDERATIONS OF TOPICAL OCULAR THERAPEUTICS
Relevant Anatomy and Physiology

Cornea
Topical medications can penetrate the corneal epithelium by both the transcellular and paracellular routes.[1,2] The ability of medications to penetrate the cornea via the transcellular route is related to each medication's oil/water coefficient due to the lipophilic epithelium.[3] The paracellular route is complicated by the tight intercellular junctions (Zonula occludens), which fuse the plasma membranes of adjoining cells in numerous

Department of Clinical Studies, University of Guelph, Ontario Veterinary College, 50 Stone Road East, Guelph, Ontario N1G 2W1, Canada
* Corresponding author.
E-mail address: lizziejj@me.com

Vet Clin Small Anim 53 (2023) 473–492
https://doi.org/10.1016/j.cvsm.2022.10.008   **vetsmall.theclinics.com**
0195-5616/23/© 2022 Elsevier Inc. All rights reserved.

places and result in an intercellular space of 0.6 nm to less than 3 nm. Lipophilic medication molecules can cross through the transcellular route, whereas the tight intercellular junctions ensure that the paracellular route is only accessible to the smallest hydrophilic molecules.[4] The corneal stroma is easily penetrated by hydrophilic medications and acts as a barrier to lipophilic substances. The endothelium is easily permeable, and it has been demonstrated that there is limited resistance to the passage of lipophilic or hydrophilic medications.[5]

Conjunctiva and sclera

The conjunctiva is up to 25 times easier to penetrate than the cornea, and the most of the absorption occurs through the paracellular route.[5–7] Following penetration of the conjunctiva, the medication can then diffuse into the anterior chamber via the sclera and cornea, or pass through scleral vessels into the anterior uvea.[8] Ophthalmic preparations formulated with a mucoadhesive polymer, which promotes prolonged contact time with the bulbar conjunctiva, will favor this noncorneal route of topical medication absorption.[9]

Medications penetrate the sclera 10 times more easily than the cornea.[5,7,10] The ability for a medication to penetrate the sclera is largely based on its molecular radius, and hydrophilic medications can cross more easily than lipophilic.[5,7,10] The amount of absorption, which occurs through the scleral route versus the corneal route has been demonstrated to be significant for certain medications.[8]

Administration of Topical Medications

Interactions with tear film and volume

Once applied, topical medications mix with the tear film on the ocular surface and within the conjunctival sac. The median basal tear volume has been reported to be 65 μL in dogs and 32 μL in cats,[11] and the average volume of a drop of an ophthalmic preparation is 40 μL (range of 25–70 μL).[12] Consequently, the tear film significantly dilutes all topical medications.[11] In dogs and cats, the rate of continuous tear film turnover is 11% to 12% per minute.[11] As a result, the volume of topical medication that reaches the ocular surface, and does not immediately overflow the eyelid margin or into the nasolacrimal puncta, is estimated to be completely removed within 10 minutes following administration.[11]

Factors influencing the nasolacrimal drainage of topical ocular medications include the volume of the drop administered, the viscosity of the ophthalmic preparation, and the rate of blinking. A loss of between 80% and 90% of the medication occurs either via the nasolacrimal system or by directly overflowing the eyelids following administration.[13,14] Studies have demonstrated that providing a larger volume of a drop only increases the rate of nasolacrimal drainage.[13,14] Administering more drops of topical medication increases nasolacrimal drainage and eyelid spillage in a manner that is proportional to the time between installation of these additional drops.[8] This is why a period of at least 5 to 10 minutes between applications of one drop of serial topical ocular medications is recommended.[13–15]

Composition of ophthalmic preparations

Topical ocular medications consist of solutions, suspensions, ointments, and gels. Solutions are composed of molecules completely dissolved in a solvent, which is usually suspended in aqueous but occasionally lipid based. In addition to the aqueous base, most solutions will have organic or inorganic carriers, buffers, emulsifiers, or wetting agents to enhance the stability and sterility of the medication.[16] Advantages of solutions are ease of administration and minimal associated discomfort after application, therefore often superior owner compliance. Disadvantages are a shorter shelf life in comparison to other formulations, such as ointments. When the therapeutic agent is not water soluble, a suspension in acetate or alcohol may be required.[17]

A suspension is composed of solid particles of the medication (active ingredient) within liquid dispersing and suspending agents. Suspensions are harder to stabilize, and this can lead to accumulation of the suspended particles and a nonuniform dispersion. As with solutions, an advantage of suspensions is ease of administration to small animals. Another advantage is prolonged contact time in comparison to solutions, which can enhance bioavailability.[17] Disadvantages include the need for the medication to be well shaken before administration to ensure appropriate dosing, and the potential for a crystal or particle within the suspension that may cause mild ocular discomfort to the animal.[16,17]

Ointments are traditionally used when a prolonged contact time is desired. Most ointments have a white petrolatum and liquid petrolatum (mineral oil) base, with or without a water-miscible agent, that is, lanolin.[16,17] The mineral oil component ensures that the ointment melts at room temperature for ease of application, and the lanolin is used to retain water-soluble medications within the ointment. Once administered, the ointment is contained in the conjunctival sac until it melts, allowing the water-soluble medication particles to be dissolved into the tear film.[17] This prolongs the interval between administration and when peak drug concentration within the target tissue is reached, in comparison to solutions or suspensions.[17,18] Ointments are retained far longer than solutions or suspensions due to their larger molecule size, viscosity, reduced nasolacrimal drainage and interactions between ointment base and tear film.[18,19] Studies have reported that ointments can be found on the ocular surface up to 4 hours following administration.[20] Advantages of ointments include less frequent dosing due to the prolonged retention on the ocular surface and increased shelf life. A disadvantage is when multiple medications are required, the retention of the ointment on the ocular surface complicates dosing intervals and one should wait at least 20 to 30 minutes between topical ocular ointments. Ointments do not have a manufactured "dropper," therefore their dosing is less precise. When ointments are applied with solutions or suspensions, they need to be applied last.[21]

Ophthalmic gels use natural gum, hyaluronic acid, cellulosic components, or polyacrylic acids to increase the viscosity of an ophthalmic preparation.[22] These medications are ideal for hydrophilic therapeutic agents because it increases the contact time with the ocular surface through the viscosity and higher molecular weight.[23] Ophthalmic gels can be a preformed gel, or they may undergo gelation once in contact with the ocular surface under the influence of pH, temperature, and electrolyte concentrations.[22] Advantages of ophthalmic gels are increased contact time, and currently no significant adverse effects associated with the gel composition have been reported.

Regardless of the preparation, the medication should mimic the eye's natural tonicity and pH as closely as possible to minimize local irritation and discomfort.[24,25] Most ophthalmic preparations have a tonicity of approximately 300 mOsm/kg, which is based on the osmolality of human tears and close to that reported in cats and dogs.[26,27] The pH must be within the range of 4.5 to 9.0, and most ophthalmic topical medications have a pH between 7.0 and 7.7 to maximize comfort.[25] This pH range of 7.0 to 7.7 has been shown to be consistent with the pH of tears in small animals.[24] If the ophthalmic preparation is formulated in a way that causes irritation and increased lacrimation, the volume of medication lost through nasolacrimal drainage and eyelid spillage increases and this impairs absorption.[15] In dogs and cats, reflex tearing will increase the rate of tear film turnover and, therefore, excretion of topically applied medications by up to 5 times.[11]

Systemic Effects of Topical Medications

It is important to acknowledge that systemic absorption will occur with all topically applied ophthalmic medications. The conjunctiva is a major site of systemic absorption, due to the large surface area and permeability of the blood vessels of the bulbar conjunctiva and episclera.[6,28] The nasolacrimal duct epithelium has been demonstrated to absorb lipophilic medications in rabbits,[29] and the nasal and oral mucosa is thought to be a significant contributor to systemic absorption of topical medications across various species.[28,29] As topical medications exceed the volume that the conjunctival fornixes can retain, the excess medication is drained through the nasolacrimal system, where it reaches the nasopharynx,[14] and eyelid seepage occurs. Because the nasopharyngeal mucosa has similar permeability to that of conjunctiva, systemic absorption readily ensues. Because these methods of systemic absorption bypass the first-pass hepatic metabolism, their potential systemic effects have been compared with those of a slow intravenous injection,[28] and this should be considered carefully in small animals. Adverse systemic effects have been associated with topical phenylephrine; timolol; glucocorticoids and atropine in dogs, cats, and other small animals[30–35]; and for the topical nonsteroidal anti-inflammatory (NSAID) diclofenac in cats.[36] Further evidence of systemic absorption of topical medications is seen when the contralateral eye displays the effects of the medications administered such as timolol.[37,38]

COMMERCIALLY AVAILABLE TOPICAL OCULAR MEDICATIONS
Antibiotics

Bacitracin, neomycin, Polymixin-B
Bacitracin is a polypeptide bacteriostatic antibiotic, which has a mostly gram-positive spectrum of activity. It demonstrates good activity against Staphylococcus intermedius and beta hemolytic Streptococcus in dogs with bacterial keratitis.[39] Bacitracin is commercially available as a combination ointment with neomycin and polymyxin-B (BNP), which increases its spectrum of antibacterial activity.

Neomycin is a bactericidal aminoglycoside with a predominantly gram-negative spectrum and is another component of the triple-antibiotic commercial preparation with bacitracin and polymyxin B. S intermedius is highly susceptible[39] and methicillin-resistant staphylococcus aureus (MRSA) and Pseudomonas are mostly susceptible[39,40]; however, beta hemolytic Streptococcus spp are highly resistant.[39]

Polymixin-B is a bactericidal polypeptide antibiotic with a gram-negative only spectrum of activity, and good activity against Pseudomonas isolates.[39] Local hypersensitivity following topical application of bacitracin has been reported.[41] Additionally, there is a report of anaphylaxis occurring in 61 cats following topical application of polymyxin-B,[42] and this warrants caution when considering administration to cats. Because both the individual antimicrobials and the combination solutions or ointments have very limited ability to penetrate an intact cornea, BNP ointment is indicated as prophylaxis in cases of superficial ulcerative keratitis and the treatment of general superficial ocular surface infections.[43]

Aminoglycosides: gentamicin and tobramycin
Gentamicin is a bactericidal aminoglycoside, which is often used for the treatment of bacterial keratitis in veterinary ophthalmology. Studies have demonstrated some resistance from beta hemolytic Streptococcus strains in dogs, however good efficacy against Pseudomonas and S intermedius spp.[39] A recent study has also demonstrated high susceptibility of MRSA isolates.[40] Due to its narrow gram-negative spectrum, and the predominantly gram-positive ocular microflora of small animals,[44–47] gentamicin is

not generally used as a first-line agent in cases of corneal ulceration. Gentamicin has minimal ability to penetrate an intact cornea, although this is improved slightly when there is concurrent keratitis.[48,49] This antibiotic has been demonstrated to have damaging effects on corneal epithelial cell wound healing in vitro.[50–52]

Tobramycin has bactericidal activity against *Staphylococcus* and *Pseudomonas* isolates.[39] There are conflicting reports on its epithelial toxicity, with some studies demonstrating minimal effects on the healing of epithelial cells,[50,51] whereas another study showed significant prolongation of healing time in comparison to other agents.[52] Tobramycin is indicated as a first-line topical antibiotic in cases of ulcerative keratitis.

Macrolides: erythromycin and azithromycin

Macrolides are a group of antibiotics that exert their action via binding the 30s ribosomal subunit and inhibiting the peptide chain lengthening required for bacterial mRNA translation.[41] They have a mostly gram-positive spectrum of activity and are primarily bacteriostatic with bactericidal activity at high concentrations. Erythromycin, a macrolide with demonstrated efficacy against *Mycoplasma* and *Chlamydophila*, is commercially available as a 0.5% ointment. It has minimal efficacy demonstrated in dogs with aerobic ocular bacterial infections and, therefore, is not indicated as prophylaxis in cases of corneal ulceration.[53] Erythromycin's primary clinical indication is in cats with *Chlamydophila* and *Mycoplasma*-associated conjunctivitis.

Azithromycin is a newer medication with increased gram-negative coverage[41] and is available commercially in a 1% ointment and solution. Topical administration of azithromycin at varying concentrations has resulted in therapeutic levels in the conjunctiva[54] and cornea[55]; however, these levels were not reached in the AH.[54] Compared with other commercially available medications, azithromycin has been shown to be less effective against *Rickettsia rickettsii*[56] and *Bartonella*,[57] and there has been a report of resistance developing rapidly.[58]

Fusidic acid

Fusidic acid is a bacteriostatic antibiotic that has a good spectrum of activity against gram-positive organisms, especially *Staphylococcus* spp, and limited activity against gram-negative organisms.[59] It is commercially available as a 1% carbolic gel, and labeled for minor ocular surface infection, such as secondary bacterial conjunctivitis in cases of keratoconjunctivitis sicca (KCS).

Sulfonamides

Sulfonamides are bacteriostatic antibiotics that inhibit bacterial folate metabolism. Sulfonamides are commercially available as 10% ophthalmic solution. The transcorneal penetration of topical sulfonamides is highly variable, and between 96% and 100% of aerobic organisms in small animals are susceptible.[53]

Fluoroquinolones: ofloxacin, ciprofloxacin, norfloxacin, lomefloxacin, sparfloxacin, gemifloxacin, levofloxacin, gatifloxacin, moxifloxacin, and besifloxacin

Fluoroquinolones are bactericidal antibiotics that inhibit bacterial DNA gyrase. Ciprofloxacin 0.3%, ofloxacin 0.3%, norfloxacin 0.3%, and lomefloxacin 0.3% are available as commercial preparations as second-generation fluoroquinolones. These medications are broad spectrum with strong efficacy against gram-positives and *Pseudomonas* spp. The spectrum of gram-positive activity increases with each generation of fluoroquinolones.[60] In canine bacterial keratitis, 100% of *Staphylococcus* spp and *Streptococcus* spp and 35% of MRSA were susceptible to ciprofloxacin 0.3%.[39,40] Good efficacy against *Pseudomonas* (93%–100% susceptibility) has also been demonstrated in dogs.[39,61] Topical ofloxacin has been shown to reach higher, and more therapeutic, aqueous humor concentrations than topical ciprofloxacin in dogs.[62] Several third-generation fluoroquinolones, sparfloxacin 0.3%, gemifloxacin 0.3%, and levofloxacin 0.5% or 1.5%, are available as topical ophthalmic therapeutic agents. In dogs, 100% of *Pseudomonas* isolates were susceptible to levofloxacin.[61] Fourth-generation fluoroquinolones, gatifloxacin 0.3% or 0.5%, moxifloxacin 0.5%, and besifloxacin 0.6%, are also available as commercial preparations. *Pseudomonas* isolates in a canine study of bacterial keratitis demonstrated resistance to both gatifloxacin and moxifloxacin.[61] Moxifloxacin has an increased ability to penetrate the cornea and achieve intraocular therapeutic concentrations, in comparison to several other fluoroquinolones.[63] Besifloxacin was developed specifically for topical ophthalmic use, and contains a mucoadhesive polymer, which is designed to increase its contact time and enhance its ability to maintain therapeutic concentrations within the cornea and aqueous humor.[64] It is recommended that fourth-generation fluoroquinolones be reserved for complex ophthalmologic infections in dogs and cats to minimize antimicrobial resistance.[41,63] Reported adverse effects include the development of a white crystalline corneal plaque following topical levofloxacin administration.[65] Additionally, cytotoxic damage and reduced stromal keratocyte proliferation with the use of ciprofloxacin, ofloxacin, and norfloxacin has been demonstrated in vitro.[66]

Tetracyclines

Tetracyclines are another group of medications that exert their antibacterial activity by interacting with the 30S ribosomal subunit to inhibit bacterial mRNA translation.[41] These medications can be short acting (tetracycline, oxytetracycline), intermediate acting (demeclocycline), or long acting (doxycycline, minocycline). Overall, tetracyclines have broad-spectrum activity, however many bacteria have developed resistant strains.[41] Rickettsial organisms are consistently susceptible, compared with *Staphylococcus* and *Streptococcus* spp, which have resistance reported to be developing.[41,56,67] In addition to antibacterial activity, tetracyclines are reported to be reactive oxygen species scavengers, and therefore exert some anti-inflammatory effects.[68,69] This was thought to contribute to the significantly shorter healing times noted in dogs receiving topical oxytetracycline in a study of canine refractory ulcers.[69]

Antivirals

Thymidine analogs

Idoxuridine and trifluridine are both thymidine analogs that impede viral replication.[70] Idoxuridine has strongly specific activity against feline herpes virus (FHV-1); however, it does not penetrate the eye well.[71,72] It is commercially available as a 0.1% solution and is reportedly well tolerated,[73,74] although it may not be very efficacious in cats with herpetic keratitis. Trifluridine also has good in vitro specificity for FHV-1,[72] and is commercially available as a 1% solution but is poorly tolerated in cats.[73,74] Both idoxuridine and trifluridine are virostatic, and therefore require frequent dosing, with topical administration required at intervals of 4 to 6 hours.[74] Dogs with CHV-1 infections have demonstrated a good response to the treatment with 1% trifluridine and no signs of discomfort were associated with topical administration.[75]

Antifungals

Natamycin

Natamycin is currently the only topical ophthalmic antifungal approved for use and commercially available as a 5% suspension.[76] Its ability to penetrate an intact cornea is poor. An in vitro study demonstrates severe cytotoxic effects on equine keratocytes.[77] Unfortunately, there are no veterinary studies evaluating the use of natamycin topically in cats or dogs.

Anti-inflammatories

Corticosteroids

There are several commercial preparations of corticosteroids available for use in small animals. These are available in varying concentrations with either a water-soluble salt solution or lipophilic acetate or alcohol solutions. For conjunctivitis or nonulcerative keratitis, a water-soluble salt preparation may be the most suitable. For cases of intra-ocular inflammation, due to the lipophilic corneal epithelium, prednisolone acetate 1% or dexamethasone alcohol 0.1% achieves superior absorption and corneal penetration.[78,79] Frequency of dosing is based on the severity of clinical signs and ranges from hourly administration to once per day or every other day use. Previous studies have demonstrated a rebound effect of inflammation if medications are discontinued abruptly, and therefore, tapering of corticosteroid administration is recommended.[80] Use of topical steroid medications has been associated with exacerbation of ocular infection through inhibition of leukocyte migration and suppression of macrophage activity.[81] Corticosteroids applied topically also impede corneal wound healing (epithelial and stromal),[82] inhibit fibroblast formation and limbal blood vessel formation,[83] and potentiate corneal collagenase leading to keratomalacia.[84] As a result, topical corticosteroids are contraindicated in almost all cases of ulcerative keratitis except the uncommon to rare Moorens ulcers and erosive corneal dystrophies in dogs. Cataract formation has been experimentally induced in cats.[85] An elevation in intraocular pressure (IOP) has been documented in cats and dogs with glaucoma.[85–87] Lipid keratopathy has been associated with chronic use of topical steroids and systemic absorption can lead to adrenal suppression, suppression of the hypothalamic-hypophyseal-adrenal axis and hepatic pathologic condition.[30,88] Interestingly, diabetic dogs treated with a topical corticosteroid compared with a topical NSAID demonstrated no clinical differences in the control of their diabetes.[89]

Nonsteroidal anti-inflammatories

Many topical ocular preparations of NSAIDs are commercially available including bromfenac (0.07%, 0.075%, 0.09%), diclofenac (0.1%), flurbiprofen (0.03%), ketorolac (0.4%, 0.45%, 0.5%), and nepafenac (0.1%, 0.3%). Flurbiprofen has been shown to be more effective than topical prednisolone in reducing the disruption of the blood aqueous barrier (BAB) and maintaining mydriasis in the face of inflammation.[90] Diclofenac 1% was demonstrated to be superior to other topical NSAIDs (flurbiprofen, suprofen, tolmetin) in preventing BAB disruption in dogs,[91] and 0.1% diclofenac significantly decreased intraocular inflammation in cats in comparison to the less effective flurbiprofen.[92] Ocular inflammation has been shown to decrease the amount of diclofenac that reaches the anterior chamber, and this results in high corneal levels but low aqueous humor concentrations.[93] The most common adverse effect reported with the use of topical NSAIDs is a transient local irritation. They should also be used with caution in ocular infections and keratitis in rabbits.[94] Topical NSAIDs may also increase the amount of leukotrienes synthesized from arachidonic acid and lower leukocyte infiltration.[95] Furthermore, topical NSAIDs have been demonstrated to reduce epithelial healing[96,97] and have been associated with keratomalacia in human studies.[98–100] This has not been reported in the canine or feline species. Slight increases in IOP have been reported in dogs[101,102] and cats,[92] and this warrants consideration when ocular hypertension or glaucoma is present.[103] Topical flurbiprofen is reported to reduce the antiglaucoma efficacy of latanoprost.[104] Systemic absorption of topical NSAIDs also occurs, with detectable plasma levels present within 7 to

14 days of administration to healthy cats.[36,105] Despite detectable feline plasma levels, cats did not demonstrate any appreciable effects or increase in biochemical markers.[105] Caution is advised when administering topical NSAIDs when a reduction in glomerular filtration rate in volume contracted cats is present.[36]

Antiglaucoma Medications

Carbonic anhydrase inhibitors: dorzolamide and brinzolamide

In healthy dogs, 2% topical dorzolamide achieved a mean reduction in IOP of 3.1 mm Hg (18%), during 30 minutes to 6 hours following administration.[106] Dogs with normal IOP had a maximum decrease in IOP of 6 mm Hg after 5 days of treatment every 8 hours.[107] In glaucomatous eyes, dorzolamide was demonstrated to decrease IOP by mean of approximately 30%.[34] Topical 1% brinzolamide administered twice daily reduced IOP to a similar extent to dorzolamide, with the maximal effect demonstrated between 5 and 6 hours following treatment in dogs with normal IOP.[108] In this study, the mean IOP returned to its premedication value 10 to 11 hours after treatment, thus administration every 8 hours is recommended.[108] The clinical efficacy of dorzolamide has also been demonstrated in feline eyes.[109,110] Dosing twice per day in cats has been shown to be as effective as 3 times daily dosing in dogs.[106,109] In cats with congenital glaucoma, dorzolamide decreases IOP by nearly 46% with TID administration.[111] Brinzolamide administered every 12 hours did not influence IOP in feline eyes[112]; however, it did reduce IOP if given every 8 hours.[113] In normotensive cat eyes, brinzolamide reduced IOP less than dorzolamide.[113] Side effects included renal tubular acidosis in a cat,[114] and blepharitis and keratitis[115] in dogs following application of 2% dorzolamide solution.[116]

Beta-adrenergic antagonists: timolol

Timolol is commercially available as a 0.25% or 0.5% solution in a maleate salt. In healthy dogs, a mean reduction in IOP of 16% (2.5 mm Hg) was noted within 2 to 4 hours following topical administration of 0.5% timolol.[38] Dose-related decreases in IOP were found inconsistently in normotensive dogs and consistently in glaucomatous dogs when timolol administered at concentrations of 4% to 6%.[117] Glaucomatous beagle eyes had a decrease in IOP of 4 to 5 mm Hg.[118] Conflicting studies have been reported with 0.25% and 0.5% that revealed limited to no reduction in IOP in dogs with normal IOPs.[35,118] In healthy cats, a single dose of 0.5% timolol reduced IOP by 22% (4.1 mm Hg) with peak effect within 6 to 12 hours following installation.[37] Combined with dorzolamide, a significant reduction of IOP was seen in eyes of glaucomatous beagles.[34] Combination of timolol and prostaglandin analogs (PG) has been reported to further reduce IOP than either drug individually.[35] A significant reduction in pupil size is seen in canine and feline patients administered with topical timolol maleate.[37,38] This miosis is more pronounced in cats than dogs, can persist up to 1 week following discontinuing treatment.[38] Systemic absorption of topical timolol is demonstrated by a reduction in IOP and pupil diameter in the contralateral eye.[38] Additionally, a significant decrease in heart rate has been demonstrated in beagles that have normal IOP and those with glaucoma when they received topical timolol (0.5%–8%).[34,117,118] To minimize potential systemic effects, it is recommended to use 0.25% timolol instead of 0.5% in cats and small dogs (<10 kg).[119] Additionally, timolol is contraindicated in cats with asthma because it may cause bronchoconstriction.[120]

Prostaglandin analogs (PGs): latanoprost, travoprost, and bimatoprost

Prostaglandin analogs are indicated for primary glaucoma in canine patients.[119] PGs, such as latanoprost, travoprost, and bimatoprost, are commonly used topical ocular antiglaucoma medications. At a concentration of 0.005%, latanoprost significantly reduces IOP in dogs with normal eyes and those with glaucoma.[121] With once daily or twice daily dosing, topical latanoprost resulted in a 25% decrease in IOP of dogs with normal eyes and a 50% reduction in IOP of glaucomatous eyes.[121,122] A similar reduction in IOP was demonstrated in glaucomatous canine eyes with administration of 0.03% bimatoprost[121,122] and 0.004% travoprost.[123,124] Twice daily administration demonstrated less daily fluctuations in the IOP of dogs[122,123,125] and 3 times per day dosing further decreased IOP.[126,127] Concurrent use of anti-inflammatories may reduce the efficacy of PGs in glaucomatous eyes, based on some conflicting reports.[104,128] Conjunctival hyperemia, epiphora, and blepharospasm have been reported in dogs after topical administration.[121]

Prostaglandin anologues are reported to be much less effective in cats, with studies of once daily 0.005% latanoprost[121] or 0.03% bimatoprost[129] or twice daily bimatoprost,[130] all reporting no significant IOP reductions. The commercial PGs are all prostaglandin-F (FP) receptor agonists, and in the feline, the FP receptor is not significantly involved in alterations in IOP in response to administration of PGs.[131] Latanoprost 0.005% did transiently lower IOP in cats with one dose but after 3 weeks of twice daily dosing, this hypotensive effect was reduced.[132]

Lacrostimulants

KCS is prevalent in veterinary ophthalmology and often has an immune-mediated cause. Lacrostimulants used in the management of KCS exert their anti-inflammatory and lacrostimulatory effects by impeding the formation and activation of T-cell lymphocytes.[133,134] Commonly used topical medications include cyclosporine (CsA) and tacrolimus.

Cyclosporine

CsA is commercially available as a 0.2% ointment (Optimmune) and topical twice per day therapy is recommended.[135] An increase in STT of greater than 5 mm 3 to 4 weeks following the initiation of treatment is considered a positive response.[135] For dogs with an excellent response to treatment (STTs > 20 mm/min), once per day application with continued careful monitoring can be considered.[135] Studies report that 80% of KCS cases respond well to CsA,[135,136] with the STT increasing with 3 to 4 weeks after continual therapy.[136] Some dogs will require 2 to 3 months of therapy with CsA before a significant increase in STT will occur,[135] and in cases of severe or absolute KCS, the success of CsA therapy is often significantly reduced.[135] Tear production can reduce dramatically in 12 to 24 hours following discontinuation of cyclosporine, so reducing CsA therapy to once a day should warrant caution.[136]

Tacrolimus

Tacrolimus has been a recent addition in the treatment of canine KCS with promising results. There are no commercial preparations available; however, it is typically compounded in a 0.02% or 0.03% solution or ointment.[137] There have been various studies comparing the efficacy of topical tacrolimus compared with CsA. A 2003 study demonstrated that dogs treated for KCS with 0.03% tacrolimus yielded similar results to those treated with 2% CsA.[138] This finding has been supported by other studies using the same[139] and increased concentrations of tacrolimus.[140] There is also evidence that tacrolimus may be more effective in cases of KCS which did not respond to previous CsA treatment,[139] or in more severe cases of KCS.[141,142] Additionally, tacrolimus has been reported to be superior in the reduction of corneal pigmentation.[140]

It is important to note that while there are anecdotal reports of the use of CsA or tacrolimus in feline patients for KCS, there is currently no peer-reviewed evidence that these medications improve the STT values in feline patients. This subject warrants further investigation but currently the treatment of KCS in feline patients involves supplementation of tears and treatment of any underlying conditions such as feline herpes virus. There has been demonstrated efficacy of CsA in the treatment of feline eosinophilic keratitis.[143]

Mydriatics and Cycloplegics

Pharmacologic dilation of the pupil in veterinary ophthalmology allows examination of the lens and posterior segment, facilitates surgical procedures, and has therapeutic intervention in cases of iridocyclitis. Depending on the clinical situation, different pharmacologic agents will be used; however, for the purposes of this review, cholinergic antagonists will be the focus.

Cholinergic antagonists: tropicamide, atropine, scopolamine, cyclopentolate
Cholinergic antagonists reversibly block cholinergic receptors in smooth muscle resulting in pupillary dilation. Following topical application of cholinergic antagonists, salivation, and occasional vomiting can occur, attributed to the bitter taste.[144–146] A significant reduction in tear production has also been reported.[147,148] Systemic absorption also occurs, with a significant elevation in heart rate reported in dogs.[31] A preliminary ocular examination including measurement of IOP and assessment of lens position is recommended before administration of mydriatic agents because dilation of the pupil can result in a significant elevation of IOP in cats[149,150] and variable elevation in dogs.[151–153] Additionally, an unstable lens can luxate anteriorly when the pupil is dilated, potentially resulting in secondary glaucoma.[154] Commercially available topical cholinergic antagonists include tropicamide (0.5% and 1% solution), atropine sulfate (0.5%–2% solution, 1% ointment), homatropine (1%–5%), scopolamine (0.25% solution), and cyclopentolate (1% and 2% solutions).

Tropicamide has a rapid onset of action with mydriasis evident from 15 minutes after application and maximal dilation evident at 30 minutes in dogs[146] and 1 to 2 hours in cats.[144,149] The pupillary dilation is not prolonged and declines after 2 hours in dogs[146] and 4 hours in cats.[144,149] The rapid onset and return to normal pupillary diameter makes tropicamide an appropriate medication for diagnostic mydriasis, as well as presurgical pupillary dilation. However, its cycloplegic properties are not as pronounced; therefore, it is not indicated in the treatment of uveitis.[155–158] Following application, STT values were unaffected in dogs but transiently decreased in cats.[148] Cats with normal IOP and those with glaucoma demonstrated a significant elevation in IOP following administration of tropicamide.[150,159]

Atropine has strong cycloplegic properties in addition to mydriasis and, therefore, is the recommended therapeutic agent for treating the discomfort associated with iridocyclitis and reducing the chance of posterior synechiae formation. Following administration of the 1% solution, peak mydriasis is evident at 60 and 30 to 45 minutes, and lasts 96 to 120 and 60 hours in dogs[146] and cats,[144] respectively. Eyes with darkly pigmented irises may exhibit a longer duration of action due to melanin binding of atropine.[160,161] In small animals, side effects of topical atropine administration are most commonly salivation or vomiting associated with the bitter taste, and this can be reduced by using an ointment rather than solution.[144,146] Less common adverse effects include periocular dermatitis[41,154] and neurologic signs.[162]

Homatropine is rarely used in dogs and cats because it has a longer time until onset of action and does not achieve maximal pupillary dilation.[144,146] Conversely, the administration of scopolamine in canine patients results in a rapid and prolonged mydriasis.[146] Cyclopentolate is more comparable to atropine, with both mydriatic and cycloplegic properties and a similar duration of action in dogs and cats.[144,146] Maximal mydriasis is not reached until 12 hours following administration in dogs.[163] Side effects include conjunctival edema in dogs[146]; however, IOP and tear production are unaffected.[163]

SUMMARY

Topical ocular therapeutics are essential for the treatment of veterinary ophthalmic diseases. To maximize patient outcomes, a thorough understanding of ocular anatomy and physiology and factors affecting the bioavailability of topical medications is required. It is important to recognize that systemic absorption of topical medications occurs and adverse effects can arise; as such, individual patients should be carefully considered for any potential contraindications.

CLINICS CARE POINTS

- Administration of multiple consecutive drops of an ophthalmic preparation will not enhance bioavailability but rather increase the rate of nasolacrimal drainage and decrease contact time. A single drop per dose is recommended.[14]
- Wait 5 to 10 minutes between solutions or suspensions[11] and always apply ointments last.
- Consider comorbidities when prescribing topical medications, especially NSAIDs, corticosteroids and beta-blockers.[34,88,89,105,114,117]
- Topical corticosteroids are contraindicated in the presence of corneal ulceration.[96–100]
- Topical NSAIDs should be used with caution in small animals with glaucoma and the IOPs monitored.[92,101–103]

DISCLOSURE

The authors have nothing to disclose.

REFERENCES

1. Grass GM, Robinson JR. Mechanisms of corneal drug penetration. I: In vivo and in vitro kinetics. J Pharm Sci 1988;77(1):3–14.
2. Grass GM, Robinson JR. Mechanisms of corneal drug penetration. II: Ultrastructural analysis of potential pathways for drug movement. J Pharm Sci 1988;77(1): 15–23.
3. Grass GM, Cooper ER, Robinson JR. Mechanisms of corneal drug penetration III: Modeling of molecular transport. J Pharm Sci 1988;77(1):24–6.
4. Sasaki H, Yamamura K, Mukai T, et al. Enhancement of ocular drug penetration. Crit Rev Ther Drug Carrier Syst 1999;16(1):85–146.
5. Prausnitz MR, Noonan JS. Permeability of cornea, sclera, and conjunctiva: a literature analysis for drug delivery to the eye. J Pharm Sci 1998;87(12): 1479–88.
6. Ahmed I, Patton TF. Importance of the noncorneal absorption route in topical ophthalmic drug delivery. Invest Ophthalmol Vis Sci 1985;26 4:584–7.
7. Hämäläinen K, Kananen K, Auriola S, et al. Characterization of paracellular and aqueous penetration routes in cornea, conjunctiva, and sclera. Invest Ophthalmol Vis Sci 1997;38(3):627–34.

8. Schoenwald RD, Deshpande GS, Rethwisch DG, et al. Penetration into the anterior chamber via the conjunctival/scleral pathway. J Ocul Pharmacol Ther 1997; 13(1):41–59.

9. Lehr CM, Lee YH, Lee VH. Improved ocular penetration of gentamicin by mucoadhesive polymer polycarbophil in the pigmented rabbit. Invest Ophthalmol Vis Sci 1994;35(6):2809–14.

10. Ambati J, Canakis CS, Miller JW, et al. Diffusion of high molecular weight compounds through sclera. Invest Ophthalmol Vis Sci 2000;41(5):1181–5.

11. Sebbag L, Allbaugh RA, Wehrman RF, et al. Fluorophotometric assessment of tear volume and turnover rate in healthy dogs and cats. J Ocul Pharmacol Ther 2019;35(9):497–502.

12. Lederer CM, Harold RE. Drop size of commercial glaucoma medications. Am J Ophthalmol 1986;101 6:691–4.

13. Agrahari V, Mandal A, Agrahari V, et al. A comprehensive insight on ocular pharmacokinetics. Drug Deliv Transl Res 2016;6(6):735–54.

14. Sebbag L, Kirner NS, Allbaugh RA, et al. Kinetics of fluorescein in tear film after eye drop instillation in beagle dogs: does size really matter? Front Vet Sci 2019; 6(457).

15. Shell JW. Pharmacokinetics of topically applied ophthalmic drugs. Surv Ophthalmol 1982;26(4):207–18.

16. Ali Y, Lehmussaari K. Industrial perspective in ocular drug delivery. Adv Drug Deliv Rev 2006;58(11):1258–68.

17. Frangie JP. Clinical pharmacokinetics of various topical ophthalmic delivery systems. Clin Pharmacokinet 1995;29(2):130–8.

18. Hardberger R, Hanna C, Boyd CM. Effects of drug vehicles on ocular contact time. Arch Ophthalmol 1975;93(1):42–5.

19. Sasaki H, Yamamura K, Nishida K, et al. Delivery of drugs to the eye by topical application. Prog Retin Eye Res 1996;15(2):583–620.

20. Greaves J, Wilson C, Birmingham A. Assessment of the precorneal residence of an ophthalmic ointment in healthy subjects. Br J Clin Pharmacol 1993;35(2): 188–92.

21. Ellis P, Riegel M. Influence of ophthalmic ointments on the penetration of pilocarpine drops. J Ocul Pharmacol Ther 1989;5(2):119–25.

22. Weiner A, Gilger B. Advancements in ocular drug delivery. Vet Ophthalmol 2010;13:395–406.

23. Kaur IP, Smitha R. Penetration enhancers and ocular bioadhesives: two new avenues for ophthalmic drug delivery. Drug Dev Ind Pharm 2002;28(4):353–69.

24. Beckwith-Cohen B, Elad D, Bdolah-Abram T, et al. Comparison of tear pH in dogs, horses, and cattle. Am J Vet Res 2014;75(5):494–9.

25. Malmberg GJ, Lupo R. Compounding in veterinary ophthalmology. Vet Clin North Am Small Anim Pract 2004;34(3):825–38.

26. Davis K, Townsend W. Tear-film osmolarity in normal cats and cats with conjunctivitis. Vet Ophthalmol 2011;14:54–9.

27. Sebbag L, Park SA, Kass PH, et al. Assessment of tear film osmolarity using the TearLab(™) osmometer in normal dogs and dogs with keratoconjunctivitis sicca. Vet Ophthalmol 2017;20(4):357–64.

28. Urtti A, Salminen L. Minimizing systemic absorption of topically administered ophthalmic drugs. Surv Ophthalmol 1993;37(6):435–56.

29. Paulsen FP, Foge M, Thale AB, et al. Animal model for the absorption of lipophilic substances from tear fluid by the epithelium of the nasolacrimal ducts. Invest Ophthalmol Vis Sci 2002;43(10):3137–43.

30. Glaze MB, Crawford MA, Nachreiner RF, et al. Ophthalmic corticosteroid therapy: systemic effects in the dog. J Am Vet Med Assoc 1988;192(1):73–5.

31. Greenberg S, Plummer C, Maisenbacher H, et al. The effect of topical ophthalmic 1% atropine on heart rate and rhythm in normal dogs. Vet Ophthalmol 2015;18(2):105–8.

32. Herring IP, Jacobson JD, Pickett JP. Cardiovascular effects of topical ophthalmic 10% phenylephrine in dogs. Vet Ophthalmol 2004;7(1):41–6.

33. Pascoe PJ, Ilkiw JE, Stiles J, et al. Arterial hypertension associated with topical ocular use of phenylephrine in dogs. J Am Vet Med Assoc 1994;205(11):1562–4.

34. Plummer CE, MacKay EO, Gelatt KN. Comparison of the effects of topical administration of a fixed combination of dorzolamide-timolol to monotherapy with timolol or dorzolamide on IOP, pupil size, and heart rate in glaucomatous dogs. Vet Ophthalmol 2006;9(4):245–9.

35. Smith LN, Miller PE, Felchle LM. Effects of topical administration of latanoprost, timolol, or a combination of latanoprost and timolol on intraocular pressure, pupil size, and heart rate in clinically normal dogs. Am J Vet Res 2010;71(9):1055–61.

36. Hsu K, Pinard C, Johnson R, et al. Systemic absorption and adverse ocular and systemic effects after topical ophthalmic administration of 0.1% diclofenac to healthy cats. Am J Vet Res 2015;76(3):253–65.

37. Wilkie DA, Latimer CA. Effects of topical administration of timolol maleate on intraocular pressure and pupil size in cats. Am J Vet Res 1991;52(3):436–40.

38. Wilkie DA, Latimer CA. Effects of topical administration of timolol maleate on intraocular pressure and pupil size in dogs. Am J Vet Res 1991;52(3):432–5.

39. Tolar EL, Hendrix DV, Rohrbach BW, et al. Evaluation of clinical characteristics and bacterial isolates in dogs with bacterial keratitis: 97 cases (1993-2003). J Am Vet Med Assoc 2006;228(1):80–5.

40. LoPinto AJ, Mohammed HO, Ledbetter EC. Prevalence and risk factors for isolation of methicillin-resistant Staphylococcus in dogs with keratitis. Vet Ophthalmol 2015;18(4):297–303.

41. Clode A, Scott E. Antibacterial agents, antifungal agents and antiviral agents. In: Gelatt JK, editor. Vet ophthalmol. 6th edition. Hoboken, NJ: John Wiley & Sons, Inc.; 2021. p. 385–416.

42. Hume-Smith K, Groth A, Rishniw M, et al. Anaphylactic events observed within 4 h of ocular application of an antibiotic-containing ophthalmic preparation: 61 cats (1993-2010). J Feline Med Surg 2011;13(10):744–51.

43. Rowley RA, Rubin LF. Aqueous humor penetration of several antibiotics in the dog. Am J Vet Res 1970;31(1):43–9.

44. Wang L, Pan Q, Zhang L, et al. Investigation of bacterial microorganisms in the conjunctival sac of clinically normal dogs and dogs with ulcerative keratitis in Beijing, China. Vet Ophthalmol 2008;11(3):145–9.

45. McDonald PJ, Watson DJ. Microbial flora of normal canine conjunctivae. J Small Anim Pract 1976;17(12):809–12.

46. Prado MR, Rocha MF, Brito EH, et al. Survey of bacterial microorganisms in the conjunctival sac of clinically normal dogs and dogs with ulcerative keratitis in Fortaleza, Ceará, Brazil. Vet Ophthalmol 2005;8(1):33–7.

47. Urban M, Wyman M, Rheins M, et al. Conjunctival flora of clinically normal dogs. J Am Vet Med Assoc 1972;161(2):201–6.

48. Insler MS, Helm CJ, George WJ. Topical vs systemic gentamicin penetration into the human cornea and aqueous humor. Arch Ophthalmol 1987;105(7):922–4.

49. Rootman DS, Willoughby RP, Bindlish R, et al. Continuous flow contact lens delivery of gentamicin to rabbit cornea and aqueous humor. J Ocul Pharmacol 1992;8(4):317–23.

50. Hendrix DV, Ward DA, Barnhill MA. Effects of antibiotics on morphologic characteristics and migration of canine corneal epithelial cells in tissue culture. Am J Vet Res 2001;62(10):1664–9.

51. Nelson JD, Silverman V, Lima PH, et al. Corneal epithelial wound healing: a tissue culture assay on the effect of antibiotics. Curr Eye Res 1990;9(3):277–85.

52. Stern GA, Schemmer GB, Farber RD, et al. Effect of topical antibiotic solutions on corneal epithelial wound healing. Arch Ophthalmol 1983;101(4):644–7.

53. Wang AL, Ledbetter EC, Kern TJ. Orbital abscess bacterial isolates and in vitro antimicrobial susceptibility patterns in dogs and cats. Vet Ophthalmol 2009; 12(2):91–6.

54. Stewart WC, Crean CS, Zink RC, et al. Pharmacokinetics of azithromycin and moxifloxacin in human conjunctiva and aqueous humor during and after the approved dosing regimens. Am J Ophthalmol 2010;150(5):744–51.e2.

55. Kuehne JJ, Yu AL, Holland GN, et al. Corneal pharmacokinetics of topically applied azithromycin and clarithromycin. Am J Ophthalmol 2004;138(4):547–53.

56. Breitschwerdt EB, Papich MG, Hegarty BC, et al. Efficacy of doxycycline, azithromycin, or trovafloxacin for treatment of experimental Rocky Mountain spotted fever in dogs. Antimicrobial Agents Chemother 1999;43(4):813–21.

57. Biswas S, Maggi RG, Papich MG, et al. Comparative activity of pradofloxacin, enrofloxacin, and azithromycin against Bartonella henselae isolates collected from cats and a human. J Clin Microbiol 2010;48(2):617–8.

58. Biswas S, Maggi RG, Papich MG, et al. Molecular mechanisms of Bartonella henselae resistance to azithromycin, pradofloxacin and enrofloxacin. J Antimicrob Chemother 2009;65(3):581–2.

59. Yue J, Lyu JX, Si W, et al. Comparison study on sensitivity of five ophthalmic antibiotics to common drug-resistant Staphylococci on ocular surface. Chi J Ophthalmol 2020;56(8):621–5.

60. Blondeau JM. Fluoroquinolones: mechanism of action, classification, and development of resistance. Surv Ophthalmol 2004;49(Suppl 2):S73–8.

61. Ledbetter EC, Hendricks LM, Riis RC, et al. In vitro fluoroquinolone susceptibility of Pseudomonas aeruginosa isolates from dogs with ulcerative keratitis. Am J Vet Res 2007;68(6):638–42.

62. Yu-Speight AW, Kern TJ, Erb HN. Ciprofloxacin and Ofloxacin Aqueous Humor Concentrations After Topical Administration in Dogs Undergoing Cataract Surgery. Invest Ophthalmol Vis Sci 2003;44(13):1452.

63. Schlech BA, Alfonso E. Overview of the potency of moxifloxacin ophthalmic solution 0.5% (VIGAMOX). Surv Ophthalmol 2005;50(S1):S7–15.

64. Deschênes J, Blondeau J. Besifloxacin in the management of bacterial infections of the ocular surface. Can J Ophthalmol 2015;50(3):184–91.

65. Park YW, Kang BJ, Lim JH, et al. Corneal plaque containing levofloxacin in a dog. Vet Ophthalmol 2015;18(6):521–6.

66. Seitz B, Hayashi S, Wee WR, et al. In vitro effects of aminoglycosides and fluoroquinolones on keratocytes. Invest Ophthalmol Vis Sci 1996;37(4):656–65.

67. Maboni G, Gressler LT, Espindola JP, et al. Differences in the antimicrobial susceptibility profiles of Moraxella bovis, M. bovoculi and M. ovis. Braz J Microbiol 2015;46(2):545–9.

68. Griffin MO, Fricovsky E, Ceballos G, et al. Tetracyclines: a pleitropic family of compounds with promising therapeutic properties. Review of the literature. Am J Physiol Cell Physiol 2010;299(3):C539–48.

69. Chandler HL, Gemensky-Metzler AJ, Bras ID, et al. In vivo effects of adjunctive tetracycline treatment on refractory corneal ulcers in dogs. J Am Vet Med Assoc 2010;237(4):378–86.

70. De Clercq E. Antiviral drugs in current clinical use. J Clin Virol 2004;30(2): 115–33.

71. Maggs DJ, Clarke HE. In vitro efficacy of ganciclovir, cidofovir, penciclovir, foscarnet, idoxuridine, and acyclovir against feline herpesvirus type-1. Am J Vet Res 2004;65(4):399–403.

72. Nasisse MP, Guy JS, Davidson MG, et al. In vitro susceptibility of feline herpesvirus-1 to vidarabine, idoxuridine, trifluridine, acyclovir, or bromovinyldeoxyuridine. Am J Vet Res 1989;50(1):158–60.

73. Gould D. Feline herpesvirus-1: ocular manifestations, diagnosis and treatment options. J Feline Med Surg 2011;13(5):333–46.

74. Maggs DJ. Antiviral therapy for feline herpesvirus infections. Vet Clin North Am Small Anim Pract 2010;40(6):1055–62.

75. Spertus CB, Mohammed HO, Ledbetter EC. Effects of topical ocular application of 1% trifluridine ophthalmic solution in dogs with experimentally induced recurrent ocular canine herpesvirus-1 infection. Am J Vet Res 2016;77(10):1140–7.

76. O'Brien TP. Therapy of ocular fungal infections. Ophthalmol Clin North Am 1999; 12(1):33–50.

77. Mathes RL, Reber AJ, Hurley DJ, et al. Effects of antifungal drugs and delivery vehicles on morphology and proliferation of equine corneal keratocytes in vitro. Am J Vet Res 2010;71(8):953–9.

78. McGhee CN. Pharmacokinetics of ophthalmic corticosteroids. Br J Ophthalmol 1992;76(11):681–4.

79. Musson DG, Bidgood AM, Olejnik O. An in vitro comparison of the permeability of prednisolone, prednisolone sodium phosphate, and prednisolone acetate across the NZW rabbit cornea. J Ocul Pharmacol 1992;8(2):139–50.

80. Leibowitz HM, Kupferman A. Antiinflammatory medications. Int Ophthalmol Clin 1980;20(3):117–34.

81. Dannenberg AM Jr. The antinflammatory effects of glucocorticosteroids. A brief review of the literature. Inflamm Res 1979;3(3):329–43.

82. Phillips K, Arffa R, Cintron C, et al. Effects of prednisolone and medroxyprogesterone on corneal wound healing, ulceration, and neovascularization. Arch Ophthalmol 1983;101(4):640–3.

83. Boneham GC, Collin HB. Steroid inhibition of limbal blood and lymphatic vascular cell growth. Curr Eye Res 1995;14(1):1–10.

84. Brown SI, Weller CA, Vidrich AM. Effect of corticosteroids on corneal collagenase of rabbits. Am J Ophthalmol 1970;70(5):744–7.

85. Zhan G-L, Miranda OC, Bito LZ. Steroid glaucoma: Corticosteroid-induced ocular hypertension in cats. Exp Eye Res 1992;54(2):211–8.

86. Gelatt KN, Mackay EO. The ocular hypertensive effects of topical 0.1% dexamethasone in beagles with inherited glaucoma. J Ocul Pharmacol Ther 1998; 14(1):57–66.

87. Gosling AA, Kiland JA, Rutkowski LE, et al. Effects of topical corticosteroid administration on intraocular pressure in normal and glaucomatous cats. Vet Ophthalmol 2016;19(S1):69–76.

88. Eichenbaum J, Macy D, Severin G, et al. Effect in large dogs of ophthalmic prednisolone acetate on adrenal gland and hepatic function. J Am Anim Hosp Assoc 1988;24(6):705–9.

89. Rankin AJ, KuKanich KS, Schermerhorn T, et al. Evaluation of diabetes mellitus regulation in dogs treated with ophthalmic preparations of prednisolone acetate versus diclofenac sodium. Am J Vet Res 2019;80(12):1129–35.

90. Dziezyc JM N, Smith W. Effect of flurbiprofen and corticosteroids on the ocular irritative response in dogs. Vet Comp Ophthalmol 1995;5:42–5.

91. Ward DA. Comparative efficacy of topically applied flurbiprofen, diclofenac, tolmetin, and suprofen for the treatment of experimentally induced blood-aqueous barrier disruption in dogs. Am J Vet Res 1996;57(6):875–8.

92. Rankin AJ, Khrone SG, Stiles J. Evaluation of four drugs for inhibition of paracentesis-induced blood-aqueous humor barrier breakdown in cats. Am J Vet Res 2011;72(6):826–32.

93. Palmero M, Bellot JL, Alcoriza N, et al. The ocular pharmacokinetics of topical diclofenac is affected by ocular inflammation. Ophthalmic Res 1999;31(4): 309–16.

94. Trousdale MD, Dunkel EC, Nesburn AB. Effect of flurbiprofen on herpes simplex keratitis in rabbits. Invest Ophthalmol Vis Sci 1980;19(3):267–70.

95. Rao NA, Patchett R, Fernandez MA, et al. Treatment of experimental granulomatous uveitis by lipoxygenase and cyclo-oxygenase inhibitors. Arch Ophthalmol 1987;105(3):413–5.

96. Hendrix DVH, Ward DA, Barnhill MA. Effects of anti-inflammatory drugs and preservatives on morphologic characteristics and migration of canine corneal epithelial cells in tissue culture. Vet Ophthalmol 2002;5(2):127–35.

97. Hersh P, Rice B, Baer J, et al. Topical nonsteroidal agents and corneal wound healing. Arch Ophthalmol 1990;108(4):577–83.

98. Flach AJ. Corneal melts associated with topically applied nonsteroidal anti-inflammatory drugs. Trans Am Ophthalmol Soc 2001;99:205–10.

99. Guidera AC, Luchs JI, Udell IJ. Keratitis, ulceration, and perforation associated with topical nonsteroidal anti-inflammatory drugs. Ophthalmology 2001;108(5): 936–44.

100. Lin JC, Rapuano CJ, Laibson PR, et al. Corneal melting associated with use of topical nonsteroidal anti-inflammatory drugs after ocular surgery. Arch Ophthalmol 2000;118(8):1129–32.

101. Krohne SG, Gionfriddo J, Morrison EA. Inhibition of pilocarpine-induced aqueous humor flare, hypotony, and miosis by topical administration of anti-inflammatory and anesthetic drugs to dogs. Am J Vet Res 1998;59(4):482–8.

102. Millichamp NJ, Dziezyc J, Olsen JW. Effect of flurbiprofen on facility of aqueous outflow in the eyes of dogs. Am J Vet Res 1991;52(9):1448–51.

103. Lu J, English R, Nadelstein B, et al. Comparison of topically applied flurbiprofen or bromfenac ophthalmic solution on post-operative ocular hypertension in canine patients following cataract surgery. Vet Ophthalmol 2017;20(2):107–13.

104. Pirie CG, Maranda LS, Pizzirani S. Effect of topical 0.03% flurbiprofen and 0.005% latanoprost, alone and in combination, on normal canine eyes. Vet Ophthalmol 2011;14(2):71–9.

105. Lanuza R, Rankin AJ, KuKanich B, et al. Evaluation of systemic absorption and renal effects of topical ophthalmic flurbiprofen and diclofenac in healthy cats. Vet Ophthalmol 2016;19(Suppl 1):24–9.

106. Cawrse MA, Ward DA, Hendrix DV. Effects of topical application of a 2% solution of dorzolamide on intraocular pressure and aqueous humor flow rate in clinically normal dogs. Am J Vet Res 2001;62(6):859–63.

107. Kennard G, Whelan NC. The additive effect of dorzolamide and latanoprost in reducing intraocular pressure in normal dogs. Abstract presented at: 32nd Annual Meeting of the American College of Veterinary Ophthalmologists; October 10–13 2001; Sarasota, FL.

108. Whelan NC, Welch P, Pace A. A comparison of the efficacy of topical brinzola-mide and dorzolamide alone and in combination with oral methazolamide in decreasing normal canine intraocular pressure. Abstract presented at: 30th Annual Meeting of the American College of Veterinary Ophthalmologists; Nov 3–7 1997; Chicago, IL.

109. Rainbow ME, Dziezyc J. Effects of twice daily application of 2% dorzolamide on intraocular pressure in normal cats. Vet Ophthalmol 2003;6(2):147–50.

110. Rankin AJ, Crumley WR, Allbaugh RA. Effects of ocular administration of ophthalmic 2% dorzolamide hydrochloride solution on aqueous humor flow rate and intraocular pressure in clinically normal cats. Am J Vet Res 2012; 73(7):1074–8.

111. Sigle KJ, Camaño-Garcia G, Carriquiry AL, et al. The effect of dorzolamide 2% on circadian intraocular pressure in cats with primary congenital glaucoma. Vet Ophthalmol 2011;14(S1):48–53.

112. Gray HE, Willis AM, Morgan RV. Effects of topical administration of 1% brinzola-mide on normal cat eyes. Vet Ophthalmol 2003;6(4):285–90.

113. McLellan GJ, Lin T-L, Hildreth S, et al. Diurnal intraocular pressure and response to topically administered 1% brinzolamide in a spontaneous feline model of pri-mary congenital glaucoma. Invest Ophthalmol Vis Sci 2009;50(13):4059.

114. Thiessen CE, Tofflemire KL, Makielski KM, et al. Hypokalemia and suspected renal tubular acidosis associated with topical carbonic anhydrase inhibitor ther-apy in a cat. J Vet Emerg Crit Care (San Antonio) 2016;26(6):870–4.

115. Beckwith-Cohen B, Bentley E, Gasper DJ, et al. Keratitis in six dogs after topical treatment with carbonic anhydrase inhibitors for glaucoma. J Am Vet Med Assoc 2015;247(12):1419–26.

116. Willis AM, Diehl KA, Robbin TE. Advances in topical glaucoma therapy. Vet Oph-thalmol 2002;5(1):9–17.

117. Gelatt KN, Larocca RD, Gelatt JK, et al. Evaluation of multiple doses of 4 and 6% timolol, and timolol combined with 2% pilocarpine in clinically normal beagles and beagles with glaucoma. Am J Vet Res 1995;56(10):1325–31.

118. Gum G, Larocca R, Gelatt K. The effect of topical timolol maleate on intraocular pressure in normal beagles and beagles with inherited glaucoma. Prog Vet Comp Ophthalmol 1991;1:141–50.

119. Willis AM. Ocular hypotensive drugs. Vet Clin North Am Small Anim Pract 2004; 34(3):755–76.

120. McLellan GJ, Miller PE. Feline glaucoma–a comprehensive review. Vet Ophthal-mol 2011;14(S1):15–29.

121. Studer ME, Martin CL, Stiles J. Effects of 0.005% latanoprost solution on intraoc-ular pressure in healthy dogs and cats. Am J Vet Res 2000;61(10):1220–4.

122. Gelatt KN, MacKay EO. Effect of different dose schedules of latanoprost on intraocular pressure and pupil size in the glaucomatous Beagle. Vet Ophthalmol 2001;4(4):283–8.

123. Gelatt KN, MacKay EO. Effect of different dose schedules of travoprost on intraocular pressure and pupil size in the glaucomatous Beagle. Vet Ophthalmol 2004;7(1):53–7.

124. Mackay EO, McLaughlin M, Plummer CE, et al. Dose response for travoprost® in the glaucomatous beagle. Vet Ophthalmol 2012;15(S1):31–5.

125. Gelatt KN, Mackay EO. Effect of different dose schedules of bimatoprost on intraocular pressure and pupil size in the glaucomatous Beagle. J Ocul Pharmacol Ther 2002;18(6):525–34.

126. Tofflemire KL, Whitley EM, Allbaugh RA, et al. Comparison of two- and three-times-daily topical ophthalmic application of 0.005% latanoprost solution in clinically normal dogs. Am J Vet Res 2015;76(7):625–31.

127. Plummer C. Medical therapy for glaucoma. In: Gelatt JK, editor. Vet Ophthalmol. 6th edition. Hoboken, NJ: John Wiley & Sons, Inc.; 2021. p. 451–78.

128. Kahane N, Bdolah-Abram T, Raskansky H, et al. The effects of 1% prednisolone acetate on pupil diameter and intraocular pressure in healthy dogs treated with 0.005% latanoprost. Vet Ophthalmol 2016;19(6):473–9.

129. Bartoe JT, Davidson HJ, Horton MT, et al. The effects of bimatoprost and unoprostone isopropyl on the intraocular pressure of normal cats. Vet Ophthalmol 2005;8(4):247–52.

130. Regnier A, Lemagne C, Ponchet A, et al. Ocular effects of topical 0.03% bimatoprost solution in normotensive feline eyes. Vet Ophthalmol 2006;9(1):39–43.

131. Bhattacherjee P, Williams BS, Paterson CA. Responses of intraocular pressure and the pupil of feline eyes to prostaglandin EP1 and FP receptor agonists. Invest Ophthalmol Vis Sci 1999;40(12):3047–53.

132. McDonald JE, Kiland JA, Kaufman PL, et al. Effect of topical latanoprost 0.005% on intraocular pressure and pupil diameter in normal and glaucomatous cats. Vet Ophthalmol 2016;19(S1):13–23.

133. Fischer G, Wittmann-Liebold B, Lang K, et al. Cyclophilin and peptidyl-prolyl cis-trans isomerase are probably identical proteins. Nature (London) 1989; 337(6206):476–8.

134. Handschumacher RE, Harding MW, Rice J, et al. Cyclophilin: a specific cytosolic binding protein for cyclosporin A. Science (New York, NY) 1984; 226(4674):544–7.

135. Morgan RV, Abrams KL. Topical administration of cyclosporine for treatment of keratoconjunctivitis sicca in dogs. J Am Vet Med Assoc 1991;199(8):1043–6.

136. Kaswan RL, Salisbury M-A, Ward DA. Spontaneous canine keratoconjunctivitis sicca: a useful model for human keratoconjunctivitis sicca: treatment with cyclosporine eye drops. Arch Ophthalmol 1989;107(8):1210–6.

137. Rankin AJ. Anti-inflammatory and immunosuppressant drugs. In: Gelatt JK, editor. Vet ophthalmol. 6th edition. John Wiley & Sons, Inc.; 2021. p. 417–34, chap 8.3.

138. Adkins E.A., An Investigation of the Safety and Efficacy Of Topical Ophthalmic Application Of Tacrolimus In Dogs. proceedings of 34th Annual Meeting of the American College of Veterinary Ophthalmologists: Coeur D'Alene, ID, 2003.

139. Hendrix DVH, Adkins EA, Ward DA, et al. An Investigation Comparing the Efficacy of Topical Ocular Application of Tacrolimus and Cyclosporine in Dogs. Vet Med Int 2011;2011:487592–5.

140. John C, Gopinathan A, Singh K, et al. Clinical evaluation of topical tacrolimus ointment usage in different stages of keratoconjunctivitis sicca in dogs. Turkish J Vet Anim Sci 2018;42(4):259–68.

141. Berdoulay A, English RV, Nadelstein B. Effect of topical 0.02% tacrolimus aqueous suspension on tear production in dogs with keratoconjunctivitis sicca. Vet Ophthalmol 2005;8(4):225–32.

142. Radziejewski K, Balicki I. Comparative clinical evaluation of tacrolimus and cyclosporine eye drops for the treatment of canine keratoconjunctivitis sicca. Acta veterinaria Hungarica (Budapest 1983) 2016;64(3):313–29.

143. Spiess AK, Sapienza JS, Mayordomo A. Treatment of proliferative feline eosinophilic keratitis with topical 1.5% cyclosporine: 35 cases. Vet Ophthalmol 2009; 12(2):132–7.

144. Gelatt KN, Boggess TS, Cure TH. Evaluation of mydriatics in the cat. Anim Hosp 1973;9:283–7.

145. Lynch R, Rubin LF. Salivation induced in dogs by conjunctival instillation of atropine. J Am Vet Med Assoc 1965;147(5):511–3.

146. Rubin LF, Wolfes RL. Mydriatics for canine ophthalmoscopy. J Am Vet Med Assoc 1962;140:137–41.

147. Hollingsworth SR, Canton DD, Buyukmihci NC, et al. Effect of topically administered atropine on tear production in dogs. J Am Vet Med Assoc 1992;200(10): 1481–4.

148. Margadant DL, Kirkby K, Andrew SE, et al. Effect of topical tropicamide on tear production as measured by Schirmer's tear test in normal dogs and cats. Vet Ophthalmol 2003;6(4):315–20.

149. Stadtbäumer K, Frommlet F, Nell B. Effects of mydriatics on intraocular pressure and pupil size in the normal feline eye. Vet Ophthalmol 2006;9(4):233–7.

150. Stadtbäumer K, Köstlin RG, Zahn KJ. Effects of topical 0.5% tropicamide on intraocular pressure in normal cats. Vet Ophthalmol 2002;5(2):107–12.

151. Kovalcuka L, Ilgazs A, Bandere D, et al. Changes in intraocular pressure and horizontal pupil diameter during use of topical mydriatics in the canine eye. Open Vet J 2017;7(1):16–22.

152. Wallin-Håkanson N, Wallin-Håkanson B. The effects of topical tropicamide and systemic medetomidine, followed by atipamezole reversal, on pupil size and intraocular pressure in normal dogs. Vet Ophthalmol 2001;4(1):3–6.

153. Taylor NR, Zele AJ, Vingrys AJ, et al. Variation in intraocular pressure following application of tropicamide in three different dog breeds. Vet Ophthalmol 2007; 10(Suppl 1):8–11.

154. Herring IP. Mydriatics/cycloplegics, anesthetics, and tear substitutes and stimulators. In: Gelatt JK, editor. Vet Ophthalmol. 6th edition. Hoboken, NJ: John Wiley and Sons, Inc.; 2021. p. 435–50.

155. Egashira SM, Kish LL, Twelker JD, et al. Comparison of cyclopentolate versus tropicamide cycloplegia in children. Optom Vis Sci 1993;70(12):1019–26.

156. Gettes BC, Belmont O. Tropicamide: comparative cycloplegic effects. Arch Ophthalmol 1961;66(3):336–40.

157. Hiatt RL, Jerkins G. Comparison of atropine and tropicamide in esotropia. Ann Ophthalmol 1983;15(4):341–3.

158. Lovasik JV. Pharmacokinetics of topically applied cyclopentolate HCl and tropicamide. Am J Optom Physiol Opt 1986;63(10):787–803.

159. Gomes FE, Bentley E, Lin TL, et al. Effects of unilateral topical administration of 0.5% tropicamide on anterior segment morphology and intraocular pressure in normal cats and cats with primary congenital glaucoma. Vet Ophthalmol 2011; 14(Suppl 1):75–83.

160. Salazar M, Patil PN. An explanation for the long duration of mydriatic effect of atropine in eye. Invest Ophthalmol 1976;15(8):671–3.

161. Salazar M, Shimada K, Patil PN. Iris pigmentation and atropine mydriasis. J Pharmacol Exp Ther 1976;197(1):79–88.

162. Ward DA. Clinical pharacology and therapeutics. Part 3. In: Gelatt JK, editor. Vet ophthalmol. 3rd edition. Philadelphia, PA: Lippincott Williams and Wilkins; 1999. p. 336–54.

163. Costa D, Leiva M, Coyo N, et al. Effect of topical 1% cyclopentolate hydrochloride on tear production, pupil size, and intraocular pressure in healthy Beagles. Vet Ophthalmol 2016;19(6):449–53.

Moving?

Make sure your subscription moves with you!

To notify us of your new address, find your **Clinics Account Number** (located on your mailing label above your name), and contact customer service at:

Email: journalscustomerservice-usa@elsevier.com

800-654-2452 (subscribers in the U.S. & Canada)
314-447-8871 (subscribers outside of the U.S. & Canada)

Fax number: 314-447-8029

Elsevier Health Sciences Division
Subscription Customer Service
3251 Riverport Lane
Maryland Heights, MO 63043

*To ensure uninterrupted delivery of your subscription, please notify us at least 4 weeks in advance of move.